SECOND EDITION

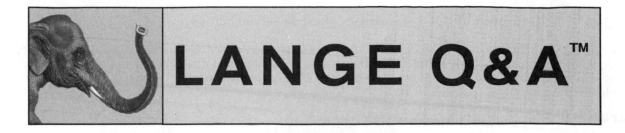

LANGE Q&A™

EMT-PARAMEDIC (P)
Self-Assessment
& Review

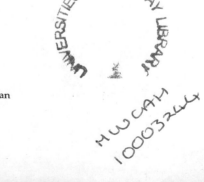

Editors

Richard E.J. Westfal, MD, FACEP
Attending Physician
Department of Medicine
Norwalk Hospital
Norwalk, Connecticut
Formerly Associate Director
Department of Emergency Medicine
Saint Vincent's Hospital
New York, New York

Gregory Santa Maria, NREMT-P, IC
Manager
Prehospital Care and Emergency Preparedness
Sioux Valley Hospital USD Medical Center
Sioux Falls, South Dakota
Formerly Paramedic Manager and Paramedic Program Director
Saint Vincent's Hospital
New York, New York

McGraw-Hill
Medical Publishing Division

New York Chicago San Francisco Lisbon London Madrid Mexico City Milan
New Delhi San Juan Seoul Singapore Sydney Toronto

Lange Q&A™: EMT-Paramedic (P): Self-Assessment & Review, Second Edition

1 2 3 4 5 6 7 8 9 0   QPD/QPD   0 9 8 7 6

Set ISBN-13: 978-0-07-147014-8
Set ISBN-10: 0-07-147014-X
Book ISBN-13: 978-0-07-148263-9
Book ISBN-10: 0-07-148263-6
CD ISBN-13: 978-0-07-148264-6
CD ISBN-10: 0-07-148264-4

Notice

Medicine is an ever-changing science. As new research and clinical experience broaden our knowledge, changes in treatment and drug therapy are required. The authors and the publisher of this work have checked with sources believed to be reliable in their efforts to provide information that is complete and generally in accord with the standards accepted at the time of publication. However, in view of the possibility of human error or changes in medical sciences, neither the authors nor the publisher nor any other party who has been involved in the preparation or publication of this work warrants that the information contained herein is in every respect accurate or complete, and they disclaim all responsibility for any errors or omissions or for the results obtained from use of the information contained in this work. Readers are encouraged to confirm the information contained herein with other sources. For example and in particular, readers are advised to check the product information sheet included in the package of each drug they plan to administer to be certain that the information contained in this work is accurate and that changes have not been made in the recommended dose or in the contraindications for administration. This recommendation is of particular importance in connection with new or infrequently used drugs.

This book was set in Palatino by International Typesetting and Composition.
The editors were Michael Brown and Christie Naglieri.
The production supervisor was Sherri Souffrance.
Project management was provided by International Typesetting and Composition.
Quebecor World was printer and binder.

This book is printed on acid-free paper.

Cataloging-in-Publication data is on file for this title with the Library of Congress.

We would like to dedicate this edition to the Paramedics of Saint Vincent's Hospital Manhattan. Their dedication to the field of prehospital emergency medicine is not measured by the events of one day, but of a lifetime of selfless and heroic acts.

Their perseverance and passion for preserving the gift of life has been an inspiration to us all. They are truly an immeasurable asset to the EMS world, the City of New York, and the people of Greenwich Village.

Richard E.J. Westfal, MD, FACEP
Gregory Santa Maria, NREMT-P, IC

Contents

Preface

This second edition of *Lange Q&A™: EMT-Paramedic (P): Self-Assessment & Review* has been revised and designed to prepare paramedics, whether entry level or seasoned veterans, for their certification examination. The book is also designed to assist medical directors and program coordinators in the appropriate evaluation of their prospective graduates.

This book is based on the 1994 U.S. Department of Transportation paramedic national standard curriculum. The National Registry of Emergency Medical Technicians bases its examination questions on this national standard. In addition to the standard examination administered by the National Registry, many states also require a paramedic to successfully complete a state paramedic examination.

The 1994 curriculum is divided into the following major modules: preparatory, airway management and ventilation, patient assessment, trauma emergencies, medical emergencies, special populations (pediatrics, neonates, geriatrics), and special operations, such as response to mass casualty and hazardous materials incidents. This text is divided into sections which correspond to each of the major modules.

In addition to the revision of the existing sections, the authors also included a section on response to chemical, biological, radiological, nuclear, and explosive (CBRNE) incidents. This new chapter covers an awareness level in regard to these incidents. This new section fills a substantial void in this much-needed area of knowledge. The full text contains over 775 review questions. The questions are distributed among all of the study subjects, but emphasis in this edition, as in the first, is placed on critical emergencies. It is these sections in which the paramedic will need to be highly proficient. It is also these sections that are intense areas of concentration in the paramedic classrooms. A CD-ROM for practice testing is available for the first time with this book.

The questions are presented in the A-type, multiple-choice format. This format is the most frequently used in state and national certifying examinations. There is one correct answer and three distracters for each question. A brief rationale for the correct answer is given for each question. The questions are referenced to information included in the following textbooks:

> Bledsoe BE, Porter RS, Shade BR. *Brady's Paramedic Care: Principles and Practice*, 2nd ed. Vol. 1–5. Upper Saddle River, NJ: Prentice-Hall, 2006.
> Sanders MJ. *Mosby's Paramedic Textbook*, 3rd ed. St. Louis, MO: Elsevier, 2005.

For each answer and rationale, there is a chapter reference that will lead the student to the correct area of the corresponding textbook for additional review.

It is the goal of the authors to provide the paramedic student with the most productive review process available. By providing a solid educational process, we ensure that a well-rounded paramedic is developed. This will result in the highest quality results where they are needed the most, at the patient's bedside.

Acknowledgments

A special note of thanks goes to my wife, Debbie, for all of her help and support and particularly for her patience while attempting to improve my "limited" computer skills.

But most of all for simply always being there for me.

Richard E.J. Westfal

Nobody walks through life alone; some people have to look for those who walk with them; others, like myself, are fortunate enough to have those people walking alongside them.

To my wife Denise, you have always supported me without question and I would never have achieved the goals I have without your love and support. To Dominick and Samantha, who persevered through long days and nights, while I was at work during New York's darkest hours, only to outshine that by taking a blind leap of faith with me and starting our new life in South Dakota.

Thanks to Monica and Rosemary for going for it, and to Cindy and Tom, my new "partners in crime," for your energetic and unwavering support. I would like to extend a special thanks to my friend Joyce Little Thunder for working with me to try and save the world, and with any luck, we'll get that done real soon.

Gregory Santa Maria

NOTE

The bibliographic citations following each answer cite the publisher of the book first (Brady, *Paramedic Care* or *Mosby, Paramedic Textbook*) and the section or chapter (e.g., Patient Assessment or Trauma) in that book in which relevant information can be found. For full book information on each citation, please see the Bibliography, on page 239

Preparatory

The following topics are covered in Section I:

- Emergency Medical Services (EMS) Systems—Roles and Responsibilities of the Paramedic
- Well-being of the Paramedic
- Medical/Legal Issues
- Ethics in Advanced Prehospital Care
- Pharmacology
- Venous Access and Medication Administration

Questions

EMS SYSTEMS—ROLES AND RESPONSIBILITIES OF THE PARAMEDIC

DIRECTIONS: Each item below contains four suggested responses. Select the one best response to each item.

1. Match the following terms with the correct definitions:

   (A) EMS systems _____
   (B) licensure _____
   (C) professionalism _____
   (D) certification _____
   (E) profession _____
   (F) ethics _____
   (G) protocols _____
   (H) medical direction _____

   1. rules and standards that govern conduct
   2. conduct that characterizes a practitioner
   3. government agency verification of competency
   4. legal framework for Paramedics to act for doctors
   5. entity made up of personnel, equipment, and resources
   6. particular field or occupation
   7. standardized approach to common patient problems
   8. agency recognition of predetermined qualifications

2. Which of the following is *not* a national group that is involved in future development of EMS?

   (A) National Association of EMS Physicians (NAEMSP)
   (B) New York State Ambulance Association
   (C) National Association of Emergency Medical Technicians (NAEMT)
   (D) National Association of Search and Rescue (NASAR)

3. Which of the following is *not* a nationally recognized level of EMS responder?

    (A) First Responder
    (B) EMT-Basic
    (C) EMT-Cardiac Technician
    (D) EMT-Paramedic

4. Prior to beginning practice as a Paramedic, it is essential that you acquire which of the following?

    (A) national licensure
    (B) state certification and/or licensure
    (C) Paramedic course completion
    (D) county certification

5. In order to retain one's level of certification, a Paramedic can participate in all of the following continuing medical education (CME) activities *except*:

    (A) membership in national associations
    (B) conferences and seminars
    (C) independent study and journal review
    (D) certification and recertification programs

6. All of the following are functions of the National Registry of Emergency Medical Technicians (NREMT) *except*:

    (A) prepare and administer standardized tests for First Responder, EMT-Basic, EMT-Intermediate, and EMT-Paramedic
    (B) assists in developing and evaluating EMS training programs
    (C) provides national licensure
    (D) works to establish a national standard of competency for all levels of EMS providers

7. Match all of the following examples of Paramedic professional behavior with the correct definition:

    (A) integrity _____
    (B) self-motivation _____
    (C) communications _____
    (D) time management _____
    (E) self-confidence _____
    (F) respect _____
    (G) diplomacy _____
    (H) patient advocacy _____

    1. arriving to work on time and ready to go
    2. presenting a case on telemetry
    3. introducing yourself to each patient
    4. persisting in having an emergently ill patient seen in the emergency department
    5. calming your partner during argument with police
    6. documenting your treatment on the call report
    7. rapid airway, breathing, and circulation (ABCs) assessment of the trauma victim
    8. verbally taking control of treating an elderly patient with emotionally upset family members

8. You are dispatched to the scene where a 45-year-old female pedestrian has been hit by a car. In addition to your ambulance, a fire department engine company was also dispatched with another level of EMS professional to assist in provision of treatment. Which of the following *best* defines this person's role?

    (A) family member
    (B) school nurse
    (C) EMT-Intermediate
    (D) First Responder

9. Which of the following is *not* categorized as a Paramedic's responsibility?

   (A) scene size-up, communicating with dispatch
   (B) direct communications with medical control physicians
   (C) initiating advanced life support and performing invasive procedures
   (D) following patient care instructions from the first arriving EMT-Basic

10. All of the following are correct statements concerning medical control *except*:

   (A) includes providing reviewing calls with Paramedics and overseeing CME
   (B) provides the legal framework for Paramedics to act on behalf of doctors
   (C) involves only direct online communications with the Paramedic
   (D) establishes and maintains prehospital protocols in conjunction with state and local laws

11. Of the following, which is the main focus in providing quality improvement for an EMS system?

   (A) ambulance maintenance
   (B) billing procedures
   (C) quality of supplies
   (D) ensuring competent and appropriate patient care efforts

12. All of the following are correct concerning EMS research *except*:

   (A) It is performed only by EMS physicians.
   (B) It is an important part of any EMS system.
   (C) Many Paramedic protocols and procedures have been instituted based on the outcomes of EMS research.
   (D) A research study consists of a hypothesis, literature review, study design, patient consent, and data collection, analysis, and statistical relevance.

WELL-BEING OF THE PARAMEDIC

DIRECTIONS: Each item below contains four suggested responses. Select the one best response to each item.

13. Which of the following *best* defines wellness?

   (A) the practice of treating patients and making them well
   (B) good health
   (C) the concept that encourages people to take responsibility for their health
   (D) a sense of feeling good

14. Which of the following is *not* an example of wellness?

   (A) physical well-being
   (B) spiritual well-being
   (C) mental and emotional well-being
   (D) financial well-being

15. All of the following are examples of wellness programs *except*:

   (A) computer course
   (B) weight reduction
   (C) stress management
   (D) smoking cessation

16. Which of the following is *not* one of the stages of a stress reaction?

   (A) alarm
   (B) resistance
   (C) exhaustion
   (D) nervous breakdown

17. Which of the following would *not* normally trigger a stress reaction?

   (A) death of a loved one
   (B) personal injury
   (C) complimentary letter
   (D) job stress

18. A Paramedic may experience all of the following symptoms of acute or chronic stress *except*:

    (A) fluttering in the chest
    (B) nausea, vomiting, and abdominal cramps
    (C) high, persistent fever
    (D) night sweats

19. You are dispatched to an 18-year-old female who is emotionally disturbed and is in possible possession of a weapon. You are the first to arrive at the scene and can see through the front window of the house that the patient is upset and has a large knife in her hand. All of the following are parts of the approach to dealing with this patient *except*:

    (A) Enter the house, introduce yourself, and begin to softly calm the patient down.
    (B) Avoid verbal confrontation with the patient and try to listen to her.
    (C) Do not let the patient block your exit.
    (D) Before attempting to restrain a patient, make sure that adequate help is available.

20. Of the following, which would be the least likely to be used as a defense mechanism that the Paramedic would use to deal with a stressful event?

    (A) denial
    (B) rationalization
    (C) isolation
    (D) crying

21. You have been working for your EMS service for the past 9 years. Recently, you notice that one of your coworkers has been steadily demonstrating classic signs of "burnout." He has been less interested in patient care, arrives late to work frequently, complains about every call, began drinking after work, and has been having increased difficulty dealing with his friends and family. How would you define his condition?

    (A) cumulative stress
    (B) acute stress reaction
    (C) critical incident stress
    (D) delayed stress

22. You are sent to an explosion at a nearby elementary school. As you arrive, you are told that the scene is currently safe. Additional information confirms over 50 serious injuries and several deaths. As you and other First Responders begin to enter the scene, an incident commander is already beginning to plan to assist all responders with the critical incident stress associated with this disaster. Which of the following would be the least likely on-scene critical incident stress debriefing (CISD) intervention?

    (A) briefing rescuers about what to expect before deployment to the scene
    (B) providing 15- to 20-minute breaks every 2 hours, away from the scene
    (C) calling all of the emergency responders together 1 hour into the event for a 30-minute talk
    (D) ensuring that maximum exposure on the scene does not exceed 12 hours

23. When intervening in a stressful event, which of the following is *not* used by CISD teams?

    (A) debriefing
    (B) demobilization
    (C) referral
    (D) denial

24. All of the following are stages of the grieving process *except*:

    (A) denial
    (B) anger
    (C) depression
    (D) exhilaration

25. Which of the following would have the least effect on the Paramedic's attitude toward death and dying?

    (A) religious and cultural understanding
    (B) prejudices
    (C) prior experiences
    (D) your grandmother's death, before you were born

MEDICAL/LEGAL ISSUES

DIRECTIONS: Each item below contains four suggested responses. Select the one best response to each item.

26. Your unit is assigned to a call for a patient with asthma. On your arrival, you find a 50-year-old male complaining of severe difficulty in breathing. You begin your advanced life support care. While you are treating this patient, your partner becomes excited and states that the police are calling for an ambulance for a shooting only three blocks away. You and your partner pack up your equipment and tell the patient that he will be OK and respond to the shooting. Later you find out that the patient called for another ambulance an hour later and was transported in critical condition. In addition to abandonment, you may also be charged with which of the following?

    (A) negligence
    (B) assault
    (C) slander
    (D) libel

27. You are assigned to an unconscious diabetic patient. After your assessment, you administer oxygen and 50% dextrose intravenously (IV). The patient awakens and is transported to the hospital without incident. You initially treated this patient under which type of consent?

    (A) informed
    (B) assumed
    (C) involuntary
    (D) implied

28. Match the following statements with their definitions:

    (A) abandonment _____
    (B) battery _____
    (C) assault _____
    (D) libel _____
    (E) slander _____
    (F) false imprisonment _____

    1. damaging a patient's character by using false or malicious spoken terms
    2. damaging a patient's character by using false or malicious written terms
    3. committing an act that places the patient in fear of bodily harm
    4. termination of a patient's care prior to ensuring a continuation of proper care
    5. touching a patient against his or her consent
    6. intentionally and unjustifiably detaining a patient against his or her will

29. The Paramedic may be required to report all of the following types of cases to the proper authorities *except*:

    (A) child abuse
    (B) stab wounds
    (C) rape
    (D) myocardial infarction in a 58-year-old male

30. You are treating a 57-year-old female whose family called 911 because the patient was experiencing chest pain. The patient is in obvious distress. The patient states that she has been in the hospital too much lately and will not go back. You make numerous attempts to convince the patient to go to the hospital, and she adamantly refuses. All of the following should be documented on your call report *except*:

    (A) patient's name, address, and date of birth
    (B) vital signs and Paramedic interventions
    (C) nothing should be written on the report, since the patient is refusing transport
    (D) attempts to convince the patient to change her mind

ETHICS IN ADVANCED PREHOSPITAL CARE

DIRECTIONS: Each item below contains four suggested responses. Select the one best response to each item.

31. Which of the following *best* defines ethics?

    (A) the study of standards, conduct, and moral judgment that governs the conduct of members of a particular group
    (B) simple compliance to peer pressure
    (C) following orders, right or wrong
    (D) religious teachings that affect any given person

32. Which of the following is the *best* premise for the Paramedic's ethical decisions?

    (A) Follow your partner's decisions on any difficult situation.
    (B) Intervene only when you feel that it is correct to do so.
    (C) Follow the family's wishes regardless of your protocols or state statutes.
    (D) Place the welfare of the patient ahead of all other considerations.

33. You are dispatched to the scene of a 77-year-old female who lost consciousness. As you walk into the home, a crying family member informs you that the patient has been chronically ill for the past 6 months with metastatic cancer. As you approach the patient, you note that she is breathing eight times per minute, her pulse is 20 beats per minute, and her blood pressure is not palpable. There are no signs of trauma and no indications of foul play. Which of the following is the most reasonable approach to this patient?

    (A) Immediately intubate, force IV fluids, and consider an external pacemaker.
    (B) Knowing your state law and your EMS system rules and regulations concerning advanced directives, inquire of the patient's family members whether there are any such advanced directives in effect, and proceed according to a combination of the laws, rules, and directives.
    (C) Do not treat this patient until you have personally spoken to her physician and your own medical control physician.
    (D) Follow your heart and try to avoid any treatment of this patient at any cost.

PHARMACOLOGY

DIRECTIONS: Each item below contains four suggested responses. Select the one best response to each item.

34. The description of a drug using its chemical composition and molecular structure is the

    (A) trade name
    (B) chemical name
    (C) official name
    (D) brand name

35. MS Contin is an example of a(an)

    (A) chemical name
    (B) generic name
    (C) trade name
    (D) official name

36. Which of the following drugs is derived from a plant?

    (A) lidocaine hydrochloride
    (B) magnesium sulfate
    (C) digitalis
    (D) penicillin

37. Lidocaine and procainamide are examples of medications derived from

    (A) synthetics
    (B) minerals
    (C) animals
    (D) plants

38. All of the following are accepted publications on drug information *except*:

    (A) *The Merck Manual*
    (B) American Medical Association (AMA) drug evaluation
    (C) medication package inserts
    (D) *Physicians' Desk Reference*

39. A controlled substance that is classified as schedule I is defined as a drug with

    (A) high abuse potential and accepted medical uses
    (B) moderate abuse potential and accepted medical uses
    (C) high abuse potential and no medical uses
    (D) low abuse potential and accepted medical uses

40. You respond to an unconscious patient in a park. On your arrival you find a 17-year-old male who is unresponsive. His friend states that the patient had injected heroin and "ate some Valium" prior to losing consciousness. The history provided by his companion leads you to conclude that the patient has overdosed on medications classified as

    (A) schedule II and schedule IV
    (B) schedule III and schedule I
    (C) schedule IV and schedule II
    (D) schedule I and schedule IV

41. Pharmacokinetics is defined as

    (A) a drug's affect on the receptor
    (B) a drug's mechanism of action on the body
    (C) the entry of medications into the body and their elimination
    (D) the use of medications in trauma patients

42. Pharmacodynamics is defined as

    (A) biotransformation to convert a drug into an active form
    (B) the crossing of a medication through the blood-brain barrier
    (C) the elimination of a drug through metabolism
    (D) the process in which the desired biochemical response is achieved

43. All of the following are pharmacokinetic factors *except*:

    (A) therapeutic index
    (B) distribution
    (C) elimination
    (D) absorption

44. A beta agonist is a medication that

    (A) inhibits beta activity by blocking receptor sites
    (B) stimulates an increase in beta activity, creating a desired drug effect
    (C) biotransforms beta medications
    (D) energizes target tissues

45. Your patient is suspected of taking an overdose of an opiate. In order to reverse this overdose, you should administer a

    (A) narcotic agonist
    (B) benzodiazepine agonist
    (C) narcotic antagonist
    (D) benzodiazepine antagonist

46. Your 55-year-old patient has overdosed on diazepam and is unconscious. Flumazenil is administered, and the patient becomes more oriented to his/her surroundings. Flumazenil is an example of a

    (A) beta agonist
    (B) beta antagonist
    (C) benzodiazepine agonist
    (D) benzodiazepine antagonist

47. Liquid penicillin is an example of which drug form?

    (A) emulsion
    (B) fluid extract
    (C) suspension
    (D) elixir

48. Your patient has self-administered sublingual nitroglycerin for his chest pain. Nitroglycerin is an example of which type of solid drug?

    (A) pill
    (B) powder
    (C) tablet
    (D) capsule

49. Elixirs, emulsions, suspensions, and solutions are all examples of which form of drug?

    (A) solid
    (B) liquid
    (C) parenteral
    (D) spirits

50. Potentiation is used to describe

    (A) the enhancement of the effect of one drug by another drug
    (B) the effect gained by taking multiple doses of a single drug
    (C) an effect in which the absence of a drug causes physical or emotional disturbances
    (D) two drugs, administered together, the total effect of which equals the sum of the effects of each individual agent

51. A side effect of a drug that produces an outcome harmful to the patient is called a

    (A) contraindication
    (B) depressant
    (C) untoward effect (reaction)
    (D) therapeutic action

52. Most drugs have known and expected side effects. However, in certain patients, a drug may have a side effect that is neither known nor expected. This circumstance is defined as

    (A) tolerance
    (B) synergism
    (C) potentiator
    (D) idiosyncratic reaction

53. The administration of a drug in several doses, causing an increased effect due to a buildup of the drug in the blood, is called

    (A) antagonism
    (B) therapeutic action
    (C) idiosyncratic reaction
    (D) cumulative action

54. Your patient has been taking a medication for 8 years. He tells you that over the years his physician has increased the dosage. This adjustment in dosage is in response to a condition known as

    (A) habituation
    (B) synergism
    (C) antagonism
    (D) tolerance

55. The process by which a drug is converted into an active form in the blood or body tissue is called

    (A) absorption
    (B) biotransformation
    (C) distribution
    (D) elimination

56. Which of the following is *not* responsible for the excretion of drug metabolites?

    (A) kidneys
    (B) liver
    (C) intestines
    (D) thyroid

57. You administer 1000 mg of a medication with a half-life of 2 hours. How many hours will it take for the medication to be excreted to less than 1 mg?

    (A) 12 hours
    (B) 14 hours
    (C) 18 hours
    (D) 20 hours

58. A medication that would produce the same effect as that of the sympathetic nervous system is known as

    (A) parasympathomimetic
    (B) sympatholytic
    (C) sympathomimetic
    (D) parasympatholytic

59. Which of the following medications is *not* a sympathomimetic?

    (A) lidocaine
    (B) epinephrine
    (C) dopamine
    (D) norepinephrine (Levophed)

60. _____ is *not* classified as a benzodiazepine.

    (A) Flumazenil
    (B) Lorazepam
    (C) Diazepam
    (D) Midazolam

61. All of the following medications are antidysrhythmics with the exception of _____.

    (A) lidocaine
    (B) procainamide
    (C) magnesium sulfate
    (D) bretylium tosylate

62. Which is *not* a parenteral route of medication administration?

    (A) IV
    (B) endotracheal
    (C) intramuscular
    (D) rectal

63. The rates of drug absorption for different routes of drug administration from the fastest to the slowest are

    (A) intramuscular
    (B) endotracheal
    (C) IV
    (D) sublingual
    (E) oral
    (F) subcutaneous

    1. 1, 4, 2, 3, 6, 5
    2. 2, 4, 3, 1, 6, 5
    3. 3, 2, 1, 6, 4, 5
    4. 4, 6, 3, 1, 2, 5

VENOUS ACCESS AND MEDICATION ADMINISTRATION

DIRECTIONS: Each item below contains four suggested responses. Select the one best response to each item.

64. Endotracheal administration is *not* indicated in which of the following medications?

    (A) lidocaine
    (B) furosemide
    (C) epinephrine
    (D) atropine

65. You are ordered to administer 10 mL of a 4% medication. How many milligrams should you administer to the patient?

    (A) 40 mg
    (B) 100 mg
    (C) 200 mg
    (D) 400 mg

66. Your medical control physician orders you to administer 20 mg of furosemide. Furosemide is supplied in vials that contain 40 mg in 4 mL. How many milliliters should you administer?

    (A) 2 mL
    (B) 4 mL
    (C) 6 mL
    (D) 8 mL

67. The medical control physician orders the administration of 1 mg of naloxone to an unconscious patient. Naloxone is supplied in a solution concentration of 0.4 mg/mL. How many milliliters should you administer?

    (A) 1.5 mL
    (B) 2.5 mL
    (C) 5.5 mL
    (D) 7.0 mL

68. A physician orders you to administer 0.3 mg of epinephrine 1:1000 solution to an asthmatic. How many milliliters should you administer?

    (A) 0.03 mL
    (B) 30 mL
    (C) 3 mL
    (D) 0.3 mL

69. Your unconscious patient requires 100 mg of thiamine prior to the administration of dextrose. Thiamine is supplied 50 mg/mL. How many milliliters should you administer?

    (A) 2 mL
    (B) 4 mL
    (C) 6 mL
    (D) 8 mL

70. You must mix a bag of lidocaine to achieve a 4:1 solution concentration. You have a 500-mL bag of solution. How many milligrams of lidocaine should be added to the bag to create a 4:1 concentration?

    (A) 500 mg
    (B) 1000 mg
    (C) 1500 mg
    (D) 2000 mg

71. You are ordered to administer a lidocaine drip to a patient. The drip will be administered at 3 mg/min. You add 2 g lidocaine to an IV bag that contains 500 mL of solution. Then you attach a drip set capable of administering 60 gtt/mL. What is your drip rate?

    (A) 15 gtt/min
    (B) 30 gtt/min
    (C) 45 gtt/min
    (D) 60 gtt/min

72. You respond to the scene of a 50-year-old male in cardiac arrest. When you hook up the monitor, you see that he is in ventricular fibrillation. After several unsuccessful attempts to defibrillate the patient, the first medication to be administered is epinephrine 1 mg of a 1:10,000 solution. How many milliliters should you administer?

    (A) 10 mL
    (B) 5 mL
    (C) 1 mL
    (D) 0.2 mL

73. A patient has been ordered to receive 300 mL of normal saline solution over the next 2 hours. Using a 500-mL bag of solution and a macro drip set (10 gtt/mL), what drip rate should the Paramedic use in order to achieve this administration?

    (A) 20 gtt/min
    (B) 25 gtt/min
    (C) 30 gtt/min
    (D) 35 gtt/min

74. The physician has ordered the patient's infusion in the preceding question increased to 500 mL over the next 2 hours. Using a 500-mL bag of solution and macro drip set (10 gtt/mL), what should you set the drip rate at in order to properly increase the infusion rate?

    (A) 40 gtt/min
    (B) 42 gtt/min
    (C) 44 gtt/min
    (D) 46 gtt/min

75. You must administer 1000 mL of normal saline to a patient over a period of 6 hours, using a 1000-mL bag of solution and a 10-gtt/min drip set. How many drops per minute should you administer to deliver this amount?

    (A) 28 gtt/min
    (B) 30 gtt/min
    (C) 42 gtt/min
    (D) 44 gtt/min

76. You are working on an unconscious diabetic. Your partner hands you a syringe and tells you that it contains 100 mg of thiamine in 2 mL of solution. After you push the medication, your partner informs you that he mistakenly filled up the syringe with diphenhydramine. In this situation, what should you, the Paramedic do?

    (A) Ignore the error. The diphenhydramine will probably have no ill effects.
    (B) Administer the thiamine and bring the patient to the hospital, making no mention of your error.
    (C) Immediately contact the medical control physician and advise them of your error, monitor your patient for ill effects of the medication during transport, document your error, and advise hospital staff on your arrival.
    (D) Discuss the situation with your partner after the call, and tell him that you will not cover for him again.

77. You are administering a subcutaneous injection to a patient. What is the most appropriate needle size and angle of insertion to be used?

    (A) 25 gauge and 90 degrees
    (B) 25 gauge and 45 degrees
    (C) 18 gauge and 90 degrees
    (D) 18 gauge and 45 degrees

78. What are the correct needle size and insertion angle for an intramuscular injection?

    (A) 25 gauge and 90 degrees
    (B) 21 gauge and 45 degrees
    (C) 21 gauge and 90 degrees
    (D) 25 gauge and 45 degrees

79. You are ordered to administer an endotracheal dose of epinephrine. In administering endotracheal medications, the normal IV dose should be increased. What should the endotracheal dose be if the normal IV dose is 1.0 mg?

    (A) 5–10 mg
    (B) 2–2.5 mg
    (C) 10–15 mg
    (D) 15–20 mg

80. Which of the following is *not* a narcotic analgesic?

    (A) morphine sulfate
    (B) meperidine
    (C) oxycodone
    (D) diazepam

81. Parasympatholytic medications can be expected to produce which of the following effects?

    (A) blocks the actions of the parasympathetic nervous system
    (B) blocks the actions of the sympathetic nervous system
    (C) mimics the actions of the parasympathetic nervous system
    (D) mimics the actions of the sympathetic nervous system

82. Atropine sulfate is classified under which of the following medication categories?

    (A) parasympathomimetic
    (B) parasympatholytic
    (C) sympathomimetic
    (D) sympatholytic

83. Epinephrine is classified as a

    (A) parasympathomimetic
    (B) parasympatholytic
    (C) sympathomimetic
    (D) sympatholytic

84. Which of the following is *not* a beta$_1$ response?

    (A) increased force of cardiac contraction
    (B) increased bronchodilation
    (C) increased heart rate
    (D) increased conduction velocity

Answers and Explanations

EMS SYSTEMS—ROLES AND RESPONSIBILITIES OF THE PARAMEDIC

1. **The answers are: (A) 5, (B) 3, (C) 2, (D) 8, (E) 6, (F) 1, (G) 7, (H) 4.** *(Brady, Paramedic Care 2e, Principles and Practice, Volume 1—Roles and Responsibilities. Mosby, Paramedic Textbook 3e, EMS Systems/Roles and Responsibilities.)*

2. **The answer is B.** Even though the organization in (B) may be involved in EMS education and development using national standards, it is not a national group. (A), (B), and (C) are national groups involved in EMS development. *(Brady, Paramedic Care 2e, Principles and Practice, Volume 1—Roles and Responsibilities. Mosby, Paramedic Textbook 3e, EMS Systems/Roles and Responsibilities.)*

3. **The answer is C.** (A), (B), EMT-Intermediate, and (D) are the four nationally recognized levels of EMS training and education. In some areas, (C) was a level of EMS certification; it has since been replaced by EMT-Intermediate. *(Brady, Paramedic Care 2e, Principles and Practice, Volume 1—Roles and Responsibilities. Mosby, Paramedic Textbook 3e, EMS Systems/Roles and Responsibilities.)*

4. **The answer is B.** Certification and/or licensure to practice as a Paramedic is granted at the state level. Many states require the Paramedic to pass a state examination. However, many states accept the candidate's results on the NREMT examination as an alternative. Most states also require recertification every 2–3 years. This may include a certain number of hours of CME to retain certification and/or licensure as well. *(Brady, Paramedic Care 2e, Principles and Practice, Volume 1—Roles and Responsibilities. Mosby, Paramedic Textbook 3e, EMS Systems/Roles and Responsibilities.)*

5. **The answer is A.** (B), (C), and (D), lectures and workshops, quality-improvement case reviews, skill laboratories, and certain approved computer Internet courses are some of the widely accepted methods of acquiring CME for maintaining Paramedic competency. (A) is not a component of acceptable continuing education. Participation in national associations is considered to be professionally important but does not constitute CME in and of itself. *(Brady, Paramedic Care 2e, Principles and Practice, Volume 1—Roles and Responsibilities. Mosby, Paramedic Textbook 3e, EMS Systems/Roles and Responsibilities.)*

6. **The answer is C.** In (A), (B), and (D), the NREMT develops and conducts standardized EMS testing and serves as a widely accepted format for providing reciprocity for EMS professionals seeking to practice in a new state. (C) is not a function of the NREMT because licensure and certification are granted on the state level. However, many states accept the NREMT certification to qualify applicants for reciprocity. *(Brady, Paramedic Care 2e, Principles and Practice, Volume 1—Roles and Responsibilities. Mosby, Paramedic Textbook 3e, EMS Systems/Roles and Responsibilities.)*

7. **The answers are: (A) 6, (B) 1, (C) 2, (D) 7, (E) 8, (F) 3, (G) 5, (H) 4.** *(Brady, Paramedic Care 2e, Principles and Practice, Volume 1—Roles and Responsibilities. Mosby, Paramedic Textbook 3e, EMS Systems/Roles and Responsibilities.)*

8. **The answer is D.** (A), (B), and (C) are incorrect. (D) A First Responder best defines this role.

With proper training, any of the other individuals could act in this capacity, however, they would not be dispatched to the scene. *(Brady, Paramedic Care 2e, Principles and Practice, Volume 1—Roles and Responsibilities. Mosby, Paramedic Textbook 3e, EMS Systems/Roles and Responsibilities.)*

9. **The answer is D.** In (A), (B), and (C), a Paramedic is responsible for conducting patient assessments, communicating with other team members, assessing the results of treatment, directing and coordinating transport, and maintaining rapport with the patient, support agencies, and the hospital. (D) is incorrect. The Paramedic has the highest level of training, and is therefore responsible to assign patient care priorities. However, a good Paramedic will utilize the capabilities of all emergency personnel on the scene. *(Brady, Paramedic Care 2e, Principles and Practice, Volume 1—Roles and Responsibilities. Mosby, Paramedic Textbook 3e, EMS Systems/Roles and Responsibilities.)*

10. **The answer is C.** Statement (C) is incorrect. Medical control involves direct online medical control. However, it also involves many off-line responsibilities, including quality assurance and continuing quality improvement, providing call-review sessions, arranging and providing CME, participating with local prehospital community committees, and in-servicing telemetry physicians. (A), (B), and (D) are correct statements. *(Brady, Paramedic Care 2e, Principles and Practice, Volume 1—Roles and Responsibilities. Mosby, Paramedic Textbook 3e, EMS Systems/Roles and Responsibilities.)*

11. **The answer is D.** (A), (B), and (C) are incorrect. These are some of the areas to follow in assessing quality improvement, however, (D) patient satisfaction is truly the top priority. *(Brady, Paramedic Care 2e, Principles and Practice, Volume 1—EMS Systems. Mosby, Paramedic Textbook 3e, EMS Systems/Roles and Responsibilities.)*

12. **The answer is A.** (B), (C), and (D) are correct statements. Statement (A) is incorrect, because, even though EMS physicians may be involved in EMS research, prehospital providers consistently participate in EMS research, with or without EMS physician oversight. *(Brady, Paramedic Care 2e, Principles and Practice, Volume 1—EMS Systems. Mosby, Paramedic Textbook 3e, EMS Systems/Roles and Responsibilities.)*

WELL-BEING OF THE PARAMEDIC

13. **The answer is C.** Wellness is based on the premise that people have control over their health behaviors. (A), (B), and (D) are incorrect. *(Brady, Paramedic Care 2e, Principles and Practice, Volume 1—The Well being of the Paramedic. Mosby, Paramedic Textbook 3e, The Well being of the Paramedic.)*

14. **The answer is D.** (A), (B), and (C) are components of wellness. (D) is not. *(Brady, Paramedic Care 2e, Principles and Practice, Volume 1—The Well being of the Paramedic. Mosby, Paramedic Textbook 3e, The Well being of the Paramedic.)*

15. **The answer is A.** (B), (C), (D), cholesterol and blood pressure screening, nutrition, physical fitness, and safety education are examples of wellness programs. (A) is not. *(Brady, Paramedic Care 2e, Principles and Practice, Volume 1—The Well being of the Paramedic. Mosby, Paramedic Textbook 3e, The Well being of the Paramedic.)*

16. **The answer is D.** (A), (B), and (C) are the classic three stages of stress. (D) is not part of the stress reaction. *(Brady, Paramedic Care 2e, Principles and Practice, Volume 1—The Well being of the Paramedic. Mosby, Paramedic Textbook 3e, The Well being of the Paramedic.)*

17. **The answer is C.** (A), (B), (D), and any major life events are some examples of stress triggers. (C) is not a stress trigger because a complimentary letter usually brings about a positive and comforting feeling. *(Brady, Paramedic Care 2e, Principles and Practice, Volume 1—The Well being of the Paramedic. Mosby, Paramedic Textbook 3e, The Well being of the Paramedic.)*

18. **The answer is C.** (A), (B), (D), rapid or difficult breathing, dry mouth, chest tightness, sweating,

flushing, urinary frequency, and muscle or joint aches are some of the symptoms of anxiety. (C) is not a symptom of anxiety because, even though anxiety may trigger fluctuations in body temperature, it should not produce a persistently high fever. A physical examination looking for a possible infectious cause would be in order. *(Brady, Paramedic Care 2e, Principles and Practice, Volume 1—The Well being of the Paramedic. Mosby, Paramedic Textbook 3e, The Well being of the Paramedic.)*

19. **The answer is A.** (B), (C), and (D) are all correct. (A) is incorrect because, at any violent scene, your safety must first be established. It would be a serious and possibly deadly mistake to enter the home of this emotionally disturbed patient before the police have secured the premises. *(Brady, Paramedic Care 2e, Principles and Practice, Volume 1—The Well being of the Paramedic. Mosby, Paramedic Textbook 3e, The Well being of the Paramedic.)*

20. **The answer is D.** (A), (B), (C), compensation, reaction formation, substitution, sublimation, regression, repression, and projection are all some of the defense mechanisms used to deal with stress. (D) is incorrect. Crying may be an expression of stress but is not considered a defense mechanism. *(Brady, Paramedic Care 2e, Principles and Practice, Volume 1—The Well being of the Paramedic. Mosby, Paramedic Textbook 3e, The Well being of the Paramedic.)*

21. **The answer is A.** Cumulative stress reactions result from experience with multiple individual stressors occurring over time. Physical and emotional exhaustion and negative attitudes characterize it. (B), (C), and (D) are incorrect. An acute stress reaction is incident specific and usually easily isolated to a single event. Critical incident stress is the reaction that many emergency responding individuals have to a disaster or multicasualty incident. Delayed stress reactions are also the result of a specific incident, but the Paramedic may not experience symptoms until days, months, or years later. *(Brady, Paramedic Care 2e, Principles and Practice, Volume 1— The Well being of the Paramedic. Mosby, Paramedic Textbook 3e, The Well being of the Paramedic.)*

22. **The answer is C.** (A), (B), (D), allowing completion of tasks before changing assignments, integrating veterans to teach newcomers how to perform the task, providing meals and snacks, maintaining normal working groups, and providing decaffeinated beverages are some of the skills used to deal with critical incident stress. (C) is not used because it would be unwise and impossible to remove all emergency responders together from the event in order to talk to them. During the event, such a response may result in more casualties and would add to the critical incident stress for the responders. *(Brady, Paramedic Care 2e, Principles and Practice, Volume 1—The Well being of the Paramedic. Mosby, Paramedic Textbook 3e, The Well being of the Paramedic.)*

23. **The answer is D.** (A), (B), (C), and defusing are some of the techniques used. (D) is incorrect. Denial is one of the defense mechanisms an individual may use to deal with stress, it is not a technique used by critical incident stress management teams. Rather, the correct approach is to try to assist the EMS responder with expressing his or her feelings concerning the entire experience. *(Brady, Paramedic Care 2e, Principles and Practice, Volume 1—The Well being of the Paramedic. Mosby, Paramedic Textbook 3e, The Well being of the Paramedic.)*

24. **The answer is D.** (A), (B), (C), anger, denial, depression, bargaining, and acceptance are all stages of the grieving process. (D) is incorrect. *(Brady, Paramedic Care 2e, Principles and Practice, Volume 1—The Well being of the Paramedic. Mosby, Paramedic Textbook 3e, The Well being of the Paramedic.)*

25. **The answer is D.** (A), (B), and (C) play an integral part in affecting each Paramedic's attitude toward death and dying. (D) does not because your grandmother's death would have little affect on your own personal feelings toward death and dying because you did not experience the event. *(Brady, Paramedic Care 2e, Principles and Practice, Volume 1—The Well being of the Paramedic. Mosby, Paramedic Textbook 3e, The Well being of the Paramedic.)*

MEDICAL/LEGAL ISSUES

26. **The answer is A.** On the scenario, you and your partner have met four criteria to be charged with negligence: (1) You were being compensated for your treatment (paid Paramedic) and since you were assigned to the call, you had a duty to act. (2) Your conduct was not reasonable or expected behavior. (3) Leaving the patient without further assessment or transport caused additional damage to the patient's condition. (4) Your abandonment of this patient was the proximate cause of his deterioration. Although it may be argued that you did not injure the patient, inappropriate treatment was the cause of this patient's deterioration. (A), (C), and (D) are incorrect. *(Brady, Paramedic Care 2e, Principles and Practice, Volume 1—Medical/Legal Aspects of Advanced Prehospital Care. Mosby, Paramedic Textbook 3e, Medical/Legal Issues.)*

27. **The answer is D.** (D) is correct, since the patient was unconscious. The definition of *implied consent* states that the patient would have allowed you to initiate treatment, if he or she was conscious and able to agree to care. (A) Informed consent applies to the conscious patient who makes a decision to be treated after an explanation of the diagnosis and the possible treatments. (C) Involuntary consent usually involves a court order to initiate care of the patient. (B) is incorrect. *(Brady, Paramedic Care 2e, Principles and Practice, Volume 1—Medical/Legal Aspects of Advanced Prehospital Care. Mosby, Paramedic Textbook 3e, Medical/Legal Issues.)*

28. **The answers are: (A) 4, (B) 5, (C) 3, (D) 2, (E) 1, (F) 6.** *(Brady, Paramedic Care 2e, Principles and Practice, Volume 1—Medical/Legal Aspects of Advanced Prehospital Care. Mosby, Paramedic Textbook 3e, Medical/Legal Issues.)*

29. **The answer is D.** Paramedics may be required by law to report all types of injuries that may be the result of assaults or other criminal activity. All of the answers are correct with the exception of (D). A 58-year-old male having a myocardial infarction is not a reportable incident. Paramedics may also be required to report certain instances of illness and/or communicable diseases. *(Brady, Paramedic Care 2e, Principles and Practice, Volume 1—Medical/Legal Aspects of Advanced Prehospital Care. Mosby, Paramedic Textbook 3e, Medical/Legal Issues.)*

30. **The answer is C.** Many lawsuits arise out of patients' refusal of care. Paramedics need to be especially careful about the documentation of these patients. All patient interactions are thoroughly documented. (A), (B), and (D) are all pertinent pieces of information that must be documented. In addition, the Paramedic should have the refusal signed by the patient and witnessed by family members or a member of law enforcement. EMS providers should keep in mind that lawsuits go to trial many years after a call. The only reference that the provider may have is a neatly written comprehensive patient care report. *(Brady, Paramedic Care 2e, Principles and Practice, Volume 1—Medical/Legal Aspects of Advanced Prehospital Care. Mosby, Paramedic Textbook 3e, Medical/Legal Issues.)*

ETHICS IN ADVANCED PREHOSPITAL CARE

31. **The answer is A.** (B), (C), and (D) are incorrect because, even though each may play a part in the practice of the Paramedic, none is a part of the definition of ethics. *(Brady, Paramedic Care 2e, Principles and Practice, Volume 1—Ethics in Advanced Prehospital Care. Mosby, Paramedic Textbook 3e, Ethics.)*

32. **The answer is D.** All EMS providers completely reduce their risk of participating in unethical behavior by always placing the welfare of the patient ahead of all other considerations. (A), (B), and (C) are incorrect. *(Brady, Paramedic Care 2e, Principles and Practice, Volume 1—Ethics in Advanced Prehospital Care. Mosby, Paramedic Textbook 3e, Ethics.)*

33. **This answer is B.** In trying to keep the patient's best interests in mind, you must be familiar with your state law and your EMS system rules and regulations concerning advanced directives. If the present situation is a little confusing,

you may choose to contact medical control in order to have additional input on how to proceed. In the meantime, even if you have been directed to honor any advanced directives, you should still provide comfort care for the patient and emotional support for the family member(s). If no advanced directives exist, in most cases you will be required to provide the appropriate care. *(Brady, Paramedic Care 2e, Principles and Practice, Volume 1—Ethics in Advanced Prehospital Care. Mosby, Paramedic Textbook 3e, Ethics.)*

PHARMACOLOGY

34. **The answer is B.** (B) The chemical name of a drug is the description of its chemical composition and molecular structure. Although (A), (C), and (D) are also used to describe drugs. Trade names are the copyrighted names given by the drug manufacturer, official names are the listings in the U.S. Pharmacopoeia or National Formulary, and brand name, the proprietary name, is another term for trade name. *(Brady, Paramedic Care 2e, Principles and Practice, Volume 1—Pharmacology. Mosby, Paramedic Textbook 3e, Pharmacology.)*

35. **The answer is C.** (C) MS Contin is the trade name for morphine sulfate. It is a potent narcotic analgesic. The trade name is the copyrighted name given by the drug manufacturer. (A), (B), and (D) are incorrect. *(Brady, Paramedic Care 2e, Principles and Practice, Volume 1—Pharmacology. Mosby, Paramedic Textbook 3e, Pharmacology.)*

36. **The answer is C.** (C) Digitalis is a derivative of the foxglove plant. There are five classifications of drug derivatives: plants (e.g., atropine sulfate, digitalis, and morphine sulfate), chemical substances (e.g., lidocaine), minerals (e.g., sodium bicarbonate and calcium chloride), microorganisms (e.g., penicillin), and animals and humans (e.g., insulin and epinephrine). *(Brady, Paramedic Care 2e, Principles and Practice, Volume 1—Pharmacology. Mosby, Paramedic Textbook 3e, Pharmacology.)*

37. **The answer is A.** (A) Lidocaine and procainamide are all synthetic medications. These medications have been developed in drug laboratories and are not natural derivatives. (B), (C), and (D) are incorrect. *(Brady, Paramedic Care 2e, Principles and Practice, Volume 1—Pharmacology. Mosby, Paramedic Textbook 3e, Pharmacology.)*

38. **The answer is A.** (A) *The Merck Manual* describes medical conditions and although it may contain some drug information, it does not contain comprehensive descriptions. (B) The AMA drug evaluation, (C) medication package inserts, and (D) the *Physicians' Desk Reference* are considered good resources of drug information for the Paramedic. The Hospital Formulary is also a good reference for drug information. *(Brady, Paramedic Care 2e, Principles and Practice, Volume 1—Pharmacology. Mosby, Paramedic Textbook 3e, Pharmacology.)*

39. **The answer is C.** Schedule I drugs are classified as illegal drugs of abuse (e.g., heroin, mescaline, and lysergic acid diethylamide [LSD]); they have high abuse potential and no accepted medical uses. Schedule II drugs (e.g., opiates and amphetamines) have high abuse potential but positive medical benefits. Schedule III drugs, which contain limited quantities of schedule II drugs, have a lower abuse potential than do schedule I and II medications. Schedule IV drugs (e.g., phenobarbital and diazepam) have a lower abuse potential than do schedule I, II, and III drugs. Schedule V drugs contain limited quantities of certain opioids and are generally used in cough or diarrhea control. *(Brady, Paramedic Care 2e, Principles and Practice, Volume 1—Pharmacology. Mosby, Paramedic Textbook 3e, Pharmacology.)*

40. **The answer is D.** Heroin is a schedule I drug with no accepted medical uses, while diazepam (Valium) is a schedule IV medication with accepted medical uses. Schedule I medications are not available by prescription. Schedule IV medications are available by a physician's prescription only. These prescriptions have strict guidelines that control the amount of refills as well as the length that the prescription may be refilled. All schedule II, III, and IV medications

must carry warning labels that alert the user to their abuse potential. *(Brady, Paramedic Care 2e, Principles and Practice, Volume 1—Pharmacology. Mosby, Paramedic Textbook 3e, Pharmacology.)*

41. **The answer is C.** (C) Pharmacokinetics is the study of how a drug enters the body and reaches its site of action. It includes absorption, distribution, biotransformation, and subsequent elimination through metabolism. (A), (B), and (D) are incorrect. *(Brady, Paramedic Care 2e, Principles and Practice, Volume 1—Pharmacology. Mosby, Paramedic Textbook 3e, Pharmacology.)*

42. **The answer is D.** (D) Pharmacodynamics is the process in which a drug binds to a receptor on the cell membrane and initiates a biochemical reaction, creating the desired response. (A), biotransformation, is the process by which a drug is made active or inactive. (C), the elimination of a drug, is part of the metabolic process of the body (pharmacokinetics). (B), the crossing of the blood-brain barrier, is part of the distribution process (pharmacokinetics). *(Brady, Paramedic Care 2e, Principles and Practice, Volume 1—Pharmacology. Mosby, Paramedic Textbook 3e, Pharmacology.)*

43. **The answer is A.** (A) The therapeutic index is the difference between the toxic and the effective dose of a medication. Therapeutic index is a factor of pharmacodynamics (the induction of a biochemical response). (B), (C), and (D) are all pharmacokinetic factors. *(Brady, Paramedic Care 2e, Principles and Practice, Volume 1—Pharmacology. Mosby, Paramedic Textbook 3e, Pharmacology.)*

44. **The answer is B.** (B) A beta agonist attaches to the cell's receptor site (a protein on the cell that allows a drug to bind to it) to create its desired effect. The process described in (A), the inhibition of the binding of one drug by another, is called antagonism. (C) and (D) are also incorrect. *(Brady, Paramedic Care 2e, Principles and Practice, Volume 1—Pharmacology. Mosby, Paramedic Textbook 3e, Pharmacology.)*

45. **The answer is C.** (C) To reverse the effects of an opioid derivative, the Paramedic should administer an opioid antagonist, in this case, naloxone. Naloxone competes for the opiate receptor sites and eliminates the effects of the opiate. (A) A narcotic agonist would stimulate receptors, thereby increasing the opioid effect. (B) A benzodiazepine agonist would potentiate the effects of the opioid by adding its sedative-hypnotic effect to the opioid overdose. (D) A benzodiazepine antagonist would have no effect on an opioid. *(Brady, Paramedic Care 2e, Principles and Practice, Volume 1—Pharmacology. Mosby, Paramedic Textbook 3e, Pharmacology.)*

46. **The answer is D.** (D) Flumazenil is a benzodiazepine receptor antagonist. A receptor antagonist blocks the receptor site of certain drugs, rendering their mechanism of action ineffective. (A) A beta agonist would attach to a beta receptor and stimulate a beta effect. (B) A beta antagonist will not block the receptor sites for benzodiazepines or narcotics. (C) A benzodiazepine receptor agonist would be an actual benzodiazepine, such as diazepam or lorazepam; this patient has overdosed on this type of agonist. *(Brady, Paramedic Care 2e, Principles and Practice, Volume 1—Pharmacology. Mosby, Paramedic Textbook 3e, Pharmacology.)*

47. **The answer is C.** (C) A suspension is a drug (usually a powder) that is added to a liquid to facilitate oral administration. Penicillin, although available in solid form, is commonly administered to children in a liquid form. Suspensions have a tendency to separate and therefore require shaking before administration. (A) Emulsions are usually oil-and-water mixtures that are used, for example, as lubricants. (B) A fluid extract is a drug that is readily soluble in a particular fluid. (D) An elixir is a syrup with the addition of alcohol. *(Brady, Paramedic Care 2e, Principles and Practice, Volume 1—Pharmacology. Mosby, Paramedic Textbook 3e, Pharmacology.)*

48. **The answer is C.** (C) Nitroglycerin comes in several forms, but only (C) is correct in this instance. (A), (B), and (D) are incorrect. (A) Pills are drugs shaped in an easy-to-swallow form. (B) Powders are drugs that have been crushed and combined with other powders to form a mixture. (D) Capsules are gelatin containers that hold a dose of medication, usually in powder form. *(Brady, Paramedic Care 2e, Principles and Practice,*

Volume 1—Pharmacology. Mosby, Paramedic Textbook 3e, Pharmacology.)

49. **The answer is B.** (B) Liquid drugs include solutions, tinctures, suspensions, spirits, emulsions, elixirs, and syrups. (A) Solid drugs include pills, powders, capsules, tablets, and suppositories. (C) Parenteral drugs are liquid drugs that are administered through intramuscular, subcutaneous, or intravenous routes. (D) Spirits are considered a liquid drug. (Brady, Paramedic Care 2e, Principles and Practice, Volume 1—Pharmacology. Mosby, Paramedic Textbook 3e, Pharmacology.)

50. **The answer is A.** (A) Potentiation is the enhancement of a drug's effect when concurrently administered with another drug (e.g., alcohol and barbiturates). (B), (C), and (D) are incorrect; they describe drug dependency, cumulative action, and synergism, respectively. (Brady, Paramedic Care 2e, Principles and Practice, Volume 1—Pharmacology. Mosby, Paramedic Textbook 3e, Pharmacology.)

51. **The answer is C.** (C) An untoward effect (reaction) is a side effect that produces a harmful outcome for the patient. Certain harmful side effects may be listed as contraindications. (A) A contraindication is a condition that could result in a dangerous outcome with the administration of the medication. (B) Depressants decrease body functions and activities. (D) Therapeutic action is the desired effect of a given drug. (Brady, Paramedic Care 2e, Principles and Practice, Volume 1—Pharmacology. Mosby, Paramedic Textbook 3e, Pharmacology.)

52. **The answer is D.** (D) An idiosyncratic reaction is an individual reaction to a drug that is not a usually expected reaction. (A), (B), and (C) are incorrect. (Brady, Paramedic Care 2e, Principles and Practice, Volume 1—Pharmacology. Mosby, Paramedic Textbook 3e, Pharmacology.)

53. **The answer is D.** (D) Cumulative action occurs when a drug is administered in several doses; the buildup of the drug in the bloodstream causes an increased therapeutic effect. (A), (B), and (C) are incorrect. (Brady, Paramedic Care 2e,

Principles and Practice, Volume 1—Pharmacology. Mosby, Paramedic Textbook 3e, Pharmacology.)

54. **The answer is D.** (D) Tolerance is the effect that occurs when a patient taking a long-term medication needs to have its dosage increased to maintain the therapeutic effect. Tolerance is caused by a decreased physiologic response to a drug administered long term. (A) Habituation is physical or psychologic dependence on a drug. (B) Synergism is the combined action of two drugs that exceeds the sum of the actions of each individual drug. (C) Antagonism is opposition between the effects of two agents in which one overtakes the receptor sites of the other, creating a drug blockade. (Brady, Paramedic Care 2e, Principles and Practice, Volume 1—Pharmacology. Mosby, Paramedic Textbook 3e, Pharmacology.)

55. **The answer is B.** (B) Biotransformation occurs when a drug is administered and it is converted into an active or inactive form. This usually occurs in the blood or body tissues. (A) Absorption refers to the absorption of drugs into the capillary beds. (C) Distribution is the delivery of a drug to its proper receptor site via the bloodstream. (D) Elimination is the breakdown of a drug and its subsequent elimination from the body, usually in the form of metabolites. (Brady, Paramedic Care 2e, Principles and Practice, Volume 1—Pharmacology. Mosby, Paramedic Textbook 3e, Pharmacology.)

56. **The answer is B.** (B) The liver, although responsible for the metabolism of many medications, is not directly responsible for their excretion. The (A) kidneys and (C) intestines, accomplish drug metabolite excretion. Sweat and salivary glands are also responsible for drug metabolite excretion, but at a lesser level of importance. (D) Thyroid is incorrect. (Brady, Paramedic Care 2e, Principles and Practice, Volume 1—Pharmacology. Mosby, Paramedic Textbook 3e, Pharmacology.)

57. **The answer is D.** (C) Twenty hours is correct. To figure out the excretion rate of this medication, you would divide the dosage in half at every 2-hour interval. In this case, it would take 20 hours for the medication to drop below 1 mg. (A), (B), and (C) are incorrect.

(Brady, Paramedic Care 2e, Principles and Practice, Volume 1—Pharmacology. Mosby, Paramedic Textbook 3e, Pharmacology.)

58. **The answer is C.** (C) Sympathomimetics are drugs or other substances that produce effects like those of the sympathetic nervous system. (A) Parasympathomimetics cause effects like those of the parasympathetic nervous system. (B) Sympatholytics are drugs or other substances that block the sympathetic nervous system. (D) Parasympatholytics are drugs or other substances that block the parasympathetic nervous system (e.g., atropine). *(Brady, Paramedic Care 2e, Principles and Practice, Volume 1—Pharmacology. Mosby, Paramedic Textbook 3e, Pharmacology.)*

59. **The answer is A.** (A) Lidocaine is classified as an antidysrhythmic medication. (B) Epinephrine, (C) dopamine, and (D) norepinephrine (Levophed) are all classified as sympathomimetics or sympathetic agonists. *(Brady, Paramedic Care 2e, Principles and Practice, Volume 1—Pharmacology. Mosby, Paramedic Textbook 3e, Pharmacology.)*

60. **The answer is A.** (A) Flumazenil is a benzodiazepine antagonist and is commonly administered to counteract an overdose of benzodiazepines. (B) Lorazepam (Ativan), (C) diazepam (Valium), and (D) midazolam (Versed) are all benzodiazepines. These medications are also known as sedative-hypnotics. *(Brady, Paramedic Care 2e, Principles and Practice, Volume 1—Pharmacology. Mosby, Paramedic Textbook 3e, Pharmacology.)*

61. **The answer is C.** (C) Magnesium sulfate, although used in the treatment of dysrhythmias, is classified as an electrolyte and/or central nervous system depressant. It is an essential element in many of the biochemical reactions that occur in the body. (A) Lidocaine, (B) procainamide, and (D) bretylium tosylate are all classified as antidysrhythmics. *(Brady, Paramedic Care 2e, Principles and Practice, Volume 1—Pharmacology. Mosby, Paramedic Textbook 3e, Pharmacology.)*

62. **The answer is D.** (D) The rectal route of drug administration is called an enteral route. Enteral routes include oral, gastric, small intestinal, and rectal. Enteral routes are the safest routes of drug administration; they are also the most unreliable. (A) Intravenous, (B) endotracheal, and (C) intramuscular are all parenteral routes. *(Brady, Paramedic Care 2e, Principles and Practice, Volume 1—Pharmacology. Mosby, Paramedic Textbook 3e, Pharmacology.)*

63. **The answer is C.** (C) 3, 2, 1, 6, 4, 5 is the correct order of absorption. The actual order, including all routes of administration, is intracardiac, intravenous, endotracheal, inhalation, sublingual, intramuscular, subcutaneous, rectal, oral, and topical. *(Brady, Paramedic Care 2e, Principles and Practice, Volume 1—Pharmacology. Mosby, Paramedic Textbook 3e, Pharmacology.)*

VENOUS ACCESS AND MEDICATION ADMINISTRATION

64. **The answer is B.** (B) Furosemide (Lasix) is not readily absorbed through the bronchial membranes and therefore is *not* a drug to be administered endotracheally. (A) Lidocaine, (C) epinephrine, and (D) atropine are all easily absorbed through the bronchial membranes. Naloxone and diazepam (Valium) are also easily absorbed and are commonly administered endotracheally. The mnemonic NAVEL (referring to naloxone, atropine, ventolin, epinephrine, and lidocaine) will assist the Paramedic in remembering which drugs are absorbed through the bronchial membranes. *(Brady, Paramedic Care 2e, Principles and Practice, Volume 1—Medication Administration. Mosby, Paramedic Textbook 3e, Venous Access and Medication Administration.)*

65. **The answer is D.** You must look at a few variables to arrive at 400 mg. The number before the percent sign (%) denotes how many grams are added to 100 mL (constant) of solution (e.g., 2% indicates that 2 g of drug is added to 100 mL of solution). Once you have the percent solution broken down into grams, it is easy to figure out the solution concentration of the drug. You have 4 g in 100 mL (i.e., 4000 mg). Therefore, your solution concentration is 40 mg/1 mL. Therefore, if

you administer 10 mL, you will be administering 400 mg of medication. *(Brady, Paramedic Care 2e, Principles and Practice, Volume 1—Medication Administration. Mosby, Paramedic Textbook 3e, Venous Access and Medication Administration.)*

66. **The answer is A.** In order to complete this calculation, you must transfer the amount of drug into a volume to be administered. If furosemide is supplied 40 mg/4 mL, then your solution concentration will be 10 mg/1 mL. Therefore, you will deliver 2 mL for a correct dose of 20 mg. *(Brady, Paramedic Care 2e, Principles and Practice, Volume 1—Medication Administration. Mosby, Paramedic Textbook 3e, Venous Access and Medication Administration.)*

67. **The answer is B.** To arrive at the correct calculation, you would be required to know the desired dose (1 mg) and the dose on hand (0.4 mg/mL). You would divide the dose on hand by the desired dose, in this case 1 mg/(0.4 mg/mL), which would be equal to 2.5 mL. (A), (C), and (D) are incorrect. *(Brady, Paramedic Care 2e, Principles and Practice, Volume 1—Medication Administration. Mosby, Paramedic Textbook 3e, Venous Access and Medication Administration.)*

68. **The answer is D.** This calculation is based on the same mathematic formula used in percent solutions. In this instance, a 1:1000 solution equals 1 g in 1000 mL of solution (1000 mg/1000 mL = 1 mg/mL). Divide the desired dose by the dose on hand, and you arrive at 0.3 mL. *(Brady, Paramedic Care 2e, Principles and Practice, Volume 1—Medication Administration. Mosby, Paramedic Textbook 3e, Venous Access and Medication Administration.)*

69. **The answer is A.** This calculation uses the formula: desired dose divided by dose on hand. Therefore, the equation is 100 mg/(50 mg/mL) = 2 mL. (B), (C), and (D) are incorrect. *(Brady, Paramedic Care 2e, Principles and Practice, Volume 1—Medication Administration. Mosby, Paramedic Textbook 3e, Venous Access and Medication Administration.)*

70. **The answer is D.** 2000 mg (2 g) should be added to the 500-mL bag to create a 4:1 concentration. This concentration means that in every 1 mL of solution, you have 4 mg of lidocaine. This is achieved by multiplying the size of your bag of solution by 4 (use 4 because your desired concentration is 4:1). That would equal 2000 mg. *(Brady, Paramedic Care 2e, Principles and Practice, Volume 1—Medication Administration. Mosby, Paramedic Textbook 3e, Venous Access and Medication Administration.)*

71. **The answer is C.** In this situation, you have to determine the amount of lidocaine in the bag per milliliter. If you have a 500-mL bag and have added 2 g of lidocaine, this would make your concentration 4:1. Now that you have the concentration, you must figure out the drip rate. This is done by dividing the desired dose by the dose on hand: (3 mg/min)/(4 mg/mL) = 0.75. Then multiply 0.75 by the rate of the drip set (60 gtt/min) to be used: 0.75 × 60 = 45 gtt/min. (A), (B), and (D) are incorrect. *(Brady, Paramedic Care 2e, Principles and Practice, Volume 1—Medication Administration. Mosby, Paramedic Textbook 3e, Venous Access and Medication Administration.)*

72. **The answer is A.** Epinephrine 1:10,000 solution (injection) equals 1 g in 10,000 mL of solution. This is equal to 1000 mg/10,000 mL. In order to calculate the number of milliliters needed to deliver 1 mg, you must further break down the concentration to 1 mg/10 mL. If you need to administer 1 mg, then you should administer 10 mL of epinephrine 1:10,000. *(Brady, Paramedic Care 2e, Principles and Practice, Volume 1—Medication Administration. Mosby, Paramedic Textbook 3e, Venous Access and Medication Administration.)*

73. **The answer is B.** In order to administer volume over time, you must have the following information: volume to be administered, time period of administration, and number of drops per milliliter your infusion set is capable of delivering. To calculate the infusion rate, you must multiply the volume to be administered by the number of drops per milliliter delivered by the solution set (300 × 10 = 3000). Then you must divide that by the time of administration (in minutes, in this case, 120). You should set your drip rate at 25 gtt/min to deliver 300 mL over the next 2 hours. *(Brady, Paramedic Care 2e, Principles and Practice, Volume 1—Medication Administration. Mosby, Paramedic Textbook 3e, Venous Access and Medication Administration.)*

74. **The answer is B.** Use the following information: volume to be administered, time period of administration, and number of drops per milliliter your infusion set is capable of delivering. Calculate the infusion rate. Multiply the volume to be administered by the number of drops per milliliter delivered by the solution set ($500 \times 10 = 5000$). Then divide that by the time of administration (in minutes, in this case, 120). You will set your drip rate at 41.6 gtt/min (rounded to the next highest number, 42) to deliver 500 mL over the next 2 hours. *(Brady, Paramedic Care 2e, Principles and Practice, Volume 1—Medication Administration. Mosby, Paramedic Textbook 3e, Venous Access and Medication Administration.)*

75. **The answer is A.** Using the formula (volume to be administered times administration set divided by time in minutes of infusion), you should come out with 27.777 gtt/min, which is rounded off to 28 gtt/min. (B), (C), and (D) are incorrect. *(Brady, Paramedic Care 2e, Principles and Practice, Volume 1—Medication Administration. Mosby, Paramedic Textbook 3e, Venous Access and Medication Administration.)*

76. **The answer is C.** Medication errors may have serious adverse effects on your patient. As a professional, you must immediately report this error to medical control. They may be able to advise you of certain side effects you should look for based on the patient's history. You must closely monitor the patient for adverse reactions and report your error to the receiving hospital. After the call, you must document the error on the run sheet. You should discuss with your partner different ways to avoid this type of event in the future. (A), (B), and (D) are incorrect. You should never ignore a medication error or try to cover up an error with omissions in your report. *(Brady, Paramedic Care 2e, Principles and Practice, Volume 1—Medication Administration. Mosby, Paramedic Textbook 3e, Venous Access and Medication Administration.)*

77. **The answer is B.** Subcutaneous injections are administered into the subcutaneous tissue, which is relatively superficial. These injections are for small amounts of solution (usually less than 0.5 mL). The proper needle is 23–25 gauge and no longer than 5/8 inches. The insertion is done with the bevel up and at a 45-degree angle. (A), (C), and (D) are incorrect. *(Brady, Paramedic Care 2e, Principles and Practice, Volume 1—Medication Administration. Mosby, Paramedic Textbook 3e, Venous Access and Medication Administration.)*

78. **The answer is C.** The correct needle size for an intramuscular injection is between 19 and 21 gauge and 1–11/2 inches. The insertion angle is 90 degrees. Intramuscular injections go deep into muscle and therefore require a longer needle. The muscle tissue can usually accommodate up to 5 mL of fluid from an intramuscular injection. (A) and (B) give an incorrect angle and needle size, respectively. (D) gives both an incorrect angle and an incorrect needle size. *(Brady, Paramedic Care 2e, Principles and Practice, Volume 1—Medication Administration. Mosby, Paramedic Textbook 3e, Venous Access and Medication Administration.)*

79. **The answer is B.** Endotracheal medications are absorbed through the pulmonary capillaries by way of bronchial tissue. The normal absorption is almost as fast as IV administration. However, you must increase your dose 2–2.5 times the IV dose. In addition, endotracheal medications should be diluted in 10 mL of solution to facilitate absorption. (A), (C), and (D) are incorrect, the dosages are too high. *(Brady, Paramedic Care 2e, Principles and Practice, Volume 1—Medication Administration. Mosby, Paramedic Textbook 3e, Venous Access and Medication Administration.)*

80. **The answer is D.** (D) Diazepam (Valium) is classified as a sedative-hypnotic. There are two major groups of sedative-hypnotics: benzodiazepines and barbiturates. Diazepam is a benzodiazepine. (A) Morphine sulfate, (B) meperidine (Demerol), and (C) oxycodone (Percocet or Percodan) are all classified as narcotic analgesic agents. *(Brady, Paramedic Care 2e, Principles and Practice, Volume 1—Medication Administration. Mosby, Paramedic Textbook 3e, Venous Access and Medication Administration.)*

81. **The answer is A.** (A) A parasympatholytic produces a blocking effect on the parasympathetic nervous system. Parasympatholytics are also known as cholinergic blockers.

(B) Sympatholytics (adrenergic blockers) block the actions of the sympathetic nervous system. (C) Parasympathomimetics (cholinergic drugs) mimic the actions of the parasympathetic nervous system. (D) Sympathomimetics (adrenergic drugs) mimic the actions of the sympathetic nervous system. *(Brady, Paramedic Care 2e, Principles and Practice, Volume 1—Medication Administration. Mosby, Paramedic Textbook 3e, Venous Access and Medication Administration.)*

82. **The answer is B.** (B) Atropine (an anticholinergic) is a parasympatholytic. It acts by blocking the actions of the parasympathetic nervous system by occupying muscarinic receptor sites. (A), (C), and (D) are incorrect. *(Brady, Paramedic Care 2e, Principles and Practice, Volume 1—Medication Administration. Mosby, Paramedic Textbook 3e, Venous Access and Medication Administration.)*

83. **The answer is C.** (C) Epinephrine is a sympathomimetic (adrenergic drug) that mimics the actions of the sympathetic nervous system. It is considered a nonselective adrenergic drug, which means that it has beta$_1$, beta$_2$, and alpha effects. It increases heart rate and contractility (beta$_1$), as well as vasoconstriction systemically (alpha). (A), (B), and (D) are incorrect. *(Brady, Paramedic Care 2e, Principles and Practice, Volume 1—Medication Administration. Mosby, Paramedic Textbook 3e, Venous Access and Medication Administration.)*

84. **The answer is B.** (B) Bronchodilation is a beta$_2$ response; the lungs are one of the beta$_2$ effector organs. Other beta$_2$ effector organs include the blood vessels, gastrointestinal tract, and liver. (A) Increased force of cardiac contraction, (C) increased heart rate, and (D) increased conduction velocity are all beta$_1$ effects. *(Brady, Paramedic Care 2e, Principles and Practice, Volume 1—Medication Administration. Mosby, Paramedic Textbook 3e, Venous Access and Medication Administration.)*

Airway Management and Ventilation

The following topic is covered in Section II:

- Airway and Ventilation

Questions

AIRWAY AND VENTILATION

DIRECTIONS: Each item below contains four suggested responses. Select the one best response to each item.

85. Which is straighter, right or left mainstem bronchi?

    (A) right
    (B) left

86. A 60-year-old female is found in pulmonary edema. She is sitting upright in a chair, laboring to breathe. You would expect her Po_2 to be

    (A) low
    (B) high
    (C) normal

87. Which of the following is the average normal tidal volume for an adult at rest:

    (A) 250 mL
    (B) 500 mL
    (C) 750 mL
    (D) 1000 mL

88. A patient has a Pco_2 of 20 mmHg. If his tidal volume is normal, what can you assume about his respiratory rate?

    (A) It is normal.
    (B) It is faster than normal.
    (C) It is slower than normal.
    (D) It can be any of the above.

89. Blind insertion airways should not be used in

    (A) unconscious patients
    (B) conscious patients
    (C) spinal injury patients
    (D) caustic ingestions

90. When using a MacIntosh laryngoscope blade, the tip of the blade should be placed

    (A) between the epiglottis and vocal cords
    (B) on the right tonsil
    (C) on the epiglottis
    (D) between the epiglottis and the base of the tongue

91. A patient with inspiratory stridor, tracheal tugging, and intercostal retractions is most likely suffering from

    (A) upper airway obstruction
    (B) asthma
    (C) chronic obstructive pulmonary disease (COPD)
    (D) pulmonary edema

92. You are assessing your patient and you find that she has absent breath sounds. This could be an indication of

    (A) pneumothorax
    (B) pneumonia
    (C) severe asthma
    (D) all of the above

93. _____ is caused by air that passes through a narrowed bronchiole.

    (A) Wheezing
    (B) Rhonchi
    (C) Rales
    (D) A bronchial sound

94. An increase in respiratory effort when lying flat is known as

    (A) asthma
    (B) eupnea
    (C) orthopnea
    (D) hyperpnea

95. Hyperventilation can be commonly seen in which of the following?

    (A) anxiety
    (B) pulmonary embolism
    (C) asthma
    (D) any of the above

96. CO_2 is transported in the blood

    (A) in solution
    (B) through interaction with the buffer system
    (C) in combination with hemoglobin
    (D) all of the above

97. All of the following structures of the respiratory system components contain dead air space except:

    (A) bronchioles
    (B) alveoli
    (C) pharynx
    (D) trachea

98. Which of the following statements is true based on the response of hemoglobin to oxygen?

    (A) A P_{O_2} of 60 mmHg produces nearly as much hemoglobin saturation as does a P_{O_2} of 90 mmHg.
    (B) A P_{O_2} of 40 mmHg produces significantly more hemoglobin saturation than does a P_{O_2} of 20 mmHg.
    (C) Both A and B are correct.
    (D) Neither A nor B is correct.

99. Which of the following blood gas values are normal for blood that has completed internal respiration?

    (A) P_{CO_2} 45 mmHg, P_{O_2} 100 mmHg
    (B) P_{CO_2} 40 mmHg, P_{O_2} 45 mmHg
    (C) P_{CO_2} 40 mmHg, P_{O_2} 100 mmHg
    (D) P_{CO_2} 40 mmHg, P_{O_2} 40 mmHg

100. Which of the following is not a component of the alveolar-capillary membrane except:

    (A) basement membrane
    (B) endothelium
    (C) smooth muscle
    (D) septal cells

101. Which of the following structures secrete surfactant?

    (A) septal cells
    (B) endothelium
    (C) alveolar basement membrane
    (D) goblet cells

102. _____ give(s) the trachea its structure.

   (A) The thyroid cartilage
   (B) Smooth muscle
   (C) Cartilaginous rings
   (D) Basement membrane

103. Bronchioles are composed of

   (A) cartilaginous rings
   (B) alveolar ducts
   (C) smooth muscle
   (D) septal cells

Questions 104–107 are based on the following scenario.

A 34-year-old woman is complaining of numbness around her mouth, dizziness, and cramps in the extremities. You note that she is breathing very deeply at 36 times per minute.

104. You can assume that her P_{CO_2} is

   (A) lower than normal
   (B) higher than normal

105. If this is the case, her arterial pH is

   (A) higher than normal
   (B) lower than normal

106. Thus, she is developing respiratory

   (A) acidosis
   (B) alkalosis

107. From the situation described above, you can assume that the patient's P_{O_2} is

   (A) normal
   (B) above normal
   (C) below normal
   (D) no determination about the P_{O_2} can be inferred from the above information

108. An oropharyngeal airway may be used to maintain airway in conscious patients.

   (A) false
   (B) true

109. When assessing a patient with dyspnea, you can be confident that she is adequately oxygenated if she does not have cyanosis.

   (A) false
   (B) true

110. Confusion and agitation are key signs of _____.

   (A) hypoxia
   (B) hyperventilation
   (C) high P_{CO_2}
   (D) all of the above

111. All patients in respiratory distress should receive oxygen.

   (A) true
   (B) false

112. The vocal cords are located in the

   (A) bronchi
   (B) carina
   (C) larynx
   (D) pharynx

Questions 113 and 114 are based on the following scenario.

You are dining at a restaurant when you notice a woman at another table who appears to be in severe distress. She is completely silent and pushes herself away from the table and staggers toward the rest room. You ask her what is wrong but she is unable to speak.

113. The most likely diagnosis in this case is

   (A) acute pulmonary edema
   (B) foreign-body airway obstruction
   (C) asthma
   (D) a heart attack

114. You should immediately

    (A) give her some water to drink
    (B) deliver four back blows
    (C) perform several abdominal thrusts
    (D) do nothing

115. Oxygen and carbon dioxide are exchanged in the lung by

    (A) diffusion
    (B) active transport
    (C) facilitated transport
    (D) osmosis

116. Infants and toddlers are best intubated with which type of laryngoscope blade?

    (A) fiber optic
    (B) MacIntosh
    (C) curved
    (D) Miller

117. The cuff of an endotracheal tube should be inflated with how many milliliters of air?

    (A) 1–2 mL
    (B) 15–20 mL
    (C) 5–10 mL
    (D) 25–30 mL

118. The appropriately sized endotracheal tube for a child may be determined by comparing the diameter of the endotracheal tube with the diameter of the child's

    (A) thumb
    (B) little finger
    (C) forefinger
    (D) nares

119. The correct landmark for a cricothyrotomy is

    (A) just above the thyroid cartilage
    (B) just above the cricoid cartilage
    (C) just below the cricoid cartilage
    (D) between the second and third tracheal rings

120. The Paramedic should limit his or her attempts at intubation to no longer than _____ seconds?

    (A) 5
    (B) 10
    (C) 30
    (D) 60

121. Which of the following is the most appropriate method of measuring an oropharyngeal airway?

    (A) from the nose to the chin
    (B) from the corner of the mouth to the ear lobe
    (C) from the nose to the ear lobe
    (D) from the chin to the ear lobe

122. The narrowest part of the airway of an infant or a toddler is the

    (A) cricoid cartilage
    (B) thyroid cartilage
    (C) oropharynx
    (D) nasopharynx

123. _____ is the most secure form of airway control.

    (A) Endotracheal intubation
    (B) Esophageal gastric tube airway
    (C) Modified jaw thrust
    (D) Oropharyngeal airway

124. The primary advantage of nasotracheal intubation is

    (A) It may be accomplished more quickly than orotracheal intubation.
    (B) It requires no skill at all.
    (C) It is easy to perform on a nonbreathing patient
    (D) It may be performed without moving the patient's head or neck.

Answers and Explanations

85. **The answer is A.** The right mainstem bronchus is straighter and larger as it leaves the carina. As a result, an endotracheal tube that is advanced too far is more likely to be placed in the right mainstem bronchus than in the left. *(Brady, Paramedic Care 2e, Principles and Practice, Volume 1— Airway Management and Ventilation. Mosby, Paramedic Textbook 3e, Airway Management and Ventilation.)*

86. **The answer is A.** Pulmonary edema fills the lungs with excess fluid and interferes with the oxygen exchange across the alveolar membrane. As a result, the partial pressure of oxygen in the patient's arterial blood falls, leading to hypoxemia. *(Brady, Paramedic Care 2e, Principles and Practice, Volume 1—Airway Management and Ventilation. Mosby, Paramedic Textbook 3e, Airway Management and Ventilation.)*

87. **The answer is B.** Although there is some variation according to patient size, the average tidal volume of air exchanged by an adult with each breath at rest is 500 mL. *(Brady, Paramedic Care 2e, Principles and Practice, Volume 1—Airway Management and Ventilation. Mosby, Paramedic Textbook 3e, Airway Management and Ventilation.)*

88. **The answer is B.** The partial pressure of carbon dioxide is inversely proportional to the amount of ventilation. As the patient's ventilation increases, the P_{CO_2} falls. The normal P_{CO_2} is 40 mmHg. In order to increase ventilation to achieve a P_{CO_2} of 20 mmHg, the respiratory rate must be increased. *(Brady, Paramedic Care 2e, Principles and Practice, Volume 1—Airway Management*

and Ventilation. Mosby, Paramedic Textbook 3e, Airway Management and Ventilation.)

89. **The answer is B.** The blind insertion airways (combitube and pharyngeal tracheal lumen [PTL]) would cause severe gagging and retching in a patient who was conscious and had an intact gag reflex. *(Brady, Paramedic Care 2e, Principles and Practice, Volume 1—Airway Management and Ventilation. Mosby, Paramedic Textbook 3e, Airway Management and Ventilation.)*

90. **The answer is D.** The tip of the MacIntosh (curved) laryngoscope blade is placed in the area between the epiglottis and the base of the tongue. This area is known as the *vallecula*. The tongue is then lifted to provide visualization of the glottic opening. The Miller (straight) laryngoscope blade is placed beneath the epiglottis, and the blade is used to lift the epiglottis directly. *(Brady, Paramedic Care 2e, Principles and Practice, Volume 1—Airway Management and Ventilation. Mosby, Paramedic Textbook 3e, Airway Management and Ventilation.)*

91. **The answer is A.** Inspiratory stridor is created as air passes through a restricted upper airway. As the negative pressure in the lungs cannot be readily equalized, tracheal tugging and intercostal retractions appear. The Paramedic should always consider stridorous respirations a result of upper airway obstruction. In the case of pulmonary edema, the patient has rapid respirations with rales heard in the chest. In asthma, the chest appears hyperinflated, and wheezes are heard in the chest. COPD patients generally have diminished breath sounds, with some scattered wheezes. *(Brady, Paramedic Care 2e, Principles*

and Practice, Volume 1—Airway Management and Ventilation. Mosby, Paramedic Textbook 3e, Airway Management and Ventilation.)

92. **The answer is D.** Breath sounds are created as air moves in and out of the air passages in the lungs. In a pneumothorax, a portion of the lung is collapsed. Breath sounds may not be heard over the area formerly occupied by the collapsed area of the lung. In pneumonia, areas of the lung are filled with fluid and pus. Air may not be able to pass through these areas to produce breath sounds. In severe asthma, the bronchoconstriction may prevent enough air from moving in and out of the lungs to produce breath sounds. *(Brady, Paramedic Care 2e, Principles and Practice, Volume 1—Airway Management and Ventilation. Mosby, Paramedic Textbook 3e, Airway Management and Ventilation.)*

93. **The answer is A.** As air moves through a narrowed bronchiole, a high-pitched musical sound known as *wheeze* is produced. This is most commonly seen in asthmatics. Rales are a fine crackling sound that is produced by fluid in the alveoli. Rhonchi are coarser sounds produced by fluid and mucous in some of the larger air passages in the lungs. Bronchial sounds are hollow tubular sounds heard near the center of the chest. *(Brady, Paramedic Care 2e, Principles and Practice, Volume 1—Airway Management and Ventilation. Mosby, Paramedic Textbook 3e, Airway Management and Ventilation.)*

94. **The answer is C.** Many patients who suffer from respiratory diseases experience increased distress while lying flat. This sign, known as orthopnea, is most commonly seen in patients with pulmonary edema. Asthma is a disease caused by a narrowing of the bronchioles. Eupnea is normal breathing. Hyperpnea is an increase in the depth and rate of respiration. *(Brady, Paramedic Care 2e, Principles and Practice, Volume 1—Airway Management and Ventilation. Mosby, Paramedic Textbook 3e, Airway Management and Ventilation.)*

95. **The answer is D.** Hyperventilation is an increase in the rate and depth of respiration that results in lowered P_{CO_2} levels. It is most commonly associated with anxiety, but hyperventilation may be a response to hypoxia. A pulmonary embolism, for instance, may interfere with the exchange of oxygen. Ventilation is increased in response to the lowered oxygen levels. *(Brady, Paramedic Care 2e, Principles and Practice, Volume 1—Airway Management and Ventilation. Mosby, Paramedic Textbook 3e, Airway Management and Ventilation.)*

96. **The answer is D.** Most of the carbon dioxide is present as carbonic acid, which is a product of the bicarbonate buffer system. Some is bound to the hemoglobin in the red blood cells, and a small amount is in solution with the blood plasma. *(Brady, Paramedic Care 2e, Principles and Practice, Volume 1—Airway Management and Ventilation. Mosby, Paramedic Textbook 3e, Airway Management and Ventilation.)*

97. **The answer is B.** Dead space consists of areas of the respiratory system where air moves with ventilation but gas exchange does not occur. Gas exchange occurs primarily in the alveoli and to some extent in the alveolar ducts. *(Brady, Paramedic Care 2e, Principles and Practice, Volume 1—Airway Management and Ventilation. Mosby, Paramedic Textbook 3e, Airway Management and Ventilation.)*

98. **The answer is C.** The affinity of hemoglobin for oxygen begins to level off dramatically after the P_{CO_2} reaches 50 mmHg. Below this level, small increases in P_{CO_2} will yield large increases in the percentage of oxygen saturation. The hemoglobin is already nearly completely saturated when the P_{CO_2} reaches 60 mmHg, and further increases in P_{CO_2} will yield only small increases in saturation. *(Brady, Paramedic Care 2e, Principles and Practice, Volume 1—Airway Management and Ventilation. Mosby, Paramedic Textbook 3e, Airway Management and Ventilation.)*

99. **The answer is D.** When arterial blood has completed gas exchange in the alveoli (external respiration), the P_{O_2} is approximately 100 mmHg, and the P_{CO_2} is approximately 45 mmHg. After the blood completes its exchange of gases with the cells (internal respiration), the P_{O_2} has fallen to approximately 40 mmHg, and the P_{CO_2} has risen to approximately 40 mmHg. *(Brady,*

Paramedic Care 2e, Principles and Practice, Volume 1—Airway Management and Ventilation. Mosby, Paramedic Textbook 3e, Airway Management and Ventilation.)

100. **The answer is C.** The alveolar-capillary membrane consists of a basement membrane to give structure and an endothelial lining across which gas exchange may occur. There are septal cells that secrete surfactant to decrease surface tension and keep the alveoli open. Smooth muscle is found primarily in the bronchioles. *(Brady, Paramedic Care 2e, Principles and Practice, Volume 1—Airway Management and Ventilation. Mosby, Paramedic Textbook 3e, Airway Management and Ventilation.)*

101. **The answer is A.** The septal cells of the alveolar-capillary membrane secrete surfactant. They are present in the alveolar-capillary membrane, along with the basement membrane and the endothelium. Goblet cells are found in the trachea and other airways. *(Brady, Paramedic Care 2e, Principles and Practice, Volume 1—Airway Management and Ventilation. Mosby, Paramedic Textbook 3e, Airway Management and Ventilation.)*

102. **The answer is C.** The trachea structure is maintained by a series of cartilaginous rings. These are not complete rings, but are open at the posterior. Without these rings, the trachea would collapse on inspiration. The thyroid cartilage gives shape to the larynx and provides support for the vocal cords. Smooth muscle and a basement membrane are present in the trachea but do not contribute to its structure. *(Brady, Paramedic Care 2e, Principles and Practice, Volume 1—Airway Management and Ventilation. Mosby, Paramedic Textbook 3e, Airway Management and Ventilation.)*

103. **The answer is C.** The bronchioles are composed primarily of smooth muscle. This allows the bronchioles to open or close in response to respiratory demands. In reactive airway diseases, such as asthma, the smooth muscle may cause bronchospasm, which will create a lower airway obstruction. Cartilaginous rings maintain the structure of the trachea. Alveolar ducts connect the alveoli with the respiratory bronchioles. The septal cells are found in the alveolar-capillary membrane and secrete surfactant to keep the alveoli from collapsing.

(Brady, Paramedic Care 2e, Principles and Practice, Volume 1—Airway Management and Ventilation. Mosby, Paramedic Textbook 3e, Airway Management and Ventilation.)

104. **The answer is A.** See rationale in question 107. *(Brady, Paramedic Care 2e, Principles and Practice, Volume 1—Airway Management and Ventilation. Mosby, Paramedic Textbook 3e, Airway Management and Ventilation.)*

105. **The answer is A.** See rationale in question 107. *(Brady, Paramedic Care 2e, Principles and Practice, Volume 1—Airway Management and Ventilation. Mosby, Paramedic Textbook 3e, Airway Management and Ventilation.)*

106. **The answer is B.** See rationale in question 107. *(Brady, Paramedic Care 2e, Principles and Practice, Volume 1—Airway Management and Ventilation. Mosby, Paramedic Textbook 3e, Airway Management and Ventilation.)*

107. **The answer is D.** This patient is suffering from a hyperventilation syndrome. Prolonged rapid and deep respirations will result in increased ventilation resulting in an increase of arterial carbon dioxide. A decrease in carbon dioxide will cause the arterial pH to rise and the blood to become more alkaline. This respiratory alkalosis will create a relative hypocalcemia in the tissues. Numbness and spasms of the hands and feet are seen as a result. The rate of respiration and apparent level of carbon dioxide give no indication of the state of oxygenation. A normal patient who hyperventilates would be expected to have a normal or slightly elevated P_{O_2}. Some patients may hyperventilate in response to a decreased P_{O_2}. The pitfall is that patients who hyperventilate are often assumed to have normal oxygenation. *(Brady, Paramedic Care 2e, Principles and Practice, Volume 1—Airway Management and Ventilation. Mosby, Paramedic Textbook 3e, Airway Management and Ventilation.)*

108. **The answer is A.** The oropharyngeal airway will cause severe gagging and retching in conscious patients with an intact gag reflex. Alternative methods of airway control, such as manual positioning or a nasopharyngeal airway, should be considered for conscious patients. (*Brady, Paramedic Care 2e, Principles and Practice, Volume 1—Airway Management and Ventilation. Mosby, Paramedic Textbook 3e, Airway Management and Ventilation.*)

109. **The answer is A.** Cyanosis is generally a late sign of hypoxia and it may be difficult to detect in patients with dark skin or poor lighting conditions. Pulse oximetry may be a more sensitive method of determining oxygenation, but it is not 100% reliable. Patients who exhibit signs of respiratory distress should receive high-concentration oxygen regardless of the absence of cyanosis. (*Brady, Paramedic Care 2e, Principles and Practice, Volume 1—Airway Management and Ventilation. Mosby, Paramedic Textbook 3e, Airway Management and Ventilation.*)

110. **The answer is A.** Patients who are hypoxic present as confused and agitated. Most patients exhibit significant distress as they struggle to get more oxygen. A high P_{CO_2} is often seen later in respiratory failure. A high P_{CO_2} will cause the patient to become lethargic. This is an ominous sign in a patient with respiratory disease. (*Brady, Paramedic Care 2e, Principles and Practice, Volume 1—Airway Management and Ventilation. Mosby, Paramedic Textbook 3e, Airway Management and Ventilation.*)

111. **The answer is A.** Supplemental oxygen should never be withheld in a patient with respiratory distress. Respiratory depression secondary to oxygen drive in COPD patients is a rare phenomenon and the Paramedic should never withhold oxygen from a patient with a history of COPD. Sufficient oxygen should be supplied to correct hypoxia, and the patient should be closely monitored for hypoventilation. (*Brady, Paramedic Care 2e, Principles and Practice, Volume 1—Airway Management and Ventilation. Mosby, Paramedic Textbook 3e, Airway Management and Ventilation.*)

112. **The answer is C.** The vocal cords are found within the superior opening of the larynx. (*Brady, Paramedic Care 2e, Principles and Practice, Volume 1—Airway Management and Ventilation. Mosby, Paramedic Textbook 3e, Airway Management and Ventilation.*)

113. **The answer is B.** See rationale in question 114. (*Brady, Paramedic Care 2e, Principles and Practice, Volume 1—Airway Management and Ventilation. Mosby, Paramedic Textbook 3e, Airway Management and Ventilation.*)

114. **The answer is C.** Patients who develop sudden distress while eating may be the victims of a foreign-body airway obstruction. This condition may easily be mistaken for a heart attack or other medical problem. The term "café coronary" is used to describe patients who have succumbed to an airway obstruction after being misdiagnosed as having a primary cardiac event. The key to diagnosing airway obstruction is the patient's inability to speak. This indicates that no air is able to pass the glottis. In an unresponsive and apneic patient, the inability to ventilate would lead to the diagnosis of airway obstruction. Several abdominal thrusts, also known as Heimlich maneuvers, should be administered to the patient until the obstruction is relieved. (*Brady, Paramedic Care 2e, Principles and Practice, Volume 1—Airway Management and Ventilation. Mosby, Paramedic Textbook 3e, Airway Management and Ventilation.*)

115. **The answer is A.** Oxygen diffuses from an area of high concentration in the alveoli to an area of lower concentration in the blood. At the same time, carbon dioxide moves from an area of high concentration in the blood to an area of lower concentration in the alveoli. The specialized alveolar-capillary membrane allows this exchange to occur. (*Brady, Paramedic Care 2e, Principles and Practice, Volume 1—Airway Management and Ventilation. Mosby, Paramedic Textbook 3e, Airway Management and Ventilation.*)

116. **The answer is D.** The larynx in infants and toddlers is more superior and anterior than that of adults. In addition, the epiglottis is larger in proportion to the other structures of the airway. For these reasons, a Miller or straight laryngoscope blade is preferred over a MacIntosh or curved blade. A fiber-optic blade may sometimes deliver a brighter light and may be easier to decontaminate, but it offers no specific advantage for pediatric patients. (*Brady, Paramedic Care 2e, Principles and Practice, Volume 1—Airway*

Management and Ventilation. Mosby, Paramedic Textbook 3e, Airway Management and Ventilation.)

117. **The answer is C.** Most endotracheal tube cuffs should be inflated with 5–10 mL of air. However, there may be a variation due to the difference in interior diameter of the trachea. Inflating with too little air may create an air leak and also allow foreign material to enter the trachea. Too much air and the pressure may damage the inside lining of the trachea. It is best to fill the cuff until significant air leakage just stops. *(Brady, Paramedic Care 2e, Principles and Practice, Volume 1—Airway Management and Ventilation. Mosby, Paramedic Textbook 3e, Airway Management and Ventilation.)*

118. **The answer is B.** One acceptable way of determining the appropriately sized endotracheal tube for a child is to compare the diameter of the tube with the diameter of the child's little finger. Other methods include the use of age-based or length-based charts, such as the Broselow tape. There are also acceptable mathematical formulas. Regardless of the method used, there may be a significant difference in the calculated size of the trachea and the actual diameter. As these methods are not foolproof, it is always important to have a range of tube sizes immediately available. *(Brady, Paramedic Care 2e, Principles and Practice, Volume 1—Airway Management and Ventilation. Mosby, Paramedic Textbook 3e, Airway Management and Ventilation.)*

119. **The answer is B.** A cricothyrotomy should be performed at the cricothyroid membrane. The membrane lies above the cricoid cartilage and below the thyroid cartilage in the anterior neck. *(Brady, Paramedic Care 2e, Principles and Practice, Volume 1—Airway Management and Ventilation. Mosby, Paramedic Textbook 3e, Airway Management and Ventilation.)*

120. **The answer is C.** Attempts at endotracheal intubation should be limited to less than 30 seconds. Hypoxia during prolonged intubation attempts is a significant complication of endotracheal intubation. Patients should be hyperventilated prior to intubation attempts in order to optimize oxygenation. Pulse oximetry should be employed when available to monitor the status of the patient's oxygen saturation. A good rule of thumb is to take a breath and hold it before beginning your intubation attempt. When the Paramedic needs to take a breath, its time to ventilate the patient before making another attempt at intubation. *(Brady, Paramedic Care 2e, Principles and Practice, Volume 1—Airway Management and Ventilation. Mosby, Paramedic Textbook 3e, Airway Management and Ventilation.)*

121. **The answer is B.** An appropriately sized oropharyngeal airway reaches from the corner of the patient's mouth to the ear lobe. When properly positioned, the flange rests against the teeth. *(Brady, Paramedic Care 2e, Principles and Practice, Volume 1—Airway Management and Ventilation. Mosby, Paramedic Textbook 3e, Airway Management and Ventilation.)*

122. **The answer is A.** The airway of an infant or a toddler is more or less funnel shaped, with the narrowest point being at the cricoid membrane. Endotracheal tubes used for infants and toddlers are not cuffed. A properly sized tube will create its own seal at the narrowest point of the airway. *(Brady, Paramedic Care 2e, Principles and Practice, Volume 1—Airway Management and Ventilation. Mosby, Paramedic Textbook 3e, Airway Management and Ventilation.)*

123. **The answer is A.** An endotracheal tube provides the most secure form of airway control. A cuffed endotracheal tube isolates the trachea and prevents the entry of foreign material while assuring that all inspired gas is delivered to the lungs. Manual methods, such as the modified jaw thrust, and simple devices, such as the oropharyngeal airway, cannot prevent the aspiration of gastric contents. The esophageal gastric tube airway will prevent the release of gastric contents but will not protect from blood or other material that may enter the upper airway, and this device is limited to a select group of patients. *(Brady, Paramedic Care 2e, Principles and Practice, Volume 1—Airway Management and Ventilation. Mosby, Paramedic Textbook 3e, Airway Management and Ventilation.)*

124. **The answer is D.** A definite plus for the treatment of trauma patients, nasotracheal intubation

can be performed without moving the patient's head or neck. It usually takes a longer time to perform nasotracheal intubation because the tube must be advanced carefully through the nose in order to avoid trauma and bleeding. Since this procedure is only performed on patients who are spontaneously breathing, this is not a significant problem. While nasotracheal intubation is a blind procedure, some skill and experience is necessary to ensure success. (Brady, Paramedic Care 2e, Principles and Practice, Volume 1—Airway Management and Ventilation. Mosby, Paramedic Textbook 3e, Airway Management and Ventilation.)

Patient Assessment

The following topics are covered in Section III:

- Patient Assessment: History
- Patient Assessment: Physical Examination Techniques
- Patient Assessment: Patient Assessment in the Field
- Patient Assessment: Communications
- Patient Assessment: Documentation

Questions

PATIENT ASSESSMENT: HISTORY

DIRECTIONS: Each item below contains four suggested responses. Select the one best response to each item.

125. The most important source for obtaining information on the patient's history is

    (A) the patient
    (B) the patient's family
    (C) witnesses at the scene
    (D) the patient's personal physician

126. Which of the following is an example of an "open-ended" question?

    (A) Do you have any allergies?
    (B) Have you been hospitalized recently?
    (C) What type of pain are you experiencing?
    (D) Are you under the care of a physician?

127. The patient's "chief complaint" is described as which of the following components of the medical history?

    (A) the patient's use of medications
    (B) previous episodes of illness
    (C) the results of your physical examination
    (D) the reason that the patient has called for assistance

128. All of the following are components of the history of present illness *except*:

    (A) onset of symptoms
    (B) past medical history
    (C) quality of pain
    (D) severity of pain

129. Your 68-year-old male patient is complaining of severe substernal chest pain radiating to his left arm. He is cool, pale, and diaphoretic. As you begin treatment, your patient tells you that the last time he had this type of pain his doctor told him he had a "bad" heart attack. The information concerning his previous heart attack is part of which component of the patient history?

    (A) chief complaint
    (B) past medical history
    (C) family history
    (D) history of present illness

130. Your 42-year-old female patient is complaining of a squeezing chest pain and difficulty breathing. She has no prior history and no other predisposing factors (e.g., smoking). Your evaluation of the patient includes an electrocardiogram (ECG), which reveals elevated S-T segments. When asked, the patient informs you that her mother "passed away" at the age of 47 from a massive heart attack. Her mother's cardiac history is an important piece of information from which component of the medical history?

    (A) past medical history
    (B) family history
    (C) history of present illness
    (D) allergies

131. You respond to an elderly patient with an altered mental status. On your arrival, you notice that the apartment is very cold, and you find your patient shivering and exhibiting early signs of hypothermia. Your evaluation of the patient's status based on the living conditions falls into which component of the patient history?

    (A) history of present illness
    (B) past medical history
    (C) social history
    (D) chief complaint

132. In questioning your patient with chest pain, he states that he has no difficulty breathing and no nausea. In addition, you notice that he has no jugular venous distention or peripheral edema. These findings should be documented as

    (A) pertinent negatives
    (B) pertinent positives
    (C) symptomatic findings
    (D) they should not be documented because they do not offer any clues as to the patient's condition

133. All of the following are components of the past medical history except:

    (A) onset of pain
    (B) medications taken
    (C) events preceding the illness or injury
    (D) patient allergies

PATIENT ASSESSMENT: PHYSICAL EXAMINATION TECHNIQUES

DIRECTIONS: Each item below contains four suggested responses. Select the one best response to each item.

134. All of the following are accepted tools for evaluating airway and breathing in the conscious patient during the primary assessment except:

    (A) inspection
    (B) end-tidal CO_2 detection
    (C) auscultation
    (D) palpation

135. All of the following pulse points are generally accepted in the determination of a pulse rate in an adult except:

    (A) femoral
    (B) radial
    (C) brachial
    (D) carotid

136. You are on the scene of a shooting, and your patient is a 46-year-old male who has been shot once in the right upper quadrant of the abdomen. He is hypovolemic during your primary survey. As you assess the skin, you can expect it to appear in any of the following ways *except*:

(A) mottled

(B) cyanotic

(C) jaundiced

(D) ashen

137. In the assessment of a patient's mental status using the AVPU scale, the A stands for

(A) alive

(B) alert

(C) appropriate

(D) affect

138. Your patient is a 17-year-old male who has been stabbed in the lower right chest and is complaining of severe difficulty breathing. Examination reveals minor external bleeding, but you note diminished breath sounds on the right side. The right side of the chest is hyporesonant (dull to percussion). This may indicate

(A) hemothorax

(B) pericardial tamponade

(C) tension pneumothorax

(D) subcutaneous emphysema

139. Capillary refill is not a good indicator of hemodynamic status in adults because it can be affected by all of the following factors *except*:

(A) smoking

(B) medications

(C) cold weather

(D) hypertension

140. To examine your patient for jugular venous distention, you should elevate the body to what angle?

(A) 45 degrees

(B) 60 degrees

(C) 75 degrees

(D) 90 degrees

141. You are called to a 22-year-old male who is unresponsive on examination. You find that he has overdosed on an opioid analgesic. You would expect his pupils to be

(A) equal and reactive

(B) dilated and unresponsive

(C) constricted

(D) unequal

142. In auscultating for bowel sounds, you should listen to the patient's abdomen for no less than how many seconds?

(A) 15 seconds

(B) 30 seconds

(C) 45 seconds

(D) 120 seconds

143. Crepitation is best defined as

(A) a crackling sensation felt on palpation of the skin

(B) reddening of an area

(C) a yellowish coloration

(D) a "black-and-blue" discoloration

144. All of the following are techniques for conducting a physical examination *except*:

(A) inspection

(B) palpation

(C) percussion

(D) evaluation of mental status

145. You are examining your head-injured patient. As you turn his head, you notice that his eyes move along with the head. This type of response is known as

    (A) dysconjugate gaze
    (B) raccoon's eyes
    (C) doll's eye response
    (D) anisocoria

146. Your 15-year-old female patient is complaining of difficulty breathing from asthma. During your physical examination, you notice that her left pupil is larger than her right pupil. This condition is known as

    (A) anisocoria
    (B) dysconjugate gaze
    (C) Battle's sign
    (D) raccoon's eyes

PATIENT ASSESSMENT: PATIENT ASSESSMENT IN THE FIELD

DIRECTIONS: Each item below contains four suggested responses. Select the one best response to each item.

147. As an emergency medical service (EMS) provider, the Paramedic must complete a scene size-up on every call. At what point during the medical or trauma call does the scene size-up begin?

    (A) on arrival at the call
    (B) when the Paramedic receives the call
    (C) when the Paramedic makes patient contact
    (D) when police, fire, or other public-safety officials brief the Paramedic at the scene

148. Identification of potential hazards includes all of the following except:

    (A) identification of the perpetrator of a crime
    (B) ensuring that a partially collapsed building is properly shored up
    (C) surveying the scene for fuel spills
    (D) determination of the presence of carbon monoxide or other agents at a scene with multiple patients complaining of severe headaches and malaise

149. You respond to a motor vehicle accident on a major highway. On your arrival, you see that four cars are involved. What is the importance in the determination of the exact number of patients involved in this accident?

    (A) Determining the exact number of patients will assist the Paramedic in billing procedures.
    (B) Determining the exact number of patients will assist the Paramedic in knowing how much equipment will be needed.
    (C) Determining the exact number of patients will assist the Paramedic in referring patients to the police for reports.
    (D) Determining the exact number of patients will assist the Paramedic in requesting additional resources at the scene.

150. Which patient age group would most likely have a fear of strangers, therefore presenting the Paramedic with a difficult patient evaluation?

    (A) birth to 12 months
    (B) 1–3 years
    (C) 4 –10 years
    (D) adolescents

151. Patients in which age group are most likely to have a fear of disfigurement but can be expected to be fully cooperative with their examination and treatment by a Paramedic?

    (A) birth to 12 months
    (B) 1–3 years
    (C) 4–10 years
    (D) adolescents

152. You respond to a 24-year-old female asthmatic. Her breathing is shallow (tidal volume 300 mL) at 28 breaths per minute. What is her minute volume?

    (A) 7200 mL
    (B) 7400 mL
    (C) 8200 mL
    (D) 8400 mL

153. You are treating a patient with an altered mental status. He is confused and disoriented. With painful stimuli, he opens his eyes and withdraws from the stimuli. What is his score on the Glasgow coma scale?

    (A) 9
    (B) 10
    (C) 11
    (D) 12

154. The respiratory pattern that is characterized by periods of rapid, irregular breaths alternating with periods of apnea is known as

    (A) Cheyne-Stokes respirations
    (B) eupnea
    (C) central neurogenic hyperventilation
    (D) Kussmaul's respirations

155. In the assessment of the patient suffering trauma from a motor vehicle accident, which factor will have the most detrimental effect on the patient?

    (A) the speed of the vehicle on impact
    (B) the type of collision
    (C) the patient's weight
    (D) the patient's position in the vehicle

156. As part of your ongoing assessment of the unstable trauma patient, you should reassess your patient

    (A) every 5 minutes
    (B) every 10 minutes
    (C) every 15 minutes
    (D) every 20 minutes

157. You are assessing an unconscious patient who has snoring respirations. What is the most frequent cause of this type of respiration in the unconscious patient?

    (A) blood
    (B) vomit
    (C) teeth
    (D) tongue

158. While assessing your patient's airway, you find that there is a food bolus lodged in the oropharynx. Basic life support maneuvers do not clear the airway. As a Paramedic, what type of intervention should you initially attempt?

    (A) direct visualization with laryngoscope and Magill forceps
    (B) needle cricothyroidotomy
    (C) abdominal thrusts
    (D) orotracheal suctioning

159. Your 55-year-old male patient is complaining of difficult breathing. He is cyanotic and breathing 32 times per minute. What is the appropriate oxygen delivery device for this patient?

    (A) nasal cannula
    (B) nonrebreather mask
    (C) bag-valve-mask
    (D) blow-by oxygen

160. Your assessment of the trauma patient reveals a patent airway, adequate breathing, but an uncontrolled arterial bleed from the midaxillary artery. Your attempts at bleeding control are unsuccessful. You first priority should be to

    (A) apply direct pressure as well as you can and continue your assessment
    (B) apply Military Anti-Shock Trousers (MAST pants) to control shock
    (C) establish large-bore intravenous access to replace lost blood volume
    (D) transport immediately, making bleeding control your first priority

161. The average normal pulse range for a newborn is

    (A) 120–160 beats per minute
    (B) 60–100 beats per minute
    (C) 80–120 beats per minute
    (D) 80–140 beats per minute

162. All of the following are signs of respiratory distress *except*:

    (A) nasal flaring
    (B) Cheyne-Stokes respirations
    (C) intercostal retraction
    (D) tracheal tugging

163. The Glasgow coma scale uses all of the following variables to identify mental status *except*:

    (A) eye opening
    (B) respiratory rate
    (C) motor response
    (D) verbal response

PATIENT ASSESSMENT: COMMUNICATIONS

DIRECTIONS: Each item below contains four suggested responses. Select the one best response to each item.

164. Which of the following transmission modes allows the Paramedic to transmit a patient's ECG while engaging in two-way voice transmission with a telemetry base?

    (A) simplex
    (B) duplex
    (C) triplex
    (D) multiplex

165. When communicating with a telemetry base, the Paramedic should do all of the following *except*:

    (A) monitor the channel to ensure that it is not in use by another crew
    (B) protect the privacy of the patient at all times
    (C) repeat all medication orders back to telemetry to ensure the proper medication and dosage
    (D) when speaking, use slang terms to shorten the transmission

166. All of the following are the responsibility of the EMS dispatcher *except*:

    (A) directing the Paramedic to the appropriate hospital
    (B) dispatching and coordinating EMS resources
    (C) coordinating with public-safety agencies
    (D) receiving and processing EMS calls

167. The agency that develops rules and regulations for the use of all radio equipment is

    (A) Federal Communications Commission (FCC)
    (B) Department of Health
    (C) Department of Transportation
    (D) the individual EMS agency

168. Which of the following are all EMS-to-medical direction frequencies?

    (A) channels 2, 5, 7, and 9
    (B) channels 1, 3, 5, and 7
    (C) channels 1, 4, 7, and 9
    (D) channels 7, 8, 9, and 10

PATIENT ASSESSMENT: DOCUMENTATION

DIRECTIONS: Each item below contains four suggested responses. Select the one best response to each item.

169. The Paramedic should produce a written patient care report on all of the following calls *except*:

    (A) a trauma call where the patient was transferred to a helicopter crew for transport
    (B) a cardiac arrest patient who was pronounced dead at the scene and not transported
    (C) an injured patient who refused care and/or transport from the scene
    (D) a report of a motor vehicle accident that was discovered to be unfounded on arrival

170. Which of the following data types should be collected on a prehospital care report?

    (A) run data, patient data, and Paramedic personal opinion
    (B) personal data, patient data, and run data
    (C) run data, patient data, and treatment data
    (D) patient data, Paramedic personal opinion, and treatment data

171. You respond to the scene of an injury. On your arrival, you find a 29-year-old male with a laceration to his forehead from falling off a skateboard. After your assessment, you tell the patient that he needs to go to the hospital to get some stitches. The patient refuses, stating he will go to his private physician. What should you document on the patient call report?

    (A) only the patient refusal information
    (B) only the patient injury information
    (C) nothing, because the patient refused transport
    (D) all the information from your interaction with the patient

172. During your documentation, you find that you made an error on your patient call report. What is the appropriate method of correcting this error?

    (A) Place a line through the error, write the correct information above it, and then initial and date your correction.
    (B) Completely cross out the error and write the correct information above it.
    (C) Leave the error in place but explain to the emergency department staff that you made an error.
    (D) Discard the patient care report and start a new one.

173. The documentation format that follows patient care in the order it was accomplished is known as the

    (A) accepted format
    (B) consumption format
    (C) chronological format
    (D) data entry format

Answers and Explanations

PATIENT ASSESSMENT: HISTORY

125. **The answer is A.** (A) The patient is always the most qualified person from whom to elicit information. He or she will give you a comprehensive medical history and medication list as well as the symptoms of his or her current illness. (B) The patient's family is also an excellent source of patient information when the patient is unable to communicate. (C) Witnesses at the scene can be good providers of information if the patient is unconscious or has suffered injury due to trauma. (D) The patient's physician will have a wealth of information about the patient, but in emergent situations, the physician may not be readily available to relay the information. (*Brady, Paramedic Care 2e, Principles and Practice, Volume 2—The History. Mosby, Paramedic Textbook 3e, History Taking.*)

126. **The answer is C.** (C) When you ask patients about the type of pain they are experiencing, it elicits an explanatory answer. It gives patients a chance to explain how they feel, which, in turn, gives you a greater understanding of their condition. (A), (B), and (D) are all "closed-ended" questions, which generally elicit a yes-or-no response. (*Brady, Paramedic Care 2e, Principles and Practice, Volume 2—The History. Mosby, Paramedic Textbook 3e, History Taking.*)

127. **The answer is D.** (D) The patient's chief complaint is usually the reason that the EMS system has been activated. It is typically an acute change that affects the patient's normal state. (A), (B), and (C) are also important components of the patient history, but they fall into their own categories in the history. (*Brady, Paramedic Care 2e, Principles and Practice, Volume 2—The History. Mosby, Paramedic Textbook 3e, History.*)

128. **The answer is B.** (B) The past medical history, although quite an important aspect of the overall patient history, is not a component of the history of present illness. Past medical history is itself a separate component of the overall history. The history of present illness includes (A) onset of symptoms, (C) quality of pain (e.g., squeezing, pressure, or burning), and (D) severity of pain. Other components include radiation of pain as well as aggravating and alleviating factors. (*Brady, Paramedic Care 2e, Principles and Practice, Volume 2—The History. Mosby, Paramedic Textbook 3e, History.*)

129. **The answer is B.** (B) The patient's information about his last heart attack falls under past medical history. This piece of information can be significant in your diagnosis. The patient's statement about the last time he had this type of pain should be an indicator that he is suffering from a myocardial infarction. Although this is good information for confirming a diagnosis, the Paramedic should never cease further history taking based on one piece of information. (A), (C), and (D), although important components of the patient's history, are incorrect. (*Brady, Paramedic Care 2e, Principles and Practice, Volume 2—The History. Mosby, Paramedic Textbook 3e, History.*)

130. **The answer is B.** (B) Family history is an important aspect of the overall patient history. As you see in this case, the patient has no prior

medical history. The observation that her mother had a cardiac condition is a critical indicator that she may be suffering from a cardiac-related illness. (A), (C), and (D) are incorrect components of the history in this example. *(Brady, Paramedic Care 2e, Principles and Practice, Volume 2—The History. Mosby, Paramedic Textbook 3e, History.)*

131.   **answer is C.** (C) The social history may be an important factor in the determination of the patient's illness. Some other examples of social history are smoking, alcohol and drug abuse, employment, and recent travel. These could be all important factors in your diagnosis. Although (A) history of present illness may include the fact that the patient is hypothermic due to living in an unheated residence, that piece of information is obtained from the social history. (B) and (D) are incorrect. *(Brady, Paramedic Care 2e, Principles and Practice, Volume 2—The History. Mosby, Paramedic Textbook 3e, History.)*

132.   **The answer is A.** (A) Pertinent negatives are findings that you may expect to be typical of the patient's presentation but that are absent in the patient's complaint. These findings should always be documented on the run sheet. The Paramedic should document all components of the patient history and physical examination, regardless of the fact that they do not support the diagnosis. (B) Pertinent positives are positive findings that support your diagnosis. (C) Symptomatic findings is another term for pertinent positives. (D) is incorrect because all information obtained by the Paramedic should be documented. *(Brady, Paramedic Care 2e, Principles and Practice, Volume 2—The History. Mosby, Paramedic Textbook 3e, History.)*

133.   **The answer is A.** (A) Onset of pain is classified in the history of present illness component of the patient history. The onset of pain can be instrumental in the differential diagnosis of certain disease. (B), (C), and (D) are all components of the past medical history. Using the mnemonic AMPLE, the Paramedic can classify the past medical history as follows: A = allergies, M = medications, P = past medical problems, L = last oral intake, and E = events preceding the emergency. *(Brady, Paramedic Care 2e,*

Principles and Practice, Volume 2—The History. Mosby, Paramedic Textbook 3e, History.)

PATIENT ASSESSMENT: PHYSICAL EXAMINATION TECHNIQUES

134.   **The answer is B.** (B) End-tidal CO_2 detection is used commonly in intubated patients, but it has no value to the Paramedic during the primary assessment, where the determination of a secure airway and breathing is essential. (A) Inspection, (C) auscultation, and (D) palpation are all medically accepted practices in the pre-hospital care arena. These follow the same criteria as look, listen, and feel. *(Brady, Paramedic Care 2e, Principles and Practice, Volume 2—Physical Examination Techniques. Mosby, Paramedic Textbook 3e, Techniques of Physical Examination.)*

135.   **The answer is C.** (C) The brachial pulse is the primary pulse point in an infant, but it is not generally used in the assessment of the pulse in an adult. Blood pressure can be estimated by the pulse point. (A) Femoral pulses represent a blood pressure of approximately 70 mmHg, (B) radial pulses that are present represent a blood pressure above 80 mmHg, and (D) carotid pulses generally represent a blood pressure of 60 mmHg. *(Brady, Paramedic Care 2e, Principles and Practice, Volume 2—Physical Examination Techniques. Mosby, Paramedic Textbook 3e, Techniques of Physical Examination.)*

136.   **The answer is C.** (C) Jaundice is a condition of increased bilirubin in the blood and is not usually associated with hypovolemic shock. The skin of a patient who is hypovolemic can present as (A) mottled or blotchy; (B) cyanotic or blue; or (D) ashen in color. In addition, the patient may present with a pale appearance (pallor). *(Brady, Paramedic Care 2e, Principles and Practice, Volume 2—Physical Examination Techniques. Mosby, Paramedic Textbook 3e, Techniques of Physical Examination.)*

137.   **The answer is B.** (B) The AVPU scale is a standard for determination of mental status; it develops a baseline for the patient's overall

condition. A = alert or awake, V = voice responsive, P = pain responsive, and U = unconscious or unresponsive. (B), (C), and (D) are incorrect. (*Brady, Paramedic Care 2e, Principles and Practice, Volume 2—Physical Examination Techniques. Mosby, Paramedic Textbook 3e, Techniques of Physical Examination.*)

138. **The answer is A.** (A) Percussion in hemothorax will reveal a chest that is hyporesonant (dull to percussion). This is due to fluid in the chest cavity, which in this instance is blood. (B) Pericardial tamponade will not present with abnormal findings during an assessment using percussion, but it will present with muffled heart sounds during auscultation. (C) In tension pneumothorax, the chest will be hyperresonant. (D) Subcutaneous emphysema will present with palpable crackling under the skin. This condition is caused by air trapping in the subcutaneous tissues. (*Brady, Paramedic Care 2e, Principles and Practice, Volume 2—Physical Examination Techniques. Mosby, Paramedic Textbook 3e, Techniques of Physical Examination.*)

139. **The answer is D.** (A), (B), and (C) are all factors that may cause capillary refill to be delayed and create a false positive in the assessment of the patient with shock. Capillary refill is usually a good indicator in pediatric patients, but it should never be used primarily in the diagnosis of hypoperfusion. Rather, it should be considered a sign of such, and the Paramedic should then identify additional signs and symptoms. (D) Hypertension will not delay capillary refill. (*Brady, Paramedic Care 2e, Principles and Practice, Volume 2—Physical Examination Techniques. Mosby, Paramedic Textbook 3e, Techniques of Physical Examination.*)

140. **The answer is A.** (A) To examine the jugular veins for distention, the patient should be placed at a 45-degree angle. Normal jugular venous distention appears in healthy patients while they are supine. The patient who is suffering from right heart failure will present with jugular venous distention even while standing (90-degree angle). (B), (C), and (D) are incorrect. (*Brady, Paramedic Care 2e, Principles and Practice, Volume 2—Physical Examination Techniques.*

Mosby, Paramedic Textbook 3e, Techniques of Physical Examination.)

141. **The answer is C.** (C) The pupils of the patient who has overdosed on an opioid will be constricted. Constricted pupils may also be present in certain patients with head trauma and may sometimes be due to taking certain medications. (A) Equal and reactive is a normal expected response for all patients. (B) Cardiac arrest, central nervous system (CNS) injury, hypoxia, and certain medications may cause dilated and unreactive pupils. (D) Unequal pupils may be caused by CNS injury, eye trauma, and certain eye medications. (*Brady, Paramedic Care 2e, Principles and Practice, Volume 2—Physical Examination Techniques. Mosby, Paramedic Textbook 3e, Techniques of Physical Examination.*)

142. **The answer is D.** (D) In normal patients, you may hear only one or two bowel sounds in a full minute. Therefore, you should listen for 2 minutes (120 seconds) to properly determine whether the patient does have normal bowel sounds. Patients who have intestinal blockages will have hyperactive bowel sounds. In addition, patients with peritonitis will have hypoactive or no bowel sounds. (A), (B), and (C) are incorrect. (*Brady, Paramedic Care 2e, Principles and Practice, Volume 2—Physical Examination Techniques. Mosby, Paramedic Textbook 3e, Techniques of Physical Examination.*)

143. **The answer is A.** (A) Crepitation, or crepitus, is a crackling or grating sensation felt on palpation. It is an indicator of subcutaneous emphysema, a fracture when the bone ends rub together or an inflamed joint or osteoarthritis. (B), (C), and (D) are incorrect. (*Brady, Paramedic Care 2e, Principles and Practice, Volume 2—Physical Examination Techniques. Mosby, Paramedic Textbook 3e, Techniques of Physical Examination.*)

144. **The answer is D.** (D) Evaluation of mental status, although part of the primary survey, is not a technique of the physical examination. (A) Inspection, (B) palpation, (C) percussion, and auscultation are the four techniques of the physical examination used by field personnel. (*Brady, Paramedic Care 2e, Principles and Practice,*

Volume 2—Physical Examination Techniques. Mosby, Paramedic Textbook 3e, Techniques of Physical Examination.)

145. The answer is C. (C) Doll's eye response is an indicator of head injury. When the head-injured patient's head is moved, the eyes are fixed and move in the direction of the head. The normal response is for the eyes to remain fixed on an object as the head is moved. (A), (B), and (D) are incorrect. *(Brady, Paramedic Care 2e, Principles and Practice, Volume 2—Physical Examination Techniques. Mosby, Paramedic Textbook 3e, Techniques of Physical Examination.)*

146. The answer is A. (A) Anisocoria is naturally present in a good percentage of the population. It occurs naturally when one person's pupils are normally of different sizes. However, unequal pupils may be a sign of head injury in the trauma patient. (B) Dysconjugate gaze is when the patient's eyes move in different directions, usually from optic nerve damage. (C) Battle's sign is a discoloration over the mastoid process that is indicative of a basilar skull fracture. (D) Raccoon's eyes are black-and-blue discolorations of the orbits of the eyes, also indicative of a basilar skull fracture. *(Brady, Paramedic Care 2e, Principles and Practice, Volume 2— Physical Examination Techniques. Mosby, Paramedic Textbook 3e, Techniques of Physical Examination.)*

PATIENT ASSESSMENT: PATIENT ASSESSMENT IN THE FIELD

147. The answer is B. (B) The scene size-up begins as soon as the Paramedic is assigned to the call. If Paramedics do a comprehensive review of all the dispatch data, in most cases they will be able to obtain a considerable amount of information, including scene safety, patient condition, and additional resources responding or needed. (A) On arrival at the call, the Paramedic performs the 10-second scene survey. (C) When the Paramedic makes patient contact, the patient history component begins. (D) On-scene briefing by police, fire, or other public-safety officials is also part of the 10-second scene survey. *(Brady,*

Paramedic Care 2e, Principles and Practice, Volume 2— Patient Assessment in the Field. Mosby, Paramedic Textbook 3e, Patient Assessment.)

148. The answer is A. (A) Identification of perpetrators is the responsibility of the police department. Although, as a safety consideration, it is important to know that the perpetrator has left the scene, this responsibility is left to police officers. (B) Paramedics should never enter a partially collapsed building unless they are specially trained in that type of rescue. The Paramedic should ensure his or her safety by confirming the status of a building prior to entry. (C) The Paramedic should survey the scene for fuel spills that could be potentially hazardous to the patient or the Paramedic. (D) Paramedics should try to identify the causative agent at any scene where there are multiple patients complaining of similar symptoms. This will ensure their safety as well as assist in patient care. *(Brady, Paramedic Care 2e, Principles and Practice, Volume 2—Patient Assessment in the Field. Mosby, Paramedic Textbook 3e, Patient Assessment.)*

149. The answer is D. (D) As part of the initial scene survey, Paramedics must ensure that they have an accurate patient count in order to request additional resources. This will eliminate any delays in patient care due to lack of personnel. (A), (B), and (C) are incorrect. *(Brady, Paramedic Care 2e, Principles and Practice, Volume 2—Patient Assessment in the Field. Mosby, Paramedic Textbook 3e, Patient Assessment.)*

150. The answer is B. (B) Children who are 1–3 years old fear strangers and suffer from separation anxiety. These patients have little understanding of their illness and may experience emotional problems associated with their illness or injury. They are best examined and treated in the presence of a parent. (A), (C), and (D) are incorrect. *(Brady, Paramedic Care 2e, Principles and Practice, Volume 2—Patient Assessment in the Field. Mosby, Paramedic Textbook 3e, Patient Assessment.)*

151. The answer is D. (D) Adolescent patients are generally approached as adults, although they have a fear of disfigurement, disability, and death and the Paramedic should be reassuring and understanding during their care. (A), (B), and (C) reflect incorrect age groups. *(Brady, Paramedic Care 2e, Principles and Practice, Volume 2— Patient Assessment in the Field. Mosby, Paramedic Textbook 3e, Patient Assessment.)*

152. **The answer is D.** (D) To calculate minute volume, you must multiply tidal volume by respiratory rate. In this case, $300 \times 28 = 8400$. This is especially useful in the determination of the patient's oxygenation. The normal tidal volume in an adult is 500 mL, and the normal respiratory rate is 12–20 breaths per minute. Therefore, if a patient is breathing at 16 breaths per minute and the tidal volume is 500 mL, the minute volume would be $500 \times 16 = 8000$. (A), (B), and (C) are mathematically incorrect. *(Brady, Paramedic Care 2e, Principles and Practice, Volume 2— Patient Assessment in the Field. Mosby, Paramedic Textbook 3e, Patient Assessment.)*

153. **The answer is C.** (C) The Glasgow coma scale is a widely used method of evaluating a patient's level of consciousness. It is scored in three categories: eye opening, motor response, and verbal response, all to outside stimuli. The patient who opens his eyes after painful stimuli is scored a 2 in eye opening. The same patient who withdraws from painful stimuli is scored a 5 in motor response, and the patient who is confused and disoriented is scored a 4 in verbal response. The individual scores are added together to develop a baseline level of consciousness. *(Brady, Paramedic Care 2e, Principles and Practice, Volume 2—Head, Facial, and Neck Trauma. Mosby, Paramedic Textbook 3e, Head and Facial Trauma.)*

154. **The answer is A.** (A) Cheyne-Stokes respirations have a variety of neurologic or metabolic causes, some of which are reversible. They are characterized by a respiratory pattern that starts shallow, becomes deeper, and then returns to shallow. This is followed by a period of apnea, and the pattern begins again. (B) Eupnea is the term for normal breathing. (C) Central neurogenic hyperventilation is characterized by a series of rapid, deep respirations and usually indicates a serious neurologic condition. (D) Kussmaul's respirations are characterized by

rapid, deep respirations presenting in patients with diabetic ketoacidosis. *(Brady, Paramedic Care 2e, Principles and Practice, Volume 2—Physical Examination Techniques. Mosby, Paramedic Textbook 3e, Glossary.)*

155. **The answer is A.** (A) The speed of the vehicle (velocity) creates the most kinetic energy and therefore creates the greatest potential for injury. Although (B) the type of collision, (C) the patient's weight, and (D) the location of the patient in the vehicle are all factors, the single most important factor in any collision is velocity. *(Brady, Paramedic Care 2e, Principles and Practice, Volume 2—Patient Assessment in the Field. Mosby, Paramedic Textbook 3e, Trauma Systems and Mechanism of Injury.)*

156. **The answer is A.** (A) The trauma patient should be reassessed often. These patients have rapid changes in vital signs and mental status and should be reevaluated after every intervention. (B), (C), and (D) are incorrect. *(Brady, Paramedic Care 2e, Principles and Practice, Volume 2— Patient Assessment in the Field. Mosby, Paramedic Textbook 3e, Patient Assessment.)*

157. **The answer is D.** (D) The tongue is the most frequent cause of snoring respirations in the unconscious patient. The tongue can also cause a complete airway obstruction in patients who cannot control their own airway. The repositioning of the airway may be all that is needed to correct this condition. (A) Blood and (B) vomit usually cause a gurgling sound and are corrected by suctioning. (D) Teeth can cause a total airway obstruction and must also be suctioned out of the airway. *(Brady, Paramedic Care 2e, Principles and Practice, Volume 2—Patient Assessment in the Field. Mosby, Paramedic Textbook 3e, Patient Assessment.)*

158. **The answer is A.** (A) The Paramedic should attempt direct visualization with a laryngoscope and then use Magill forceps to remove the obstruction. (B) Needle cricothyroidotomy should be the last effort made. Needle cricothyroidotomy will provide an airway, but it is not an adequate airway maintenance intervention. (C) Abdominal thrusts in this situation have failed, although that would be one of the first basic life support interventions. (D) Suctioning

can be used for smaller obstructions but will not work on a lodged food bolus. *(Brady, Paramedic Care 2e, Principles and Practice, Volume 2— Patient Assessment in the Field. Mosby, Paramedic Textbook 3e, Airway Management and Ventilation.)*

159. **The answer is C.** (C) The patient with difficulty breathing who has obvious respiratory compromise and a respiratory rate of less than 10 or over 28 should be ventilated using a bag-valve-mask. This will ensure proper tidal volume. (A) The nasal cannula will not deliver an appropriate amount of oxygen to a patient with poor tidal volume. (B) The nonrebreather mask, like the nasal cannula, requires the patient to have acceptable air exchange to properly deliver oxygen. (D) Blow-by oxygen is usually used only with pediatric patients who will not tolerate a mask. *(Brady, Paramedic Care 2e, Principles and Practice, Volume 2—Patient Assessment in the Field. Mosby, Paramedic Textbook 3e, Patient Assessment.)*

160. **The answer is D.** (D) Immediate transport is indicated for all patients who have uncontrolled bleeding. There is not time for comprehensive assessments due to the large possibility of fluid loss. (A) The Paramedic should continue to apply direct pressure, but the assessment should not continue, since the priority should be to stop fluid loss. (B) Application of MAST is not indicated for patients with uncontrolled bleeding above the level of the pants. (C) Establishment of a large-bore intravenous access is indicated but is not the first priority. Replacement crystalloid can only replace at a 3:1 ratio to whole blood. Therefore, maintenance of blood volume is the highest priority. *(Brady, Paramedic Care 2e, Principles and Practice, Volume 2—Patient Assessment in the Field. Mosby, Paramedic Textbook 3e, Patient Assessment.)*

161. **The answer is A.** (A) The normal pulse rate for an infant is 120–160 beats per minute. Infants usually have higher pulse and respiratory rates but lower blood pressures than older children and adults. (B) Sixty to 100 beats per minute is the average pulse rate for an adult. (C) Eighty to 120 beats per minute is the average pulse rate for a 3-year-old child. (D) Eighty

to 140 beats per minute is the average pulse rate for a 1-year-old child. *(Brady, Paramedic Care 2e, Principles and Practice, Volume 2—Patient Assessment in the Field. Mosby, Paramedic Textbook 3e, Techniques of Physical Examination.)*

162. **The answer is B.** (B) Cheyne-Stokes respirations are a sign of metabolic or neurologic compromise, not of hypoxia or distress. (A), (C), and (D) are all common signs of respiratory distress. The Paramedic should be aware that the patient might exhibit just one or all of these signs. Additional signs of respiratory distress include tachypnea and anxiety. *(Brady, Paramedic Care 2e, Principles and Practice, Volume 2—Patient Assessment in the Field. Mosby, Paramedic Textbook 3e, Techniques of Physical Examination.)*

163. **The answer is B.** (A), (C), and (D) are all indicators used for the determination of mental status in patients. The minimum score for all patients is 3, and the maximum score (normal) is 15. (B) Respiratory rate is not measured in the Glasgow coma scale, but it is used as an indicator in the trauma score. *(Brady, Paramedic Care 2e, Principles and Practice, Volume 2—Trauma. Mosby, Paramedic Textbook 3e, Head, Facial, and Neck Trauma.)*

PATIENT ASSESSMENT: COMMUNICATIONS

164. **The answer is D.** (D) Multiplex transmissions allow two-way voice communication at the same time as transmission of an ECG. This feature is highly advantageous to patient care. (A) Simplex transmissions allow only one person to speak at a time, finish his or her transmission, and then receive a response. (B) Duplex communications allow the Paramedic to send and receive voice transmission simultaneously. This is accomplished by the use of dual frequencies. (C) Triplex communications do not exist. *(Brady, Paramedic Care 2e, Principles and Practice, Volume 2—Communications. Mosby, Paramedic Textbook 3e, Communications.)*

165. **The answer is D.** (D) The Paramedic should never use slang terms while making telemetry contact. These terms are not professionally

accepted and may cause confusion as to the patient's actual condition. (A), (B), and (C) are all appropriate techniques for telemetry communication. *(Brady, Paramedic Care 2e, Principles and Practice, Volume 2—Communications. Mosby, Paramedic Textbook 3e, Communications.)*

166. **The answer is A.** (A) The EMS dispatcher does not direct the Paramedic to the appropriate hospital. Selecting the hospital is the duty of the Paramedic. (C) In certain circumstances, the EMS dispatcher will coordinate with area hospitals to ensure that no hospitals are overloaded with patients. However, the Paramedic decides where to transport. (B) and (D) are both direct responsibilities of the EMS dispatcher. *(Brady, Paramedic Care 2e, Principles and Practice, Volume 2—Communications. Mosby, Paramedic Textbook 3e, Communications.)*

167. **The answer is A.** (A) The FCC is responsible for all regulation of radio transmissions and frequency use. The primary functions of the FCC are to license radio frequencies, establish standards for radio equipment, and establish and enforce rules and regulations regarding radio transmissions. (B) The Department of Health, (C) the Department of Transportation, and (D) the individual EMS agency all have roles regarding EMS communications. However, the FCC is the governmental regulatory agency for all EMS agencies. *(Brady, Paramedic Care 2e, Principles and Practice, Volume 2—Communications. Mosby, Paramedic Textbook 3e, Communications.)*

168. **The answer is B.** The EMS ultrahigh frequency (UHF) special emergency radio services channels consist of 10 EMS radio frequencies. Channels 1 through 8 are all EMS-to-medical direction frequencies. Channels 9 and 10 are dispatch, or steering, channels. *(Brady, Paramedic Care 2e, Principles and Practice, Volume 2—Communications. Mosby, Paramedic Textbook 3e, Communications.)*

PATIENT ASSESSMENT: DOCUMENTATION

169. **The answer is D.** Patient care reports should be completed whenever the Paramedic arrives at the scene and has an interaction with a patient. This report should be completed whether the patient is transported or not. Documentation of (A), (B), and (C) is required by all Paramedics. This documentation serves to provide the EMS agency with a historical chart of patient interaction. (D) An unfounded call is not required to be documented, but some systems require a call report on all EMS calls. *(Brady, Paramedic Care 2e, Principles and Practice, Volume 2—Documentation. Mosby, Paramedic Textbook 3e, Documentation.)*

170. **The answer is C.** (C) Paramedics should always collect run data, patient data, and treatment data on their call reports. This information has multiple uses and is primarily important in the continuation of patient care in the emergency department. There is no place for a Paramedic's personal opinion on a patient care report. Although the Paramedic's diagnosis is essential to the treatment information, personal opinions should remain off the report. (A), (B), and (D) are incorrect. *(Brady, Paramedic Care 2e, Principles and Practice, Volume 2—Documentation. Mosby, Paramedic Textbook 3e, Documentation.)*

171. **The answer is D.** (D) Every patient interaction should be documented completely. The Paramedic should obtain all call information and write it on the patient call report. This includes all patients refusing medical care and/or transport. In some cases, the Paramedic should document all attempts to convince the patient to be seen at the hospital. This report should be signed and witnessed at the scene. (A), (B), and (C) are incorrect. *(Brady, Paramedic Care 2e, Principles and Practice, Volume 2—Documentation. Mosby, Paramedic Textbook 3e, Documentation.)*

172. **The answer is A.** (A) The Paramedic who makes a documentation error can easily correct that error by drawing a line through the erroneous comment and writing the correction above it. This technique will prevent the Paramedic from being falsely accused of trying to cover up his or her error. (B), (C), and (D) are incorrect. *(Brady, Paramedic Care 2e, Principles and Practice, Volume 2—Documentation. Mosby, Paramedic Textbook 3e, Documentation.)*

173. **The answer is C.** (C) The chronological format follows the care of the patient in the order in which it was done. This is a simple, easy-to-use format in which the Paramedic documents, in time and possible abbreviations, the assessment and care of the patient. This format has the advantage of showing the patient's condition on arrival as well as the response to treatment in real time. This is an important quality assurance tool to which the Paramedic can refer when legal or call-review issues arise. (A), (B), and (D) are incorrect. *(Brady, Paramedic Care 2e, Principles and Practice, Volume 2—Documentation. Mosby, Paramedic Textbook 3e, Documentation.)*

Patient Presentations: Trauma

The following topic is covered in Section IV:

- Trauma and Trauma Systems

Questions

TRAUMA AND TRAUMA SYSTEMS

DIRECTIONS: Each item below contains four suggested responses. Select the one best response to each item.

174. In patients with spinal cord injury, a loss of sensation below the nipple line would indicate damage at what level of vertebrae?

    (A) C5
    (B) C6
    (C) T1
    (D) T4

175. In patients with spinal cord injury, loss of sensation at the umbilicus would indicate damage at what level of vertebrae?

    (A) T4
    (B) T8
    (C) T10
    (D) T12

176. In patients with head injury, _____ is the best indicator of the degree of injury?

    (A) level of consciousness (LOC)
    (B) absence of sensation
    (C) deep-tendon reflexes
    (D) respiratory pattern

177. A resulting compromise of spinal injury on the autonomic nervous system may result in

    (A) bradycardia, due to parasympathetic stimulation
    (B) low blood pressure, due to vasodilation
    (C) elevated blood pressure, due to vasoconstriction
    (D) a rise in body temperature, due to vasoconstriction

178. Rising intracranial pressure in a head injury patient would produce

    (A) rising pulse rate and rising blood pressure
    (B) falling pulse rate and rising blood pressure
    (C) falling pulse rate and falling blood pressure
    (D) rising pulse rate and falling blood pressure

179. When confronted with a head injury patient who is profoundly hypotensive, your first reaction should be to

(A) intubate and hyperventilate
(B) administer intravenous (IV) dexamethasone
(C) give 2.0 mg naloxone IV
(D) look for signs of other injuries

180. Unconscious patients with severe isolated head injury should be managed by all of the following *except*:

(A) rapid infusion of IV fluid
(B) oxygen
(C) close monitoring
(D) spinal immobilization

181. You extricate an injured female from a wrecked auto, you observe that she is in respiratory distress. Physical examination reveals an area of her left chest that moves in opposition to the rest of the chest with respiration. The most likely diagnosis is

(A) tension pneumothorax
(B) simple pneumothorax
(C) hemothorax
(D) flail chest

182. Your patient has blood in his ear canal, this could be indicative of

(A) ear infection
(B) skull fracture
(C) intracerebral bleeding
(D) ruptured eardrum

183. A 35-year-old male has been rescued from his burning basement by firefighters. The patient is now responsive to pain and has second- and third-degree burns over 40% of his body. Your most immediate concern is

(A) controlling airway and ventilation
(B) preventing infection
(C) treating for shock
(D) apply wet dressings to the burns

184. Blistered skin surrounded by a red area best describes

(A) first-degree burn
(B) second-degree burn
(C) third-degree burn
(D) radiation burn

185. An impaled object may be removed if

(A) it is impaled in the eye
(B) it is too large to easily stabilize
(C) it is impaled in the cheek
(D) it interferes with splinting

186. Which of the following fractures should *not* be straightened?

(A) elbow
(B) femur
(C) radius
(D) tibia

187. Properly applied splints should

(A) be twice as long as the fractured bone
(B) be applied very loosely
(C) immobilize the joint proximal and distal to the injured bone
(D) immobilize only the joint proximal to the injured bone

188. Which of the following is the most serious complication of a pelvic fracture?

(A) prolonged disability
(B) urinary incontinence
(C) internal bleeding
(D) urinary tract infection

189. In relationship to the fracture site, the Paramedic should check the _____ pulse.

(A) proximal
(B) distal
(C) medial
(D) lateral

190. A man was burned on the full circumference of both arms and the full circumference of his right thigh. His percentage of burns is approximately

    (A) 18%
    (B) 27%
    (C) 32%
    (D) 36%

191. Which of the following complications of burn injury would *not* be treatable in the prehospital arena?

    (A) gram-negative sepsis
    (B) airway obstruction
    (C) carbon monoxide poisoning
    (D) shock

192. A 25-year-old female has been struck in the right eye with a pipe. She has a ruptured right globe, an orbital fracture, and no other obvious injury. You should bandage

    (A) the right eye tightly
    (B) both eyes loosely
    (C) the right eye loosely
    (D) both eyes tightly

193. Emergency care for most burns caused by chemicals is to treat initially by flooding the affected area with water. Which of the following is an exception to this rule?

    (A) hydrochloric acid
    (B) sodium hydroxide solution
    (C) dry lime
    (D) gasoline

194. Your patient has an extremity fracture and has a large area of swelling, which of the following signs should you *not* elicit?

    (A) crepitus
    (B) ecchymosis
    (C) swelling
    (D) tenderness

195. Which of the following procedures is *not* acceptable in the treatment of open fractures?

    (A) pushing any protruding bone ends back under the skin
    (B) covering the open wound with a sterile dressing
    (C) immobilizing the joint above and below
    (D) checking a distal pulse prior to splinting

196. Choose the true statement regarding pelvic fractures.

    (A) No immobilization is necessary.
    (B) Pneumatic anti shock garment (PASG) is contraindicated.
    (C) Injury to the urinary tract is rare.
    (D) Patients are usually more comfortable when transported with the knees slightly flexed.

197. Which of the following is *not* a sign of pericardial tamponade?

    (A) muffled heart sounds
    (B) distended neck veins
    (C) tracheal shift
    (D) narrowed pulse pressure

198. Which of the following is the most important factor in determination of the mechanism of injury?

    (A) the direction of impact
    (B) the size of the auto involved
    (C) the weight of the victim
    (D) the speed of impact

199. Secondary collisions in a motor vehicle crash occur when

    (A) the organs collide with the interior of the occupants
    (B) the interior of the vehicle collides with the exterior
    (C) the occupants collide with the interior of the vehicle
    (D) the vehicle collides with another object

200. Which of the following types of motor vehicle collisions would most likely result in an aortic rupture?

(A) rollover
(B) frontal impact
(C) rear impact
(D) side impact

201. Fractures of the calcanei and lumbar spine are most commonly seen as a result of

(A) high-speed motor vehicle collisions
(B) falls from a height of greater than 15 feet
(C) motor vehicle-pedestrian accidents
(D) bicycle accidents

202. Which organs are most vulnerable to primary blast injury from the pressure wave of an explosion?

(A) heart
(B) liver
(C) lungs
(D) long bones

203. The wound area of tissue damage from a medium-velocity handgun bullet will usually be

(A) the same as the diameter of the bullet
(B) one-half the diameter of the bullet
(C) twice the diameter of the bullet
(D) 20 times the diameter of the bullet

204. The presence of a clearly palpable radial pulse suggests a systolic blood pressure of at least

(A) 60 mmHg
(B) 80 mmHg
(C) 100 mmHg
(D) 120 mmHg

205. A normal capillary refill time is usually

(A) less than 1 second
(B) less than 2 seconds
(C) greater than 2 seconds
(D) less than 4 seconds

206. A crackling feeling over a large area of the chest on palpation is a sign of

(A) hemothorax
(B) subcutaneous emphysema
(C) cardiac contusion
(D) aortic rupture

207. Which of the following statements is true regarding the use of bag-valve-mask to ventilate victims of multiple trauma?

(A) It rarely provides effective ventilation.
(B) It may require two persons to utilize effectively.
(C) It cannot be used in cases of thoracic trauma.
(D) It does not increase the danger of tension pneumothorax.

208. Injuries of the _____ result in referred pain to the left shoulder.

(A) liver
(B) spleen
(C) cervical spine
(D) right lung

209. In a trauma patient, distended neck veins are most likely a sign of

(A) cervical spine injury
(B) hemothorax
(C) profound shock
(D) tension pneumothorax

Questions 210–211 are based on the following scenario.

You are called to the scene of a combine accident where the driver has fallen from the machine and landed head first on a cement garage floor. On your arrival, the patient is unconscious and has blood coming from his nose. Your assessment reveals the following additional information: BP 190/130, pulse 48, respirations 32, rapid, deep, and irregular. You notice that the patient has an obvious deformity in the cervical spine.

210. Based on the information above, what would be your highest priority?

    (A) large bore IV
    (B) control any obvious bleeding
    (C) establish cervical spine immobilization
    (D) control airway

211. The patient's vital signs would be indicative of which of the following:

    (A) hypovolemic shock
    (B) head injury
    (C) basal skull fracture
    (D) airway compromise

212. The best method of maintaining an airway in a trauma patient is

    (A) triple airway maneuver
    (B) head tilt, chin lift
    (C) head tilt, neck lift
    (D) modified jaw thrust

213. The trachea will shift _____ in a patient with tension pneumothorax.

    (A) toward the injured side
    (B) toward the uninjured side
    (C) anteriorly in the neck
    (D) posteriorly in the neck

214. Your patient has suffered chest trauma and is now presenting with premature ventricular contractions, this is best treated by using

    (A) rapid infusion of IV fluid
    (B) MAST
    (C) hyperventilation
    (D) IV lidocaine

215. A patient with a flail chest segment should be treated with

    (A) positive-pressure ventilation
    (B) cricothyrotomy
    (C) manual stabilization
    (D) needle decompression

216. Your trauma patient opens his eyes to verbal stimulation, is disoriented, and localizes pain. What is his Glasgow coma score?

    (A) 13
    (B) 12
    (C) 11
    (D) 10

217. Which of the following traumatic injuries can be easily mistaken for an acute myocardial infarction?

    (A) cardiac contusion
    (B) pericardial tamponade
    (C) aortic rupture
    (D) pulmonary contusion

218. The Paramedic should spend _____ on scene with the critical trauma patient unless there are extenuating circumstances.

    (A) less than 10 minutes
    (B) more than 10 minutes
    (C) less than 20 minutes
    (D) as long as necessary to assess and treat every injury

219. _____ is the largest factor in determining expended kinetic energy.

    (A) Velocity
    (B) Mass
    (C) Sectional density
    (D) Angular momentum

220. Tenderness, guarding, rigidity, and distention of the abdomen are signs of

    (A) injury to the superficial abdominal muscles
    (B) anxiety
    (C) injury to internal abdominal organs
    (D) shock

221. Your patient presents with dyspnea, hoarseness, and facial burns after being trapped in a confined space with a fire, you should consider

(A) IV fluid replacement
(B) giving copious amounts of water by mouth
(C) endotracheal intubation
(D) sedation with diazepam

222. Choose the incorrect statement about electrical pathway burns.

(A) They are usually only superficial.
(B) There is a danger of cardiac dysrhythmia.
(C) There may be an exit wound.
(D) There may be deep-tissue damage far from the site of the surface injury.

223. The exit wound from a high velocity weapon would be

(A) the same diameter as the entrance
(B) round with a clearly defined edge
(C) larger than the entrance and irregularly shaped
(D) smaller than the entrance due to bullet fragmentation

224. The preferred method of controlling severe bleeding is

(A) vascular clamps
(B) direct pressure
(C) tourniquet
(D) elevation

225. Of the following, which is the highest priority consideration of a Paramedic treating a facial wound?

(A) hypovolemic shock
(B) disfigurement
(C) severe pain
(D) airway compromise

226. Which of the following is least useful in treating hypovolemic shock?

(A) MAST
(B) IV volume replacement
(C) bleeding control
(D) vasopressors

227. To determine the possible injuries resulting from a motor vehicle accident (MVA), the Paramedic would consider the

(A) mechanism of injury
(B) debris
(C) condition or injuries of the other occupants
(D) length of skid marks

228. How much of the "golden hour" is given to the prehospital medical care provider for scene assessment and care?

(A) 1 minute
(B) 10 minutes
(C) 20 minutes
(D) 30 minutes

229. The decision of whether to transport a patient immediately or to attempt on-scene care is one of the most critical decisions you will make during a medical emergency.

(A) true
(B) false

230. As the speed of an automobile doubles, the energy potential will

(A) reduce by one-half
(B) remain unchanged
(C) double
(D) quadruple

231. Because blunt force trauma does not penetrate the skin, there is little worry about damage to internal organs.

(A) true
(B) false

232. The anatomic region most commonly injured in the rear-end impact is the

    (A) extremities
    (B) neck
    (C) chest
    (D) head

233. The hollow-point, soft-tipped bullet is designed to increase the profile and thereby the rate of energy exchanged.

    (A) true
    (B) false

234. Your 55-year-old patient has powder burns and tattooing around an entrance wound, this would suggest

    (A) a gun used at close range
    (B) a high-powered rifle
    (C) use of a black powder
    (D) use of a "dum-dum" bullet

235. The major reason for allowing fluid to drain from the nose or ear is that

    (A) It may release intracranial pressure.
    (B) Its flow will prevent pathogens from entering the meninges.
    (C) It is impossible to stop the flow anyway.
    (D) Regeneration of cerebrospinal fluid is beneficial to the healing process.

236. In a head injury, the brain moves forward, then backward, causing injury opposite the impact, this is known as a _____ injury.

    (A) subdural hematoma
    (B) epidural hematoma
    (C) contrecoup
    (D) a concussion

237. Your patient has what appears to be a large hematoma inside her pupil and iris, this is known as

    (A) hyphema
    (B) glaucoma
    (C) retinopathy
    (D) hematoma

238. Manual spinal stabilization should be maintained until

    (A) a cervical collar is applied
    (B) the patient begins to object
    (C) the patient has no pain
    (D) the patient is immobilized with a spine board

239. Prolonged intubation attempts may cause dysrhythmias and increased intracranial pressure in the head injury patient.

    (A) true
    (B) false

240. Hyperventilating a head injury patient at 20 breaths per minute will

    (A) lower Pao_2, decreasing cerebral blood flow
    (B) lower $Paco_2$, decreasing cerebral blood flow
    (C) increase $Paco_2$, increasing cerebral blood flow
    (D) increase Pao_2, increasing cerebral blood flow

241. The best way to control severe arterial bleeding from the neck is

    (A) careful direct pressure
    (B) tourniquet
    (C) an occlusive dressing covered with a dressing
    (D) pressure dressing with tight bandage

242. A patient with a head injury should be observed for hypothermia or hyperthermia.

    (A) true
    (B) false

243. Your 55-year-old male has a metal splinter embedded in his eye, which of the following would be appropriate?

    (A) a protective cup over the eye
    (B) a tight dressing over the eye
    (C) removal of the object and bandaging of the eye
    (D) a loose dressing over the object

244. The area between the visceral and parietal pleura is

    (A) filled with air
    (B) filled with fluid
    (C) a potential space
    (D) part of the diaphragm

245. Your patient was involved in a motor vehicle collision 2 days ago. He called the ambulance today because of severe pain in the right flank and blood in his urine, you suspect injury to the

    _____.

    (A) kidney
    (B) spleen
    (C) liver
    (D) heart

246. A stab wound located at the margin of the lower ribs on the anterior of the body should be suspected of causing injury to

    (A) abdominal organs only
    (B) thoracic organs only
    (C) the spine
    (D) abdominal and thoracic organs

247. Rib fractures are not routinely immobilized, doing so may

    (A) cause severe pain
    (B) cause a flail chest
    (C) increase bleeding into the chest
    (D) increase the chances of atelectasis and pneumonia

248. Flail chest segments will present in which of the following fashions:

    (A) move in the opposite direction of the rib cage during respiration
    (B) move along with the rib cage during respiration
    (C) will not move during respiration
    (D) move when the patient is not breathing

249. Frothy blood bubbling from a chest wound is a sign of

    (A) flail chest
    (B) hemothorax
    (C) open pneumothorax
    (D) tension pneumothorax

250. A male patient fell from a ladder striking his chest on some building materials. The patient initially complained of pleuritic pain on the right side of his chest, and some crepitus could be felt over the third and fourth ribs on the right side. En route to the hospital, the patient developed severe shortness of breath and signs of shock. You should suspect

    (A) tension pneumothorax
    (B) ruptured aorta
    (C) intra-abdominal bleeding
    (D) traumatic asphyxia

251. After a traumatic injury to the chest, blood may collect in the sac around the heart, this is known as

    (A) myocardial infarction
    (B) pericardial tamponade
    (C) cardiomyopathy
    (D) congestive heart failure

252. Of the following, which is *not* a sign of pericardial tamponade?

    (A) tracheal deviation
    (B) narrowing pulse pressure
    (C) jugular vein distention
    (D) rapid thready pulse

253. In the absence of a spinal injury, a patient with a chest injury is best transported

    (A) lying on the uninjured side
    (B) lying on the injured side
    (C) in the Trendelenburg position
    (D) lying on the left side

254. The correct landmark for a pleural decompression is

    (A) second intercostal space, midclavicular
    (B) third intercostal space, midaxillary
    (C) fifth intercostal space, midclavicular
    (D) fifth intercostal space, immediately adjacent to the sternum

255. Your patient begins to exhibit difficult breathing after you place an occlusive dressing over his open chest wound, your first action should be

    (A) intubate and hyperventilate the patient
    (B) roll the patient onto the uninjured side
    (C) unseal the wound
    (D) increase the percentage of oxygen given to the patient

256. Your 55-year-old male has been in a collision. During the collision, he hit his chest against the steering wheel. He is now complaining of chest pains and has ECG changes consistent with a heart attack, this syndrome should be treated as a

    (A) tension pneumothorax
    (B) pericardial tamponade
    (C) flail chest
    (D) myocardial infarction

257. A male patient has been stabbed in the chest. The knife is impaled in the chest on your arrival. You should

    (A) remove the knife and leave the wound open to the air
    (B) stabilize the knife in place with bulky dressings
    (C) remove the knife and place an airtight dressing over the wound
    (D) perform a needle decompression of the chest

258. An abdominal wound with a loop of bowel protruding through it should be managed by

    (A) covering with a dry sterile dressing
    (B) leaving it exposed to the air
    (C) replacing the bowel carefully back through the wound
    (D) covering with a moist sterile dressing

259. A soft-tissue injury that results when a joint is moved beyond its normal range of motion is known as a

    (A) sprain
    (B) strain
    (C) dislocation
    (D) contusion

260. A suspected dislocation should be managed

    (A) by immobilizing the bone above the joint only
    (B) by immobilizing the bone below the joint only
    (C) without immobilization
    (D) by immobilizing the bones above and below the joint

261. Of the following, which fracture has the highest possibility of being a life threat?

    (A) humerus
    (B) clavicle
    (C) femur
    (D) tibia

262. The Paramedic should look for signs of _____ while treating a pelvic fracture.

    (A) paralysis
    (B) permanent deformity
    (C) injury to the bladder
    (D) severe hemorrhage

263. Prior to splinting a fractured elbow, you detected a strong distal pulse and the patient had normal motion and sensation. After splinting, you are unable to feel a distal pulse and the patient complains of numbness in his fingers. You should first

    (A) remove the splint and reapply it
    (B) remove the splint and do not attempt to reapply it
    (C) loosen the splint and recheck the pulse
    (D) transport the patient to the hospital

264. While attempting to realign an angulated fracture, you meet resistance and the patient complains of extreme pain. You should

    (A) apply more force to the limb
    (B) rotate the limb slowly while applying force
    (C) apply a traction splint
    (D) splint the fracture in its present position

265. The Paramedic should splint a dislocation _____.

    (A) after being realigned
    (B) as they are found
    (C) in an extended position
    (D) in a flexed position

266. Of the following, which is the most effective tool in splinting a fractured femur?

    (A) a traction splint
    (B) a PASG
    (C) an air splint
    (D) a rigid board splint

267. Pillow splints are suggested for which of the following injuries?

    (A) fracture of femur
    (B) ankle fractures
    (C) humerus fractures
    (D) knee fractures

268. A collection of blood under the skin is

    (A) a contusion
    (B) a hematoma
    (C) a laceration
    (D) an abrasion

269. A wound which is susceptible to infection with tetanus and other anaerobic bacteria is

    (A) incision
    (B) contusion
    (C) puncture
    (D) avulsion

270. An injury where soft tissue has been torn away is known as

    (A) a contusion
    (B) an amputation
    (C) an abrasion
    (D) an avulsion

271. A type of open wound with jagged edges caused by tearing forces is known as

    (A) an abrasion
    (B) an incision
    (C) a laceration
    (D) a puncture

272. Patients who have been trapped in an enclosed space with a combustion will most likely suffer from

    (A) cyanide poisoning
    (B) thermal burns
    (C) heat stroke
    (D) carbon monoxide poisoning

273. A third-degree burn is characterized by _____, which differentiates it from other categories of burns.

(A) lack of pain
(B) lack of blistering
(C) color
(D) oozing of fluid

274. Identify the most serious burn condition.

(A) second-degree burns to the entire left arm
(B) third-degree burns to the right lower leg
(C) first-degree burns to the entire body
(D) second-degree burns around the mouth and nose

275. Severe bleeding from the wrist may be controlled by pressure on the _____ pressure point.

(A) femoral
(B) temporal
(C) popliteal
(D) brachial

276. The IV solution most appropriate for the use in burn patients is _____.

(A) Ringer's lactate
(B) normal saline solution
(C) 1/2 normal saline solution
(D) D_5W

277. Immediate management for chemical burn injuries is

(A) a dry, sterile dressing
(B) irrigation with alcohol
(C) applying a neutralizing agent
(D) irrigation with copious amounts of water

278. Skin contaminated with phenol should be initially irrigated with which of the following?

(A) soap water
(B) water
(C) alcohol
(D) mineral oil

279. How should contamination and burns from dry lime be managed?

(A) Irrigate with alcohol.
(B) Irrigate with water immediately.
(C) Apply a baking soda solution.
(D) Brush the chemical away and then irrigate with water.

280. Of the following, which is *not* an indicator of spinal injury?

(A) a rapid pulse
(B) a large contusion on the forehead
(C) numbness and tingling in the extremities
(D) a spider crack in the windshield

281. Which of the following would *not* be a reason for immediate transport to a trauma center?

(A) suspected lumbar spine injury
(B) signs of shock
(C) unstable pelvic fracture
(D) deteriorating LOC

282. A tourniquet should always be used to control bleeding from an amputation.

(A) true
(B) false

283. In some cases of _____ , priapism in an indicator of injury.

(A) spinal injury
(B) airway obstruction
(C) hypovolemia
(D) cardiac tamponade

284. As you attempt to immobilize your patient, the patient's body does not conform as well as you are comfortable with, you should

    (A) not use a backboard and transport on the ambulance cot
    (B) use a short board
    (C) use noncompressible padding to fill the void
    (D) force the patient down to the board

285. Sandbags are not used to stabilize the head of a spinal injury patient because

    (A) Sandbags are very expensive.
    (B) Sandbags cannot hold the patient's head securely.
    (C) The patient's head may be pushed to the side by the weight of the bags.
    (D) Sandbags are very difficult to use.

286. You find a child on a playground after a fall, he is not responsive to voice or pain and has slow, snoring respirations. Your most immediate action would be to

    (A) open the airway using the head tilt, chin lift
    (B) maintain in-line stabilization and open the airway with a jaw thrust
    (C) perform endotracheal intubation while maintaining in-line stabilization
    (D) insert an esophageal obturator airway and ventilate with a bag-valve-mask

287. The Paramedic should check motor and sensory function in all extremities and document her findings before extricating a patient from a wreck.

    (A) true
    (B) false

288. A 43-year-old man was the driver in a motor vehicle crash. Examination of the patient reveals a laceration on the forehead, bruising of the chest, and a tender abdomen. The patient was the unrestrained driver of a compact car that was struck head-on by a pickup truck. The patient is responsive to voice but is disoriented. His BP is 80/50, pulse 125, and respiratory rate 16. Neck veins are flat and breath sounds are equal bilaterally. The patient's skin is pale, cool, and diaphoretic. The patient's hypotension is most likely due to

    (A) hypoxia
    (B) hypovolemia
    (C) a tension pneumothorax
    (D) pericardial tamponade

289. A 35-year-old male was struck by an auto. His right thigh is painful. Physical examination reveals tenderness in the thigh and bruising. There is also shortening and external rotation of the right leg. The most appropriate splint would be

    (A) a traction splint
    (B) a pillow splint
    (C) a sling and swathe
    (D) splinting of the uninjured leg

290. Of the following, which facial bone is the most frequently fractured?

    (A) maxilla
    (B) nose
    (C) zygoma
    (D) mandible

291. The victim of a MVA appears to be in severe distress. The patient has stridorous respirations, and subcutaneous air can be felt in the anterior neck. Which of the following is the most likely cause of this patient's presentation?

    (A) zygoma fracture
    (B) aortic disruption
    (C) fractured larynx
    (D) simple pneumothorax

292. The _____ makes up the lower third of the face.

(A) ethmoid
(B) zygoma
(C) maxilla
(D) mandible

293. _____ may be caused by a closed head injury.

(A) Tachycardia
(B) Hypotension
(C) Increased alertness
(D) Abnormal breathing patterns

294. _____ is a term to describe bilateral periorbital ecchymosis.

(A) Raccoon's eyes
(B) Cullen's sign
(C) Battle's sign
(D) McBurney's sign

295. Which of the following is *true* about Glasgow coma scale?

(A) A score of 3 is normal.
(B) A score of 15 is indicative of a poor prognosis.
(C) A score of 12 accompanies brain death.
(D) A score of 7 represents coma.

296. The best way to immobilize an injured hand is

(A) flat on a board splint
(B) in the position of function
(C) with a pillow
(D) to the other hand

297. _____ results from a patient hitting her head against the windshield during a motor vehicle crash.

(A) Distraction
(B) Whiplash
(C) Hyperflexion
(D) Axial loading

298. A possible complication of a parietal or temporal skull fracture is

(A) subarachnoid hemorrhage
(B) intraventricular hematoma
(C) subdural hematoma
(D) epidural hematoma

299. All of the following are signs of hypovolemic shock:

(A) pale skin, tachycardia, and hypotension
(B) dilated pupils, pale skin, and bounding pulse
(C) dilated pupils, bradycardia, and flushed skin
(D) bounding pulse, flushed skin, and bradycardia

300. Pregnant patients near term who have suffered significant trauma should be transported

(A) lying in the left lateral recumbent position
(B) lying supine
(C) in the Trendelenburg position
(D) in the semi-Fowler's position

301. The national standard curriculum recommends volume replacement of _____ for all trauma patients.

(A) a saline lock
(B) one IV with a small-bore catheter
(C) one IV with a large-bore catheter
(D) two IVs with large-bore catheters

302. Of the following, which IV solution set would provide the most rapid fluid infusion?

(A) 60 gtts/mL
(B) 15 gtts/mL
(C) 10 gtts/mL
(D) burette

303. Your patient is a 16-year-old male who has been struck in the abdomen with a baseball bat. On your arrival, he is lying supine and holding his abdomen. He is alert and oriented. His vital signs are: BP 100/60, pulse 110, respirations 26. His skin is cool and clammy and slightly cyanotic. Lungs are clear. You suspect

(A) hypovolemic shock
(B) pericardial tamponade
(C) tension pneumothorax
(D) undiagnosed head injury

304. Your patient in question 303 would have injuries secondary to

(A) pressure wave
(B) blunt force trauma
(C) penetrating trauma
(D) paper bag syndrome

305. Treatment of the patient in question 303 would include all of the following *except*:

(A) endotracheal intubation
(B) fluid therapy with large bore IV
(C) spinal immobilization
(D) administration of oxygen

306. You are called to the scene of a 35-year-old female with a gunshot wound. Bystanders state that there was an altercation, and as the woman was walking away, her assailant pulled a gun and shot her in the back. On your arrival, the patient is alert and oriented, complaining of pain in the area of the entry wound and dizziness. Your assessment reveals an entry wound approximately 1 cm below her left scapula with no visible exit wound. Her vital signs are: BP 110/60, pulse 100, and respirations are 28 and slightly labored. Breath sounds reveal slightly diminished sounds on the left side. Based on your findings, it is appropriate to delay transport to assess this patient further and allow police to gather appropriate information.

(A) true
(B) false

307. Based on your findings in the patient in question 306, you suspect

(A) pneumothorax
(B) pericardial tamponade
(C) hypovolemic shock
(D) hemothorax

308. You would expect to initiate the following interventions to the patient in question 306 *except*:

(A) oxygen administration
(B) IV therapy
(C) spinal immobilization
(D) needle decompression of the thorax

309. As you transport this patient, she begins to complain of severe dizziness and begins sweating. You reassess the patient and find her BP is now 60 palpable and her heart rate is 130 and thready. Auscultation of the chest continues to reveal slightly diminished breath sounds on the left, but you now also detect muffled heart sounds. You suspect

(A) tension pneumothorax
(B) hemothorax
(C) pericaridal tamponade
(D) precordial thump

310. Field treatment for pericardial tamponade would include all of the following *except*:

(A) administration of oxygen
(B) fluid therapy
(C) cardiac monitoring
(D) pericardiocentesis

Answers and Explanations

TRAUMA AND TRAUMA SYSTEMS

174. The answer is D. Spinal injuries at the level of the T4 vertebrae will cause a loss of sensation and motor ability below the nipple line. C1 injuries will cause quadriplegia and will interfere with normal respirations. T1 injuries result in loss of function at the shoulder level and below. (*Brady, Paramedic Care 2e, Principles and Practice, Volume 4—Spinal Trauma. Mosby, Paramedic Textbook 3e, Spinal Trauma.*)

175. The answer is C. Loss of sensation at the umbilicus is associated with injury to the spine at the T10 (tenth thoracic vertebrae). Injuries at this level can result in paraplegia with total loss of function in all areas below the umbilicus. (*Brady, Paramedic Care 2e, Principles and Practice, Volume 4—Spinal Trauma. Mosby, Paramedic Textbook 3e, Spinal Trauma.*)

176. The answer is A. Altered LOC is a most important sign when evaluating a patient with a head injury. Deteriorating mental status is an early sign of a rise in intracranial pressure. This is seen in serious head injury. Altered respirator patterns are often a late sign of a serious head injuries. Loss of sensation and abnormal deep-tendon reflexes are difficult to continually assess and may be to due to a spinal or local injury. (*Brady, Paramedic Care 2e, Principles and Practice, Volume 4—Head, Facial, and Neck Trauma. Mosby, Paramedic Textbook 3e, Head and Facial Trauma.*)

177. The answer is B. Injury to the sympathetic nervous system may accompany injury to the spine. Dysfunction of the sympathetic nervous system will cause vasodilation and subsequent fall in blood pressure. There is not normally any parasympathetic stimulation; therefore, bradycardia would not be present, but the dysfunction of the sympathetic nervous system would prevent tachycardia in compensation for the fall in blood pressure. The vasodilation will cause a fall in body temperature. (*Brady, Paramedic Care 2e, Principles and Practice, Volume 4—Head, Facial, and Neck Trauma. Mosby, Paramedic Textbook 3e, Head and Facial Trauma.*)

178. The answer is B. Rising blood pressure and falling pulse rate seen in serious head injuries is known as Cushing's reflex. In an attempt to counter the decrease in cerebral perfusion caused by rising intracranial pressure, the systolic blood pressure will rise. The high systolic blood pressure will activate receptors in the carotid bodies, resulting in bradycardia. (*Brady, Paramedic Care 2e, Principles and Practice, Volume 4—Head, Facial, and Neck Trauma. Mosby, Paramedic Textbook 3e, Head and Facial Trauma.*)

179. The answer is D. Hypotension is rarely a primary result of an isolated head injury. With the exception of pediatric patients, any patient who has a suspected isolated head injury with resulting hypotension should be assessed for other hidden injuries. All external bleeding should be controlled, and signs of internal bleeding should be managed with rapid transport and IV fluid replacement. (*Brady, Paramedic Care 2e, Principles and Practice, Volume 4—Head, Facial, and Neck Trauma. Mosby, Paramedic Textbook 3e, Head and Facial Trauma.*)

180. The answer is A. A rapid infusion of IV fluids may cause an increase in intracranial pressure in a patient with an isolated head injury. IV fluids should be kept at a KVO (keep vein open) rate unless the patient becomes hypotensive. The Paramedic should observe the blood pressure of the patient with isolated head injury, especially when an IV has been established. *(Brady, Paramedic Care 2e, Principles and Practice, Volume 4—Head, Facial, and Neck Trauma. Mosby, Paramedic Textbook 3e, Head and Facial Trauma.)*

181. **The answer is D.** An area of the chest moving in opposition to the rest of the chest is known as paradoxical respiration. This is seen when multiple rib fractures disrupt the integrity of the chest wall. The condition is known as flail chest. *(Brady, Paramedic Care 2e, Principles and Practice, Volume 4—Thoracic Trauma. Mosby, Paramedic Textbook 3e, Thoracic Trauma.)*

182. **The answer is B.** Basal skull fractures can cause leakage of blood and cerebrospinal fluid from the ears. A ruptured eardrum or infection may also cause blood in the ear canal. Until a skull fracture is ruled out, no other diagnosis should be considered acceptable. *(Brady, Paramedic Care 2e, Principles and Practice, Volume 4—Head, Facial, and Neck Trauma. Mosby, Paramedic Textbook 3e, Head and Facial Trauma.)*

183. **The answer is A.** Patients suffering from severe burn injury in an enclosed area are likely to have burns to the airway and respiratory tract. Airway obstruction due to edema and respiratory difficulty may develop rapidly. These must be managed immediately. Shock from burns is not likely to occur rapidly in the field, and infections are not seen in the prehospital phase. Burn dressings should be delayed until the airway is secure, and patients with extensive burns should have dry, sterile dressings. *(Brady, Paramedic Care 2e, Principles and Practice, Volume 4—Burns. Mosby, Paramedic Textbook 3e, Burns.)*

184. **The answer is B.** Partial-thickness burns, or second-degree burns, are characterized by blisters surrounded by reddened skin. Third-degree burns, also known as full-thickness burns, are characterized by dry, painless charred or brown or white skin. First-degree burns, also known as superficial burns, are characterized by reddened, painful skin. *(Brady, Paramedic Care 2e, Principles and Practice, Volume 4—Burns. Mosby, Paramedic Textbook 3e, Burns.)*

185. **The answer is C.** Impaled objects in the cheek should be removed because they may cause airway obstruction. The end of the object should be located, and the object should be gently removed from the way that it entered. Objects impaled in the eye should be stabilized in place and the other eye loosely bandaged. Large objects should be cut so they can be stabilized. *(Brady, Paramedic Care 2e, Principles and Practice, Volume 4—Head, Facial, and Neck Trauma. Mosby, Paramedic Textbook 3e, Head and Facial Trauma.)*

186. **The answer is A.** Any fracture that involves a joint should be immobilized in the position found with the exception of injuries involving neuromuscular compromise. In the cases where compromise is suspected, a single attempt to realign the joint should be made in the field. *(Brady, Paramedic Care 2e, Principles and Practice, Volume 4—Musculoskeletal Trauma. Mosby, Paramedic Textbook 3e, Musculoskeletal Trauma.)*

187. **The answer is C.** All splints should be applied so that they immobilize the joint above and below the fracture site. This will ensure that excessive movement will not occur, resulting in additional injury. A splint should be applied so as to prevent unnecessary movement, but not be too snug as to affect nerve or circulatory function. *(Brady, Paramedic Care 2e, Principles and Practice, Volume 4—Musculoskeletal Trauma. Mosby, Paramedic Textbook 3e, Musculoskeletal Trauma.)*

188. **The answer is C.** Pelvis fractures can result in massive internal hemorrhage. Unstable pelvic fractures may affect many blood vessels. The pelvic area, and the anatomy surrounding it form a bowl that can hide swelling associated with severe bleeding. *(Brady, Paramedic Care 2e, Principles and Practice, Volume 4—Musculoskeletal Trauma. Mosby, Paramedic Textbook 3e, Musculoskeletal Trauma.)*

189. **The answer is B.** Pulse, movement, and sensation should be assessed before splinting any fracture. Vascular compromise is a complication of fracture. Distal pulses should also be checked

after splinting. If a pulse is lost after splinting, the splint should be adjusted to allow for the return of circulatory function. Loss of pulses secondary to fracture can threaten the limb. *(Brady, Paramedic Care 2e, Principles and Practice, Volume 4—Musculoskeletal Trauma. Mosby, Paramedic Textbook 3e, Musculoskeletal Trauma.)*

190. **The answer is B.** Using the standard adult rule of nines, each arm is 9% and the right thigh is also 9% burnt, for a total of 27%. *(Brady, Paramedic Care 2e, Principles and Practice, Volume 4—Burns. Mosby, Paramedic Textbook 3e, Burns.)*

191. **The answer is A.** Infection is a late complication of burn injury and is not seen in the prehospital phase of acute burn injury. Infections are managed with topical and systemic antibiotics that are not available to prehospital providers. Airway obstruction is the most immediate complication of burn injury that must be managed in the field. *(Brady, Paramedic Care 2e, Principles and Practice, Volume 4—Burns. Mosby, Paramedic Textbook 3e, Burns.)*

192. **The answer is B.** Bandaging both eyes will minimize movement of the injured eye. Bandages should be applied loosely so as to prevent further damage to the eye. *(Brady, Paramedic Care 2e, Principles and Practice, Volume 4—Head, Facial, and Neck Trauma. Mosby, Paramedic Textbook 3e, Head and Facial Trauma.)*

193. **The answer is C.** Dry corrosive powders, such as lime, should be brushed away first before flooding the area with copious amounts of water. Applying water to large amounts of dry corrosive material may spread the chemical and cause further injury. Liquid corrosives should be treated initially by irrigation with water. *(Brady, Paramedic Care 2e, Principles and Practice, Volume 4—Burns. Mosby, Paramedic Textbook 3e, Burns.)*

194. **The answer is A.** Crepitus is observed when broken bone ends move against each other. While this may occur incidentally during physical examination, it is accompanied by pain and should never be elicited intentionally. Ecchymosis, swelling, and tenderness are observed passively, and are not caused by the examination. *(Brady,*

Paramedic Care 2e, Principles and Practice, Volume 4— Musculoskeletal Trauma. Mosby, Paramedic Textbook 3e, Musculoskeletal Trauma.)

195. **The answer is B.** The Paramedic should never attempt to push protruding bone ends back into place. This may cause damage to surrounding structures. Checking distal circulation, covering wounds with sterile dressings, and immobilizing both joints adjacent to the fractured bone are all appropriate treatment. *(Brady, Paramedic Care 2e, Principles and Practice, Volume 4—Musculoskeletal Trauma. Mosby, Paramedic Textbook 3e, Musculoskeletal Trauma.)*

196. **The answer is D.** Most patients with pelvic fractures will be more comfortable if transported with their knees slightly flexed. This will allow the pelvis to be better supported on the spine board. Patients with a pelvic fracture should be immobilized to ease transportation and prevent further injury. The PASG may be used to treat hypotension secondary to unstable pelvic fracture. Patients with pelvic fracture commonly have injury to the urinary bladder and urethra. *(Brady, Paramedic Care 2e, Principles and Practice, Volume 4—Musculoskeletal Trauma. Mosby, Paramedic Textbook 3e, Musculoskeletal Trauma.)*

197. **The answer is C.** Tracheal deviation is seen in tension pneumothorax when the lung is pushed away from the affected side. Muffled heart sounds, distended neck veins, and narrowed pulse pressure are classical signs of cardiac tamponade known as Beck's triad. *(Brady, Paramedic Care 2e, Principles and Practice, Volume 4— Thoracic Trauma. Mosby, Paramedic Textbook 3e, Thoracic Trauma.)*

198. **The answer is D.** The amount of energy released in a collision is what determines the severity of injury. The energy of objects in motion is calculated by the equation $E = mv^2$. The velocity (v) is the most significant factor in determining energy. The mass and size of the vehicles and victims has a lesser effect on the amount of energy released. *(Brady, Paramedic Care 2e, Principles and Practice, Volume 4—Trauma and Trauma Systems. Mosby, Paramedic Textbook 3e, Trauma Systems/Mechanism of Injury.)*

199. The answer is C. The typical motor vehicle crash is composed of three collisions that combine to produce injury. The first collision occurs when the vehicle strikes an object. The vehicle immediately undergoes a change in speed, but the occupants are still moving at the original speed until they strike the interior of the vehicle, producing the second collision. The third collision occurs when the occupants' internal organs strike each other and the internal surfaces of the body. *(Brady, Paramedic Care 2e, Principles and Practice, Volume 4—Trauma and Trauma Systems. Mosby, Paramedic Textbook 3e, Trauma Systems/ Mechanism of Injury.)*

200. The answer is B. The largest deceleration forces are caused by frontal impact collisions. Deceleration causes the aorta to be pulled and stretched to such an extent that it may tear at the ligament attachment points. *(Brady, Paramedic Care 2e, Principles and Practice, Volume 4—Thoracic Trauma. Mosby, Paramedic Textbook 3e, Thoracic Trauma.)*

201. The answer is B. Patients who fall from heights greater than 15 feet are likely to land feet first, causing injury to the heels. Fractures of the calcanei are a sign that patients have fallen from a substantial height and are likely to have other serious injuries. *(Brady, Paramedic Care 2e, Principles and Practice, Volume 4—Head, Facial, and Neck Trauma. Mosby, Paramedic Textbook 3e, Head and Facial Trauma.)*

202. The answer is C. The pressure wave from an explosion moves through the air. The organs most susceptible to this pressure wave are the hollow organs. Solid organs and bones are less likely to be injured from the pressure wave. *(Brady, Paramedic Care 2e, Principles and Practice, Volume 4— Trauma and Trauma Systems. Mosby, Paramedic Textbook 3e, Trauma Systems/Mechanism of Injury.)*

203. The answer is C. A medium-velocity handgun bullet is likely to create a wound channel that is twice the diameter of the bullet as it dissipates its energy through the tissues. A low-velocity projectile, such as a knife, will create tissue damage of the same diameter as the projectile. A high-velocity rifle bullet that contains massive amounts of energy may create tissue damage along a wound track 20 times the diameter of the bullet. *(Brady, Paramedic Care 2e, Principles and Practice, Volume 4—Trauma and Trauma Systems. Mosby, Paramedic Textbook 3e, Trauma Systems/Mechanism of Injury.)*

204. The answer is B. As a general rule, the presence of a radial pulse usually indicates a systolic blood pressure of at least 80 mmHg. *(Brady, Paramedic Care 2e, Principles and Practice, Volume 4— Hemorrhage and Shock. Mosby, Paramedic Textbook 3e, Hemorrhage and Shock.)*

205. The answer is B. Normal peripheral capillary refill should occur in less than 2 seconds. Delayed capillary refill can be a sign of circulatory compromise. The Paramedic should be aware that capillary refill can be altered by other means, such as cold exposure. Additional patient evaluation should be performed in cases where the Paramedic suspects other causes of delayed capillary refill. *(Brady, Paramedic Care 2e, Principles and Practice, Volume 4—Hemorrhage and Shock. Mosby, Paramedic Textbook 3e, Hemorrhage and Shock.)*

206. The answer is B. A collection of air under the skin, known as subcutaneous emphysema, will cause crepitus to be felt on palpation. Decreased breath sounds and dyspnea are signs of hemothorax, electrocardiographic (ECG) changes are used to diagnose cardiac contusion, and aortic rupture is seen as profound hypotension after a deceleration injury. *(Brady, Paramedic Care 2e, Principles and Practice, Volume 4—Thoracic Trauma. Mosby, Paramedic Textbook 3e, Thoracic Trauma.)*

207. The answer is B. A two-handed technique may be required to obtain an adequate mask seal while maintaining a jaw thrust without compromising spinal immobilization. This necessitates a second person to operate the bag. A patient can be ventilated very effectively with this method. The bag-valve-mask can be used on a patient with thoracic injury, but there is an increased risk of tension pneumothorax. *(Brady, Paramedic Care 2e, Principles and Practice, Volume 1— Airway Management and Ventilation. Mosby, Paramedic Textbook 3e, Airway Management and Ventilation.)*

208. The answer is B. Bleeding from a ruptured spleen causes irritation to the diaphragm on the left side, this results in referred pain to the left shoulder. Injury to the liver typically causes right upper quadrant pain, a fracture of C1 will cause neck pain near the base of the skull, and a hemothorax will cause chest pain and difficulty breathing. *(Brady, Paramedic Care 2e, Principles and Practice, Volume 4—Abdominal Trauma. Mosby, Paramedic Textbook 3e, Abdominal Trauma.)*

209. **The answer is D.** A tension pneumothorax will cause a displacement of the great veins of the chest. The resultant venous obstruction will cause distention of the neck veins. Injury to the cervical spine, hemothorax, and shock are more likely to involve an actual or relative hypovolemia, which will cause flattened neck veins. *(Brady, Paramedic Care 2e, Principles and Practice, Volume 4—Thoracic Trauma. Mosby, Paramedic Textbook 3e, Thoracic Trauma.)*

210. **The answer is C.** The patient has obviously fallen from a height and based on your findings of a deformity in the cervical spine region, you should have a high index of suspicion of cervical spinal injury. The first intervention the Paramedic should complete is to protect the cervical spine by applying manual stabilization. As airway would be your next most important intervention, you could accomplish both tasks by using the jaw-thrust maneuver. This maneuver would allow you to maintain the airway while stabilizing the spine. *(Brady, Paramedic Care 2e, Principles and Practice, Volume 4—Spinal Trauma. Mosby, Paramedic Textbook 3e, Spinal Trauma.)*

211. **The answer is B.** The patient's increased blood pressure and decreased pulse, along with the altered LOC are all indicative of closed head injury. This presentation is known as Cushing's reflex. *(Brady, Paramedic Care 2e, Principles and Practice, Volume 4—Head, Facial, and Neck Trauma Mosby, Paramedic Textbook 3e, Head and Facial Trauma.)*

212. **The answer is D.** The modified jaw thrust is the best method for initially managing the airway of a trauma patient. This method allows the airway to be maintained without significant movement of the cervical spine. The head tilt, chin lift; head tilt, neck lift; or triple airway maneuver involve tilting the head, causing significant movement of the cervical spine. *(Brady, Paramedic Care 2e, Principles and Practice, Volume 1—Airway Management and Ventilation. Mosby, Paramedic Textbook 3e, Airway Management and Ventilation.)*

213. **The answer is B.** Expansion of air in the pleural space occurs on the injured side of a tension pneumothorax. This expansion will push the structures of the mediastinum, including the trachea, toward the uninjured side. *(Brady, Paramedic Care 2e, Principles and Practice, Volume 4—Thoracic Trauma. Mosby, Paramedic Textbook 3e, Thoracic Trauma.)*

214. **The answer is D.** Cardiac contusion can mimic symptoms of cardiac disease and should be treated pharmacologically in the same way as a myocardial infarction. In the case of premature ventricular contractions, lidocaine is the drug of choice. MAST trousers and rapid infusions of IV fluids should be used with caution in cases of cardiac contusion because of the chance of heart failure. Oxygen should be administered, but ventilation should be maintained normally. *(Brady, Paramedic Care 2e, Principles and Practice, Volume 4—Thoracic Trauma. Mosby, Paramedic Textbook 3e, Thoracic Trauma.)*

215. **The answer is A.** Severe cases of flail chest, where the chest wall instability interferes with ventilation, should be managed with positive-pressure ventilation. Cricothyrotomy should only be considered in cases where an airway cannot be maintained by other means. Manual stabilization may not be effective in severe cases. Needle decompression should be used if there is a suspicion of tension pneumothorax. *(Brady, Paramedic Care 2e, Principles and Practice, Volume 4—Thoracic Trauma. Mosby, Paramedic Textbook 3e, Thoracic Trauma.)*

216. **The answer is B.** Eye opening to verbal stimulation receives 3 points for eye response. Disoriented speech receives 4 points for verbal response. Localizing pain receives 5 points for motor response. The total number of points is 12. *(Brady, Paramedic Care 2e, Principles and Practice, Volume 4—Head, Facial, and Neck Trauma. Mosby, Paramedic Textbook 3e, Head and Facial Trauma.)*

217. The answer is A. Posttraumatic cardiac contusion presents with chest pain similar to that of a myocardial infarction. Some complications of cardiac contusion are dysrhythmia and heart failure. Pulmonary contusion presents as dyspnea and lung congestion. Aortic rupture will cause profound shock or sudden death. Muffled heart sounds, distended neck veins, and narrowed pulse pressure are seen with pericardial tamponade. (*Brady, Paramedic Care 2e, Principles and Practice, Volume 4—Thoracic Trauma. Mosby, Paramedic Textbook 3e, Thoracic Trauma.*)

218. The answer is A. On-scene time should be minimized to a *maximum* of 10 minutes or less. Most trauma patients require rapid surgical intervention. Unnecessarily, long-scene times can be detrimental to patient outcome. (*Brady, Paramedic Care 2e, Principles and Practice, Volume 4—Trauma and Trauma Systems. Mosby, Paramedic Textbook 3e, Trauma Systems/Mechanism of Injury.*)

219. The answer is A. Using the formula for kinetic energy, $E = mv^2$, velocity (v) is the most significant factor. Doubling the mass (m) will double the amount of energy, but doubling the velocity will increase the amount of energy four times. (*Brady, Paramedic Care 2e, Principles and Practice, Volume 4— Trauma and Trauma Systems. Mosby, Paramedic Textbook 3e, Trauma Systems/ Mechanism of Injury.*)

220. The answer is C. Internal bleeding in the abdomen will cause irritation to the peritoneum. The patient will experience abdominal distention, tenderness, and guarding to palpation. Eventually the abdominal muscles will become rigid. Injury to the superficial abdominal wall may cause some tenderness, but not guarding or rigidity. Anxiety and shock do not normally cause abdominal pain. (*Brady, Paramedic Care 2e, Principles and Practice, Volume 4—Thoracic Trauma. Mosby, Paramedic Textbook 3e, Thoracic Trauma.*)

221. The answer is C. Dyspnea, hoarseness, and facial burns are signs of airway injury. This may lead to airway obstruction due to edema. Many patients who are trapped in confiend spaces suffer from airway burns. The Paramedic should maintain a high index of suspicion when treating a burn patient and agressivly look for signs of airway compromise. Endotracheal intubation is the appropriate immediate treatment. IV fluid replacement will not help this airway problem. Burn patients should not receive anything by mouth. Sedation with diazepam should only be used if necessary to accomplish intubation. (*Brady, Paramedic Care 2e, Principles and Practice, Volume 4—Burns. Mosby, Paramedic Textbook 3e, Burns.*)

222. The answer is A. As electricity enters the body, its natural tendency will be to exit at a ground point. There are often wounds where the electricity enters and exits the body. The burn injury will often extend deeply into the tissues of the body far from the wounds. There is a danger of cardiac dysrhythmia and respiratory paralysis as a result of electrical injury. (*Brady, Paramedic Care 2e, Principles and Practice, Volume 4—Burns. Mosby, Paramedic Textbook 3e, Burns.*)

223. The answer is C. As a high-velocity bullet moves through the tissues of the body, it builds up a shock wave and pushes tissues ahead of it. The elastic skin on the other side of the body stretches outward until it tears in an irregularly shaped wound as the bullet bursts outward. (*Brady, Paramedic Care 2e, Principles and Practice, Volume 4—Trauma and Trauma Systems. Mosby, Paramedic Textbook 3e, Trauma Systems/Mechanism of Injury.*)

224. The answer is B. Direct pressure is highly effective in the control of most external bleeding. Pressure should be applied to the wound with a dressing until all bleeding stops. Once bleeding is controlled, the dressings should be held in place with a pressure dressing. Elevating the effective limb may help. A tourniquet should be reserved as a last resort if pressure and elevation fail. (*Brady, Paramedic Care 2e, Principles and Practice, Volume 4—Hemorrhage and Shock. Mosby, Paramedic Textbook 3e, Hemorrhage and Shock.*)

225. The answer is D. Bleeding, swelling, and displaced structures are all airway threats after severe facial injury. Patients should be carefully monitored for airway patency. Shock is not common from isolated facial injuries. While they are serious problems, pain and disfigurement are not life threatening. (*Brady, Paramedic Care 2e, Principles and Practice, Volume 4—Head, Facial, and Neck Trauma. Mosby, Paramedic Textbook 3e, Head and Facial Trauma.*)

226. **The answer is D.** Bleeding control is the most important treatment for patients with signs of shock. This may be accomplished by direct pressure for external bleeding or rapid transport to the operating room for internal bleeding. IV fluid replacement should be started and MAST trousers considered for profound shock. (*Brady, Paramedic Care 2e, Principles and Practice, Volume 4—Thoracic Trauma. Mosby, Paramedic Textbook 3e, Thoracic Trauma.*)

227. **The answer is A.** Speed, deceleration rate, and direction of impact are all contributing factors in mechanism of injury. Much of this information may be gathered by examining the vehicles involved in the crash. The amount of debris, other injuries, and skid marks do not give as much information about the energy absorbed by the victims. (*Brady, Paramedic Care 2e, Principles and Practice, Volume 4—Thoracic Trauma. Mosby, Paramedic Textbook 3e, Thoracic Trauma.*)

228. **The answer is B.** Many critical trauma patients require immediate surgical management. In order to move the patient as rapidly as possible to the operating room, time spent on the scene should be minimized. Scene times of 10 minutes or less are optimal. (*Brady, Paramedic Care 2e, Principles and Practice, Volume 4—Trauma and Trauma Systems. Mosby, Paramedic Textbook 3e, Trauma Systems/ Mechanism of Injury.*)

229. **The answer is A.** The decision to move immediately or attempt on-scene care is critical. The most common preventable causes of mortality in trauma patients are asphyxia and hemorrhage. All on-scene care should be aimed at securing an airway, maintaining an airway, and controlling bleeding. (*Brady, Paramedic Care 2e, Principles and Practice, Volume 4—Trauma and Trauma Systems. Mosby, Paramedic Textbook 3e, Trauma Systems/ Mechanism of Injury.*)

230. **The answer is D.** The release of energy is what causes injury in trauma. Using the formula

$E = mv^2$, a 2000-lb car moving at 30 mph will have 900,000 units of energy. If we double the speed to 60 mph, the energy will rise to 3,600,000 units. (*Brady, Paramedic Care 2e, Principles and Practice, Volume 4—Trauma and Trauma Systems. Mosby, Paramedic Textbook 3e, Trauma Systems/Mechanism of Injury.*)

231. **The answer is B.** Internal organs will strike each other, and other internal structures in cases of blunt force trauma. This motion can cause severe damage to these organs. The solid organs that have more mass are particularly vulnerable to injury as a result of this motion. (*Brady, Paramedic Care 2e, Principles and Practice, Volume 4— Thoracic Trauma. Mosby, Paramedic Textbook 3e, Thoracic Trauma.*)

232. **The answer is B.** In rear-impact collisions, the head will hyperextend backward over the rear seat, causing neck muscle and cervical spine injury. This is especially true if the headrests are not properly adjusted. (*Brady, Paramedic Care 2e, Principles and Practice, Volume 4—Trauma and Trauma Systems. Mosby, Paramedic Textbook 3e, Trauma Systems/Mechanism of Injury.*)

233. **The answer is A.** Hollow-point and soft-tipped bullets are designed to spread out on impact, increasing the frontal profile of the bullet. This causes the wound channel to be larger and more energy to be transferred to the victim. (*Brady, Paramedic Care 2e, Principles and Practice, Volume 4— Trauma and Trauma Systems. Mosby, Paramedic Textbook 3e, Trauma Systems/Mechanism of Injury.*)

234. **The answer is A.** A victim of close range gunfire will be sprayed with gas and gunpowder. This will cause burns and "tattooing" around the wound. This is seen regardless of the type of weapon or ammunition. (*Brady, Paramedic Care 2e, Principles and Practice, Volume 4—Trauma and Trauma Systems. Mosby, Paramedic Textbook 3e, Trauma Systems/Mechanism of Injury.*)

235. **The answer is A.** If a patient has cerebrospinal fluid leaking from the ears, no intervention should be made to prevent it. Packing of the ears or nose may cause a buildup of intracranial pressure. The appropriate treatment would be

a loose dressing and rapid transport. *(Brady, Paramedic Care 2e, Principles and Practice, Volume 4— Head, Facial, and Neck Trauma. Mosby, Paramedic Textbook 3e, Head and Facial Trauma.)*

236. The answer is C. Contrecoup describes an injury that occurs when the brain strikes the inside of the skull opposite to the original impact site. An epidural hematoma is a collection of blood between the skull and dura mater. A subdural hematoma is a collection of blood between the dura mater and the brain. A concussion is a transient loss of consciousness due to a blow to the head. *(Brady, Paramedic Care 2e, Principles and Practice, Volume 4—Head, Facial, and Neck Trauma. Mosby, Paramedic Textbook 3e, Head and Facial Trauma.)*

237. The answer is A. A hyphema is a collection of blood that may be seen in front of a patient's pupil and iris due to a direct trauma to the eye. *(Brady, Paramedic Care 2e, Principles and Practice, Volume 4—Head, Facial, and Neck Trauma. Mosby, Paramedic Textbook 3e, Head and Facial Trauma.)*

238. The answer is D. Until the patient is completely secured to a longboard, the Paramedic should maintain manual stabilization. Proper stabilization should reduce pain and must be maintained. *(Brady, Paramedic Care 2e, Principles and Practice, Volume 4—Spinal Trauma. Mosby, Paramedic Textbook 3e, Spinal Trauma.)*

239. The answer is A. Multiple and prolonged intubation attempts may cause laryngospam and gagging. This can result in dysrhythmias and increased intracranial pressure. Adequate preoxygenation and sedation as necessary will help to facilitate uncomplicated airway intervention. *(Brady, Paramedic Care 2e, Principles and Practice, Volume 4—Head, Facial, and Neck Trauma. Mosby, Paramedic Textbook 3e, Head and Facial Trauma.)*

240. The answer is B. Mild hyperventilation will lower $PaCO_2$, causing cerebral vasoconstriction, thereby decreasing cerebral blood flow. This may be useful in preventing increased intracranial pressure. However, hyperventilation should be reserved for those patients showing signs of increased intracranial pressure. Reducing cerebral blood flow may be harmful for patients in the early stages of head injury. *(Brady, Paramedic Care 2e, Principles and Practice, Volume 4—Head, Facial, and Neck Trauma. Mosby, Paramedic Textbook 3e, Head and Facial Trauma.)*

241. The answer is A. Arterial bleeding from the neck should be controlled with direct pressure. Care must be taken so as not to create an airway obstruction. Tourniquets and tight bandages would cause an airway obstruction and are inappropriate in the management of neck wounds. Venous bleeding from the neck should be managed with an occlusive dressing to prevent air embolism. *(Brady, Paramedic Care 2e, Principles and Practice, Volume 4—Head, Facial, and Neck Trauma. Mosby, Paramedic Textbook 3e, Head and Facial Trauma.)*

242. The answer is A. Some head injuries affect the body's temperature-regulating mechanism. This can result in hypothermia or hyperthermia. Spinal injuries that may accompany serious head injuries may also cause hypothermia due to vasodilation from decreased sympathetic tone. *(Brady, Paramedic Care 2e, Principles and Practice, Volume 4—Head, Facial, and Neck Trauma. Mosby, Paramedic Textbook 3e, Head and Facial Trauma.)*

243. The answer is A. A protective cup should be secured over an object impaled in the eye to prevent movement and further injury. Tight dressings should be avoided because they may force the object deeper or collapse the globe. Impaled objects in the eye should never be removed. A loose dressing may not prevent movement of the object. *(Brady, Paramedic Care 2e, Principles and Practice, Volume 4—Head, Facial, and Neck Trauma. Mosby, Paramedic Textbook 3e, Head and Facial Trauma.)*

244. The answer is C. Under normal circumstances, the pressure between the visceral and parietal pleura is lower than atmospheric pressure. This causes the lungs to expand and fill the space completely. In certain types of illness or injury, air or fluid may collect in the pleural space. The diaphragm lies beneath the lungs. *(Brady, Paramedic Care 2e, Principles and Practice, Volume 4— Thoracic Trauma. Mosby, Paramedic Textbook 3e, Thoracic Trauma.)*

245. The answer is A. Kidney injury is generally accompanied by flank pain and trace or visible blood in the urine. Right upper quadrant pain is a sign of injury to the liver. Pain in the left upper quadrant referred to the left shoulder is a sign of injury to the spleen. Injury to the heart will cause pain in the anterior part of the chest. *(Brady, Paramedic Care 2e, Principles and Practice, Volume 4—Abdominal Trauma. Mosby, Paramedic Textbook 3e, Abdominal Trauma.)*

246. The answer is D. During respiration, the diaphragm rises and falls, exposing the thoracic and abdominal organs to injury from a penetration at the level of the lower rib margin. A wound may also extend through the diaphragm and cause injuries to the thoracic and abdominal organs simultaneously. It is unlikely that a stab wound to the anterior surface of the body would cause injury to the spine. *(Brady, Paramedic Care 2e, Principles and Practice, Volume 4—Abdominal Trauma. Mosby, Paramedic Textbook 3e, Abdominal Trauma.)*

247. The answer is D. The decreased expansion of the lungs that results from rib fracture immobilization will impair the exchange of air and may lead to the collapse of alveoli. This will make the patient more susceptible to respiratory infections, such as pneumonia. *(Brady, Paramedic Care 2e, Principles and Practice, Volume 4—Thoracic Trauma. Mosby, Paramedic Textbook 3e, Thoracic Trauma.)*

248. The answer is A. Paradoxical respiration will be seen as a result of flail chest. Flail segments will move opposite of the rib cage during the ventilation process. *(Brady, Paramedic Care 2e, Principles and Practice, Volume 4—Thoracic Trauma. Mosby, Paramedic Textbook 3e, Thoracic Trauma.)*

249. The answer is C. Frothy blood bubbling from a chest wound is a sign of a "sucking" chest wound. There is a direct opening for air to pass into the chest. This is an open pneumothorax. Paradoxical movement of a section of the chest wall is seen with flail chest. Diminished breath sounds at the bases of the lung fields and signs of shock are seen with hemothorax. A patient with a tension pneumothorax will have diminished breath sounds and tracheal deviation. *(Brady,*

Paramedic Care 2e, Principles and Practice, Volume 4—Thoracic Trauma. Mosby, Paramedic Textbook 3e, Thoracic Trauma.)

250. The answer is A. Tension pneumothorax will generally present with severe dyspnea and shock. The Paramedic can auscultate for diminished breath sounds and observe tracheal deviation. *(Brady, Paramedic Care 2e, Principles and Practice, Volume 4—Thoracic Trauma. Mosby, Paramedic Textbook 3e, Thoracic Trauma.)*

251. The answer is B. If blood collects in the pericardial sac surrounding the heart, it may compress the heart and prevent it from filling normally. This condition is known as pericardial tamponade. A myocardial infarction is the death of heart muscle due to a lack of oxygen. A cardiomyopathy is a nonspecific disease of heart muscle. Congestive heart failure results from a weakened heart muscle. *(Brady, Paramedic Care 2e, Principles and Practice, Volume 4—Thoracic Trauma. Mosby, Paramedic Textbook 3e, Thoracic Trauma.)*

252. The answer is A. Jugular vein distention, a narrowed pulse pressure, and a rapid thready pulse are signs of pericardial tamponade. Muffled heart sound is another sign that is commonly seen with pericardial tamponade. Tracheal deviation is seen with tension pnuemothorax because the lungs are displaced toward the uninjured side. *(Brady, Paramedic Care 2e, Principles and Practice, Volume 4—Thoracic Trauma. Mosby, Paramedic Textbook 3e, Thoracic Trauma.)*

253. The answer is B. The priority in treatment of a trauma patient is to protect the cervical spine from injury. If the Paramedic is *absolutely* sure that there is no spinal injury, a patient with a chest injury is best transported lying on the injured side. In this case, gravity will help to prevent the displacement of the heart and great vessels if a tension pneumothorax should develop. This will be a very rare transport position as it is extremely difficult to rule out cervical spine injury in the field. *(Brady, Paramedic Care 2e, Principles and Practice, Volume 4—Thoracic Trauma. Mosby, Paramedic Textbook 3e, Thoracic Trauma.)*

254. The answer is A. The landmark for pleural decompression is the midclavicular line, second intercostal space. This space is located above the third rib. The needle should always be inserted over the top of the rib, as blood vessels run at the bottom of each rib. The second intercostal space is appropriate, as there are few structures which can be damaged by a needle insertion in that area. *(Brady, Paramedic Care 2e, Principles and Practice, Volume 4—Thoracic Trauma. Mosby, Paramedic Textbook 3e, Thoracic Trauma.)*

255. The answer is C. This patient is developing a tension pneumothorax from trapped air. Unsealing the dressing will allow the air to be released. Leaving an open side to occlusive dressings may allow air to escape and prevent this problem. Intubation and hyperventilation will introduce large amounts of air into the chest and are likely to make this problem worse. Transporting a patient on the injured side may relieve some of the organ displacement that results from a tension pneumothorax. High-concentration oxygen would be helpful, but it is more important to relieve the tension pneumothorax. *(Brady, Paramedic Care 2e, Principles and Practice, Volume 4—Thoracic Trauma. Mosby, Paramedic Textbook 3e, Thoracic Trauma.)*

256. The answer is D. Blunt force trauma to the anterior chest may cause a contusion to the cardiac muscle. The injured myocardium is prone to dysrhythmias and complications similar to a myocardial infarction. Patients with suspected myocardial contusion should have continuous ECG monitoring. Dysrhythmias should be managed with the same medications as a myocardial infarction. *(Brady, Paramedic Care 2e, Principles and Practice, Volume 4—Thoracic Trauma. Mosby, Paramedic Textbook 3e, Thoracic Trauma.)*

257. The answer is B. The Paramedic should stabilize impaled objects as they are found using bulky dressings. An occlusive dressing should be placed around the bulky dressing to ensure that an open chest wound is sealed. The patient shoud be monitored for diminished breath sounds on a regular basis. *(Brady, Paramedic Care 2e, Principles and Practice, Volume 4—Thoracic Trauma. Mosby, Paramedic Textbook 3e, Thoracic Trauma.)*

258. The answer is D. "Eviscerated" organs must be protected by moist sterile dressings. Large bulky dressings soaked in saline solution will keep the organs moist. A plastic occlusive dressing should be placed over the dressing to retain moisture. Dry dressings can pull moisture from the exposed organs and result in additional injury. *(Brady, Paramedic Care 2e, Principles and Practice, Volume 4—Abdominal Trauma. Mosby, Paramedic Textbook 3e, Abdominal Trauma.)*

259. The answer is A. If a joint is moved beyond its normal range of motion, an injury to ligaments and other connective tissues that surround the joint may occur. This is known as a sprain. A strain is an injury that occurs to a muscle that has been overstressed. A dislocation occurs when the bones of joint are forced out of their normal position. A contusion is a soft-tissue injury that results from blunt force trauma. *(Brady, Paramedic Care 2e, Principles and Practice, Volume 4—Musculoskeletal Trauma. Mosby, Paramedic Textbook 3e, Musculoskeletal Trauma.)*

260. The answer is D. Dislocations should be immobilized to prevent further injury. In order to properly immobilize a joint, it is necessary to include the bone above and the bone below the joint in the immobilizaton. *(Brady, Paramedic Care 2e, Principles and Practice, Volume 4—Musculoskeletal Trauma. Mosby, Paramedic Textbook 3e, Musculoskeletal Trauma.)*

261. The answer is C. Femoral fractures can result in large amounts of blood loss. As many large blood vessels follow the femur and corresponding joints, the threat of blood loss is high. The muscular area can also hide large amounts of blood loss from the unsuspecting eye of the Paramedic. *(Brady, Paramedic Care 2e, Principles and Practice, Volume 4—Musculoskeletal Trauma. Mosby, Paramedic Textbook 3e, Musculoskeletal Trauma.)*

262. The answer is D. A pelvic fracture may involve injury to major blood vessels, and instability of the pelvis creates a large area for blood to collect. Injury to the bladder is often seen with pelvic fracture, but this is not life threatening. Severe deformities and paralysis are not common with a fractured pelvis. *(Brady, Paramedic*

Care 2e, Principles and Practice, Volume 4—Musculoskeletal Trauma. Mosby, Paramedic Textbook 3e, Musculoskeletal Trauma.)

263. **The answer is C.** The Paramedic should check pulses before and after application of a splint. If the pulse is lost after splint application, it is most likely due to a tightly applied splint. Before complete removal of the splint, the Paramedic should loosen the splint and reassess the distal pulse. *(Brady, Paramedic Care 2e, Principles and Practice, Volume 4—Musculoskeletal Trauma. Mosby, Paramedic Textbook 3e, Musculoskeletal Trauma.)*

264. **The answer is D.** If resistance is met while attempting to realign a fracture, no further attempt should be made to straighten the limb. Applying more force or further manipulation is likely to cause further injury. *(Brady, Paramedic Care 2e, Principles and Practice, Volume 4—Musculoskeletal Trauma. Mosby, Paramedic Textbook 3e, Musculoskeletal Trauma.)*

265. **The answer is B.** Dislocated joints should be splinted in the position in which they are found. An exception to this is when there is circulatory or neurologic compromise. In this case, one attempt at gentle manipulation of the limb should be made in an effort to restore circulation and neurologic function. *(Brady, Paramedic Care 2e, Principles and Practice, Volume 4—Musculoskeletal Trauma. Mosby, Paramedic Textbook 3e, Musculoskeletal Trauma.)*

266. **The answer is A.** Traction splints are the most effective means of stabilizing and immobilizing a long bone fracture. This type of splint will align bone ends and reduce muscle spasm from the injury. This can also reduce bleeding and the chance of soft-tissue injury secondary to protruding bone ends from an open fracture. It can also reduce the chance of bone ends breaking the skin and creating an open fracture. *(Brady, Paramedic Care 2e, Principles and Practice, Volume 4—Musculoskeletal Trauma. Mosby, Paramedic Textbook 3e, Musculoskeletal Trauma.)*

267. **The answer is B.** Pillow splints are a good and acceptable form of splinting for ankle injuries. The pillow should be wrapped around the ankle and secured with cravats or a bandage. A pillow will not provide adequate rigidity to splint long bones, such as the femur and humerus. *(Brady, Paramedic Care 2e, Principles and Practice, Volume 4—Musculoskeletal Trauma. Mosby, Paramedic Textbook 3e, Musculoskeletal Trauma.)*

268. **The answer is B.** When an injury to blood vessels causes a collection of blood beneath the skin, this is known as a hematoma. A contusion is an injury to soft tissue caused by blunt force trauma. A laceration is a jagged open wound caused by a tearing force applied to the skin. An abrasion is an open wound caused by friction applied to the skin. *(Brady, Paramedic Care 2e, Principles and Practice, Volume 4—Soft Tissue Trauma. Mosby, Paramedic Textbook 3e, Soft Tissue Trauma.)*

269. **The answer is C.** Puncture wounds create an injury site that does not have exposure to air to promote healing. Anerobic bacteria that are injected into the wound secondary to a puncture can thrive and cause infection. *(Brady, Paramedic Care 2e, Principles and Practice, Volume 4—Soft Tissue Trauma. Mosby, Paramedic Textbook 3e, Soft Tissue Trauma.)*

270. **The answer is C.** An avulsion is a wound where soft tissue has been torn away. An avulsion may be complete when the tissue is completely separated from the body or partial when it remains connected by a flap. A contusion is a soft-tissue injury from blunt force trauma. An abrasion is an open wound caused by friction. An amputation occurs when a portion of the body containing a bone has been torn away. *(Brady, Paramedic Care 2e, Principles and Practice, Volume 4—Soft Tissue Trauma. Mosby, Paramedic Textbook 3e, Soft Tissue Trauma.)*

271. **The answer is C.** Lacerations are jagged wounds that are caused by rough edges that tear at the skin. An incision is a wound with smooth edges created by a sharp object. An abrasion is an open wound caused by friction against the skin. A puncture is created when a pointed object protrudes deep under the skin. *(Brady, Paramedic Care 2e, Principles and Practice, Volume 4—Soft Tissue Trauma. Mosby, Paramedic Textbook 3e, Soft Tissue Trauma.)*

272. **The answer is D.** Carbon monoxide is a common product of incomplete combustion. The carbon monoxide levels in an enclosed space with a fire will rise rapidly. Most fatalities in fires result from carbon monoxide poisoning. Cyanide poisoning may result from the burning of certain plastics. Thermal burns and systemic heat stroke will not occur unless the victim is exposed for a longer period of time. *(Brady, Paramedic Care 2e, Principles and Practice, Volume 4—Burns. Mosby, Paramedic Textbook 3e, Burns.)*

273. **The answer is A.** Third-degree burns extend through the full thickness of the dermis. As a result, the nerve endings that would normally perceive pain are destroyed. First-degree burns and some second-degree burns do not involve blisters. Third-degree burns may appear brown, red, black, or white, depending on the source of the burn. The surface of a third-degree burn appears dry. *(Brady, Paramedic Care 2e, Principles and Practice, Volume 4—Burns. Mosby, Paramedic Textbook 3e, Burns.)*

274. **The answer is D.** Burns around the nose and mouth, and singed nasal hair are indicative of airway and respiratory burns. Patients who present with these indicators of respiratory burns should be throughly assessed for sign and symptoms of airway damage, as well as damage to the lower airways and respiratory system. *(Brady, Paramedic Care 2e, Principles and Practice, Volume 4—Burns. Mosby, Paramedic Textbook 3e, Burns.)*

275. **The answer is D.** Pressure on the brachial artery, located in the medial upper arm, may help to control bleeding from the area of the wrist. The femoral pressure point in the groin may be used for bleeding in the upper leg. The temporal pressure point on the skull may be used for bleeding from the scalp. The popliteal pressure point behind the knee may be used to help control bleeding in the lower leg. *(Brady, Paramedic Care 2e, Principles and Practice, Volume 4—Hemorrhage and Shock. Mosby, Paramedic Textbook 3e, Hemorrhage and Shock.)*

276. **The answer is A.** Ringer's lactate is an electrolyte solution and is indicated in the treatment of burn injuries to initiate fluid and electrolyte replacement, which is common with burn injury. Other IV fluids that are used in the field, such as normal saline, can be used for fluid replacement, but contain no electrolytes. *(Brady, Paramedic Care 2e, Principles and Practice, Volume 4—Burns. Mosby, Paramedic Textbook 3e, Burns.)*

277. **The answer is D.** The Paramedic should irrigate the area of a chemical burn with copious amounts of water for at least 20 minutes. With the exception of dry chemicals, which should be brushed away, all chemical burns and exposures need thorough irrigation. *(Brady, Paramedic Care 2e, Principles and Practice, Volume 4—Burns. Mosby, Paramedic Textbook 3e, Burns.)*

278. **The answer is C.** Phenol (carbolic acid) is a caustic substance that is not soluble in water. Irrigation with water will not be effective. Phenol is soluble in alcohol. Irrigation with alcohol will help to remove phenol from the skin. *(Brady, Paramedic Care 2e, Principles and Practice, Volume 4—Burns. Mosby, Paramedic Textbook 3e, Burns.)*

279. **The answer is D.** Dry caustic chemicals should be managed by brushing as much of the chemical away as possible prior to irrigating with water. Some dry chemicals are activated by water, and irrigating first may cause more damage. Neutralizing agents, such as baking soda, may cause a chemical reaction that will release heat and gases. Alcohol should only be used to irrigate contamination with phenol. *(Brady, Paramedic Care 2e, Principles and Practice, Volume 4—Burns. Mosby, Paramedic Textbook 3e, Burns.)*

280. **The answer is A.** Some spinal injuries will result in damage to the sympathetic nerve network or brachial plexus in the spinal cord (C5-T1). Disruption of this network will affect the sympathetic nervous system and prevent the heart rate from increasing. This will result in some spine-injured patients to present with normal or slow pulses. A spider crack in the windshield and contusion on the patient's forehead are signs of axial loading that may lead to spinal injury. Numbness and tingling of the

extremities are signs that there may be injury to the spinal cord. *(Brady, Paramedic Care 2e, Principles and Practice, Volume 4—Head, Facial, and Neck Trauma. Mosby, Paramedic Textbook 3e, Head and Facial Trauma.)*

281. The answer is A. A patient with a lumbar spine injury is not likely to deteriorate or require immediate surgery. Spinal injury patients benefit from careful, deliberate transportation. Patients with signs of shock may have internal bleeding that will benefit from immediate surgery. An unstable pelvic fracture may cause severe internal bleeding. A deteriorating mental status may indicate a severe injury to the central nervous system. *(Brady, Paramedic Care 2e, Principles and Practice, Volume 4—Spinal Trauma. Mosby, Paramedic Textbook 3e, Spinal Trauma.)*

282. The answer is B. Even though an amputation may appear to be a life threatening and difficult injury to manage, the Paramedic can usually control the bleeding with direct pressure and pressure dressings. A tourniquet may cause more of the limb to be lost and should only be considered as a last resort. *(Brady, Paramedic Care 2e, Principles and Practice, Volume 4—Musculoskeletal Trauma. Mosby, Paramedic Textbook 3e, Musculoskeletal Trauma.)*

283. The answer is A. A spinal injury may affect the nerves that suppress an erection. In these cases, a patient would have a persistent erection, known as priapism. *(Brady, Paramedic Care 2e, Principles and Practice, Volume 4—Spinal Trauma. Mosby, Paramedic Textbook 3e, Spinal Trauma.)*

284. The answer is C. You should fill any voids with a noncompressible padding, such as folding sheets, in order to better stabilize the patient. The patient will not be any more likely to conform to the short board. You should never attempt to force a patient down to the board. By doing this, you would be likely to create more injuries. *(Brady, Paramedic Care 2e, Principles and Practice, Volume 4—Spinal Trauma. Mosby, Paramedic Textbook 3e, Spinal Trauma.)*

285. The answer is C. Commercially produced head immobilization devices are indicated for good immobilization. Sandbags do not secure to a longboard effectively and will roll as the board is moved. This can result in additional damage to the spine. *(Brady, Paramedic Care 2e, Principles and Practice, Volume 4—Spinal Trauma. Mosby, Paramedic Textbook 3e, Spinal Trauma.)*

286. The answer is B. The modified jaw thrust is the most appropriate way to manage the airway of a trauma patient. This should be the primary airway maneuver that the Paramedic attempts. After securing the patient to a spine board, more advanced methods of airway management can be used, such as endotracheal intubation. *(Brady, Paramedic Care 2e, Principles and Practice, Volume 4—Head, Facial, and Neck Trauma. Mosby, Paramedic Textbook 3e, Head and Facial Trauma.)*

287. The answer is A. The Paramedic should assess and document all movement and sensation on a patient prior to beginning the extrication process. Patients complaining of numbness and tingling may require additional protection prior to extrication. *(Brady, Paramedic Care 2e, Principles and Practice, Volume 4—Head, Facial, and Neck Trauma. Mosby, Paramedic Textbook 3e, Head and Facial Trauma.)*

288. The answer is B. Abdominal tenderness and guarding can be indicative of internal bleeding. Frontal collisions are likely to cause trauma to the solid organs of the abdomen with internal bleeding. The chest examination did not reveal any signs of pulmonary compromise. Tension pneumothorax and pericardial tamponade cause distended neck veins. *(Brady, Paramedic Care 2e, Principles and Practice, Volume 4—Abdominal Trauma. Mosby, Paramedic Textbook 3e, Abdominal Trauma.)*

289. The answer is A. Pain in the right thigh with shortening and external rotation of the limb are classic signs of femur fracture. Femur fractures are best managed with a traction splint that will move the bone ends back into alignment. A pillow splint would not provide enough support for a fractured femur. A sling and swathe is used for an upper arm. If a traction splint is not available, the fractured leg may be secured to the uninjured leg. *(Brady, Paramedic Care 2e, Principles and Practice, Volume 4—Musculoskeletal Trauma. Mosby, Paramedic Textbook 3e, Musculoskeletal Trauma.)*

290. The answer is B. Blows to the face generally damage the frontal bones, which are exposed and unprotected. This will result in facial fracture. *(Brady, Paramedic Care 2e, Principles and Practice, Volume 4—Head, Facial, and Neck Trauma. Mosby, Paramedic Textbook 3e, Head and Facial Trauma.)*

291. The answer is C. The patient has signs of upper airway obstruction. A fracture of the cartilages making up the larynx will cause airway obstruction due to swelling and displacement of structures. A zygoma fracture would be seen as a deformity to the face. An aortic disruption would cause sudden and severe shock. A simple pneumothorax would cause shortness of breath and diminished breath sounds. *(Brady, Paramedic Care 2e, Principles and Practice, Volume 4—Head, Facial, and Neck Trauma. Mosby, Paramedic Textbook 3e, Head and Facial Trauma.)*

292. The answer is C. The maxilla is located in the lower third of the face and the upper jaw. The ethmoid is located in the skull, between the eyes. The mandible is the lower jaw. The zygoma is the upper and outer cheek. *(Brady, Paramedic Care 2e, Principles and Practice, Volume 4—Head, Facial, and Neck Trauma. Mosby, Paramedic Textbook 3e, Head and Facial Trauma.)*

293. The answer is D. The patient with rising intracranial pressure will present with a decrease in mental status, hypertension, and bradycardia. As the pressure increases, the patient can develop abnormal breathing patterns such as central neurogenic hyperventilation. This is the result of the body trying to lower the intercranial pressue by reducing carbon dioxide levels which will constrict arteries. If a head injury patient appears with hypotension and tachycardia, it is usually the result of bleeding somewhere else in the body. *(Brady, Paramedic Care 2e, Principles and Practice, Volume 4—Head, Facial, and Neck Trauma. Mosby, Paramedic Textbook 3e, Head and Facial Trauma.)*

294. The answer is A. Bilateral periorbital ecchymosis (two black eyes) are sometimes referred to as raccoon's eyes. This is a sign of basal skull fracture. Battle's sign is an ecchymosis behind the ear and is also a sign of basal skull fracture. Cullen's sign is ecchymosis around the navel, associated with abdominal bleeding. McBurney's sign is abdominal pain and tenderness in the right lower quadrant. *(Brady, Paramedic Care 2e, Principles and Practice, Volume 4—Head, Facial, and Neck Trauma. Mosby, Paramedic Textbook 3e, Head and Facial Trauma.)*

295. The answer is D. A score of 15 on the Glasgow coma scale is normal. A score of 3 would indicate complete unresponsiveness. Scores below 8 are recognized to represent coma. *(Brady, Paramedic Care 2e, Principles and Practice, Volume 4—Head, Facial, and Neck Trauma. Mosby, Paramedic Textbook 3e, Head and Facial Trauma.)*

296. The answer is B. The Paramedic should immobilize an injured hand in the position of function, this can be accomplished by placing roller gauze in the patient's hand while applying the splint. *(Brady, Paramedic Care 2e, Principles and Practice, Volume 4—Musculoskeletal Trauma. Mosby, Paramedic Textbook 3e, Musculoskeletal Trauma.)*

297. The answer is D. Axial loading occurs when a patient hits a windshield, or dives head first into a pool. The top of the head comes in contact with the hard surface and the shock of the impact is generated down the spine resulting in spinal injury. The Paramedic should maintain a high index of suspicion when assessing the patient and the scene for clues to the injury type. *(Brady, Paramedic Care 2e, Principles and Practice, Volume 4—Trauma and Trauma Systems. Mosby, Paramedic Textbook 3e, Trauma Systems/Mechanism of Injury.)*

298. The answer is D. Fractures of the temporal and parietal skull may cause a disruption of the middle cerebral artery. This will cause arterial bleeding between the skull and the dura mater. An intraventricular hemorrhage is a bleed that occurs deep within the brain. A subdural hematoma is a collection of venous blood between the dura mater and the brain. A subarachnoid hemorrhage is bleeding at the base of the brain that most commonly occurs as a result of the spontaneous rupture of an aneurysm at the base of the brain. *(Brady, Paramedic Care 2e, Principles and Practice, Volume 4—Head, Facial, and*

Neck Trauma. Mosby, Paramedic Textbook 3e, Head and Facial Trauma.)

299. The answer is A. Cool, moist, pale, ashen, and cyanotic skin are common signs of hypovolemic shock. Flushing is usually not a sign of hypovolemia. *(Brady, Paramedic Care 2e, Principles and Practice, Volume 4—Hemorrhage and Shock. Mosby, Paramedic Textbook 3e, Hemorrhage and Shock.)*

300. The answer is A. In cases of near-term pregnancy, the gravid uterus will press on the inferior vena cava while the patient lies supine. This may reduce the venous return to the heart and aggravate hypovolemia caused by trauma. Whenever possible, trauma patients, who are pregnant near term should be transported in the left lateral recumbent position. In addition to improving the venous return, this position allows for better circulation to the fetus. *(Brady, Paramedic Care 2e, Principles and Practice, Volume 4—Obstetrics. Mosby, Paramedic Textbook 3e, Obstetrics.)*

301. The answer is D. The appropriate treatment for the trauma patient includes establishing two large bore IV lines to initiate fluid replacement. The Paramedic should be careful not to delay transport to initiate fluid replacement. Trauma patients are in need of surgical intervention and should be transported as soon as possible. *(Brady, Paramedic Care 2e, Principles and Practice, Volume 4—Hemorrhage and Shock. Mosby, Paramedic Textbook 3e, Hemorrhage and Shock.)*

302. The answer is C. The solution set that would provide the most rapid fluid flows would be the set that could deliver 10 gtts/mL. Many trauma systems use this, as well as the 15 gtts/mL sets. Sets that deliver 60 gtts/mL are generally used for treatment of medical conditions, and a burette is used in the delivery of precise amounts of fluids, usually in pediatrics. *(Brady, Paramedic Care 2e, Principles and Practice, Volume 4—Hemorrhage and Shock. Mosby, Paramedic Textbook 3e, Hemorrhage and Shock.)*

303. The answer is A. History of trauma to the abdomen, guarding, and cool clammy skin are all signs indicative of hypovolemic shock. The patient's blood pressure and pulse rate should

alert the Paramedic to a state of compensated shock, and a red flag should motivate the Paramedic to initiate rapid transport. *(Brady, Paramedic Care 2e, Principles and Practice, Volume 4—Abdominal Trauma. Mosby, Paramedic Textbook 3e, Abdominal Trauma.)*

304. The answer is B. The history of the event would indicate that this patient was a victim of blunt force trauma. In cases of blunt force trauma such as this, the impact of the baseball bat would produce a temporary cavity that would displace the abdominal organs, resulting in damage. As the impact is released, the organs would return to normal position. Initial outward appearances may not indicate injury. The presentation of the patient, as well as the history of the event will provide enough information, combined with the clinical presentation to warrant appropriate rapid transport. *(Brady, Paramedic Care 2e, Principles and Practice, Volume 4—Trauma and Trauma Systems. Mosby, Paramedic Textbook 3e, Trauma Systems/Mechanism of Injury.)*

305. The answer is A. This patient is a trauma patient who has been diagnosed with blunt force trauma to the abdomen with compensated shock. The appropriate treatment for this patient would include spinal immobilization, oxygen administration, and fluid replacement therapy with high-volume IV solutions. Endotracheal intubation, while always an option in trauma care, is not indicated in this patient. This patient is awake and alert and does not need ventilatory support. *(Brady, Paramedic Care 2e, Principles and Practice, Volume 4—Abdominal Trauma. Mosby, Paramedic Textbook 3e, Abdominal Trauma.)*

306. The answer is B. Based on the location of the gunshot wound alone, this patient is clearly a patient that needs rapid transport to a trauma center. The mechanism of injury is such that the pathway of this bullet is located in the cardiac silhouette or the outline of the heart as it is located in the chest. The gunshot does not seem to be causing a life threat at this time, but minor indicators such as a mildly diminished left chest, should alert the Paramedic to the dangers of delayed transport. *(Brady, Paramedic*

Care 2e, Principles and Practice, Volume 4—Trauma and Trauma Systems. Mosby, Paramedic Textbook 3e, Trauma Systems/Mechanism of Injury.)

307.   **The answer is A.** The findings in the scenario would indicate a developing pneumothorax on the patient's left side. The history, mechanism of injury, and physical findings would serve to confirm this diagnosis. Rapid transport and continued aggressive assessment for deterioration of the patient's condition is indicated. A trauma stand by for surgical intervention is also indicated. *(Brady, Paramedic Care 2e, Principles and Practice, Volume 4—Thoracic Trauma. Mosby, Paramedic Textbook 3e, Thoracic Trauma.)*

308.   **The answer is D.** In treating this patient based on kinematics alone, spinal immobilization would be indicated as would oxygen administration. IV therapy would also be indicated, although the patient's blood pressure seems unaffected by the injury. A thought would be to insert two large bore IVs and maintain at a KVO rate. The patient's condition does not call for a needle decompression, as this patient is not presenting as a tension pneumothorax. In a tension pneumothorax, the patient would have decreased blood pressure, absent breath sounds on the affected side, and tracheal deviation to the unaffected side. This is clearly not the case here, so needle decompression is not

indicated. *(Brady, Paramedic Care 2e, Principles and Practice, Volume 4—Thoracic Trauma. Mosby, Paramedic Textbook 3e, Thoracic Trauma.)*

309.   **The answer is C.** As you continue to assess your patient, you find she has developed a pericardial tamponade. This is caused by blood or fluid accumulation in the pericardial sac around the heart. This is highly probable based on the history of this event. Signs and symptoms are consistent with pressure on the heart. Decreased blood pressure, increased pulse, and muffled heart sounds are clinical indicators of this condition. *(Brady, Paramedic Care 2e, Principles and Practice, Volume 4—Thoracic Trauma. Mosby, Paramedic Textbook 3e, Thoracic Trauma.)*

310.   **The answer is D.** Unfortunately, there is no field treatment for reversing pericardial tamponade. The in-hospital treatment is pericardiocentesis, which is a lifesaving intervention. This is not a skill that can easily be performed in an ambulance and not without a good amount of training. The Paramedic should continue rapid transport, oxygenation, and could elect to begin cardiac monitoring for ECG changes. A call ahead to the receiving hospital would assist in the patient's rapid care. *(Brady, Paramedic Care 2e, Principles and Practice, Volume 4—Thoracic Trauma. Mosby, Paramedic Textbook 3e, Thoracic Trauma.)*

Patient Presentations: Medical

The following topics are covered in Section V:

- Medical Pulmonary
- Medical Cardiology
- Medical Neurology
- Endocrinology
- Allergies and Anaphylaxis
- Gastroenterology
- Renal and Urology
- Toxicology
- Hematology
- Environmental Emergencies
- Infectious and Communicable Diseases
- Behavioral and Psychiatric Disorders
- Gynecology
- Obstetrics

Questions

MEDICAL PULMONARY

DIRECTIONS: Each item below contains four suggested responses. Select the one best response to each item.

311. All of the following are signs of impending respiratory failure *except*:

    (A) altered mental status
    (B) nasal flaring and tracheal tugging
    (C) respiratory rate of 18 breaths per minute
    (D) accessory muscle use

312. You begin to evaluate a 30-year-old female with a long history of asthma who is complaining of increasing difficulty breathing for the past 5 days. The patient notes that she caught a cold about a week ago and has been getting worse ever since. She is having difficulty speaking in complete sentences but does note that she has taken her inhaler medications several times a day, without improvement. Which of the following findings on auscultation is the most critical in this asthmatic?

    (A) silent chest, decreasing oxygen saturation, tachycardia
    (B) severe inspiratory and expiratory wheezing
    (C) mild expiratory wheezing and productive cough
    (D) diffuse bilateral rhonchi and fever

313. You are dispatched to a 24-year-old male who is complaining of difficulty breathing. He has a 10-year history of asthma and has been under the care of a primary care physician. He has been taking a number of medications daily yet notes that the onset of the hay fever season has played a significant part in worsening his breathing. As you assess the patient, you note that his vital signs are a blood pressure of 122/70, a pulse rate of 108 beats per minute, and a respiratory rate of 36 breaths per minute. With medical control approval, all of the following are acute emergency care treatments available to you for treating this asthmatic patient *except*:

(A) nasal oxygen at 2–3 L/min
(B) IV corticosteroids and IV magnesium sulfate
(C) subcutaneous (SC) epinephrine
(D) beta-agonist oral and ipratropium bromide inhalers

314. The pathology of the airways in asthma includes all of the following *except*:

(A) edema
(B) secretions
(C) inflammation
(D) foreign body

315. All of the following are medications that physicians commonly prescribe for the outpatient treatment of asthmatic patients *except*:

(A) the oral beta-agonist inhalers labeled albuterol, metaproterenol, isoetharine, terbutaline, and ipratropium bromide oral inhaler
(B) oral prednisone, oral prednisolone, and various steroid inhalers
(C) oral ibuprofen
(D) oral aminophylline preparations

316. Which of the following items is specifically helpful for evaluating the asthmatic patient at home, in the prehospital setting by the Paramedic, in the emergency department (ED), and in the hospital units?

(A) peak expiratory flow rate (PEFR) meter
(B) arterial blood gas determinations
(C) pulse oximetry
(D) capnography

317. All of the following are conditions associated with chronic obstructive pulmonary disease (COPD) *except*:

(A) emphysema
(B) renal failure
(C) chronic bronchitis
(D) cor pulmonale

318. You are dispatched to a 70-year-old male, at home, with difficulty breathing. As you arrive at the patient's home, the patient's wife tells you that the patient has chronic lung disease due to smoking three packs of cigarettes a day for 40 years. The patient had a cold 2 weeks ago and has been coughing up increasing amount of yellow phlegm and has been feeling more short of breath. The patient has had difficulty even walking to the bathroom and around the apartment. Last month he was able to walk a couple of blocks outside, with feeling a little short of breath but nothing as dramatic as this. On examining the patient, you note that he is sitting upright in a chair and leaning forward, appearing frightened, with his arms holding the bottom of the chair. The patient's lips and nail beds are cyanotic, and he is breathing at 40 breaths per minute, with a blood pressure of 146/82, a regular pulse rate of 96 beats per minute, supraclavicular retractions, and pursed-lip breathing. All of the following are parts of the acute management of this patient *except*:

(A) 100% oxygen by nonrebreather mask
(B) SC epinephrine 0.3 mg
(C) IV line to keep a vein open
(D) albuterol or metaproterenol oral inhaler

319. You are called to a school auditorium on the night of the school dance. As you arrive, a teacher tells you that one of the students is having difficulty breathing. The patient is a 16-year-old male who states that he had the acute onset of right-sided chest pain, which is aggravated with coughing and taking a deep breath. On your chest examination, you note that there are no breath sounds in the right chest. The patient's trachea is in the midline and his respiratory rate is 16 breaths per minute. Which of the following is the correct patient care option?

    (A) needle decompression of the chest
    (B) beta-agonist oral inhaler
    (C) 100% oxygen by nonrebreather mask
    (D) endotracheal intubation

320. Match the following pulmonary conditions with the symptoms and/or signs.

    (A) emphysema
    (B) pulmonary edema
    (C) spontaneous pneumothorax
    (D) pulmonary thromboembolism
    (E) lung cancer

    1. bilateral distant breath sounds
    2. heavy smoker, hemoptysis, weight loss
    3. deep vein thrombosis, acute pleuritic chest pain, bed rest
    4. unilateral absent breath sounds
    5. pink frothy sputum, diaphoresis

321. An acute pulmonary disease that produces noncardiogenic pulmonary edema and severe hypoxemia, and is brought about by increased capillary permeability in the pulmonary arterial system is known as

    (A) asthma
    (B) pneumonia
    (C) acute pulmonary embolism
    (D) adult respiratory distress syndrome

322. You are dispatched to the home of a 22-year-old male who is complaining of severe dizziness and is breathing rapidly. The patient's brother tells you that the patient just had a very intense argument with his girlfriend. He is dizzy, is unable to catch his breath, and feels numbness and tingling in his hands and feet. On examination, you note that the patient's lungs are bilaterally clear, without rales, rhonchi, or wheezes, and with very good aeration. The correct emergent treatment of this patient includes which of the following?

    (A) administering IV epinephrine
    (B) administering oxygen and trying to reassure the patient
    (C) administering a beta-agonist oral inhaler
    (D) allowing the patient to simply rebreathe in a paper bag

323. All of the following are medications that are prescribed by physicians for patients suffering from difficulty breathing due to various diseases except:

    (A) aminophylline tablets, oral beta-agonist inhalers, oral steroid inhalers, and oral steroid tablets
    (B) digoxin tablets; nitroglycerin tablets, spray, paste, or patches; furosemide tablets; Isordil tablets; Captopril tablets; Enalapril tablets; and aspirin
    (C) Pepcid, Zantac, Axid, Prilosec, Prevacid, and Tagamet
    (D) erythromycin, Cipro, amoxicillin

324. While driving to pick up lunch, you are dispatched to a "difficulty breathing" patient. As you enter the apartment, you are brought into the bedroom of a 24-year-old female who tells you of feeling like she had flu 2 days ago. She had fever, chills, headache, tiredness, and weakness. She tried to drink a lot of fluids and take rest in bed but for the past day she feels much worse with high fever and chills every couple of hours. She also notes that her deep cough is causing her to bring up a lot of yellow-green phlegm. This morning, when she became very short of breath, she became very worried and called for the ambulance. As you begin to examine the patient you note that the patient is hot to touch, with a respiratory rate of 32 breaths per minute, a pulse rate of 112 beats per minute, blood pressure of 112/68, and a pulse oximetric measurement of 96%. On auscultation of the lungs, you note dry crisp rales in the right lower lung base. All of the following are part of the prehospital emergency medical treatment of this patient *except*:

(A) IV fluids, ECG monitoring, and pulse oximetry
(B) opening and maintaining the airway
(C) 100% oxygen with a nonrebreather mask
(D) IV antibiotics

325. All of the following are types of pneumonia *except*:

(A) AIDS
(B) aspiration
(C) mycoplasma
(D) tuberculosis

326. As you approach the home of a "difficulty breathing" patient, a woman approaches you to mention that her husband is 58 years old and has a serious drinking problem. Just two nights ago he was drinking heavily and returned home and fell asleep on the couch. The next morning the woman stated that she found him lying on his back on the couch with vomitus around his mouth and gurgling with each breath. The next day she noted that he developed a high fever, appeared very weak, and was having difficulty breathing. She then decided to call the ambulance. All of the following are predisposing factors for developing aspiration pneumonia *except*:

(A) head injury
(B) alcohol and/or drug use
(C) smoking
(D) anesthesia

327. All of the following are correct statements concerning capnography *except*:

(A) Capnography is the measurement of carbon dioxide concentrations in exhaled air.
(B) Sudden decrease in end-tidal CO_2 may be due to esophageal intubation.
(C) Increased end-tidal CO_2 levels are found in patients in cardiac arrest, shock, and pulmonary emboli.
(D) A memory aid for $ETCO_2$ is yellow (tube is correctly placed); tan (think about it); and purple (problem; the tube is not in the trachea)

MEDICAL CARDIOLOGY

DIRECTIONS: Each item below contains four suggested responses. Select the one best response to each item.

328. You are at Thanksgiving dinner with your entire family and all of a sudden a discussion about cardiovascular disease begins and the opinions begin to fly. After all opinions are expressed, everyone turns to you for the correct answer. All of the following are correct *except*:

    (A) Uncle Billy says that almost 500,000 people die every year of coronary heart disease.
    (B) Your mother follows up by stating half of those, who die each year, will die of sudden death before they reach the hospital.
    (C) Your brother says that there are several reversible risk factors for coronary artery disease including family history of premature coronary artery disease, smoking, hypercholesterolemia, and hypertension.
    (D) Your sister chimes in that while a family history of premature coronary disease is a risk factor for coronary artery disease, it is not reversible.

329. All of the following are known to be major risk factors predisposing to coronary artery disease *except*:

    (A) older age
    (B) marijuana use
    (C) hypertension
    (D) diabetes

330. All of the following are correct statements about the anatomy of the heart *except*:

    (A) The heart is located above the diaphragm, posterior to, slightly to the left of the sternum, and anterior to the spine.
    (B) The heart is surrounded by the pericardium and is made up of the outer-layer epicardium, the middle-layer myocardium, and the inner-layer endocardium.
    (C) The four chambers of the heart consist of the right atria, right ventricle, left atria, and left ventricle.
    (D) The four valves in the heart are the tricuspid (between the right atrium and right ventricle) and the pulmonary (between the right ventricle and the pulmonary artery) on the right side of the heart and the mitral (between the left atrium and the left ventricle) and ventricular (between the left ventricle and the aorta) on the left side of the heart.

331. Which of the following is the correct sequence of flow of blood leaving the left ventricle?

    (A) arteries, aorta, arterioles, vena cavae, venules, veins, right atrium
    (B) right atrium, aorta, arteries, arterioles, venules, vena cavae, veins
    (C) arteries, aorta, arterioles, veins, vena cavae, right atrium, venules
    (D) aorta, arteries, arterioles, venules, veins, vena cavae, right atrium

332. Cardiac output is defined as the amount of blood that is pumped out of either ventricle in liters per minute. Which of the following is the correct formula for determining a patient's cardiac output?

    (A) cardiac output (millimeters per minute) = stroke volume (milliliters) × heart rate (beats per minute)
    (B) $E = mc^2$
    (C) cardiac output = venous return × respiratory rate
    (D) cardiac output = blood pressure × heart rate

333. In the normal heart, certain areas of the myocardium receive coronary artery blood supply from particular branches of the coronary arteries. All of the following are correct examples *except*:

    (A) The left anterior descending (LAD) artery supplies blood to the anterior wall of the left ventricle.
    (B) The left circumflex artery supplies blood to the lateral and posterior walls of the left ventricle.
    (C) The right coronary artery supplies blood to the inferior wall of the left ventricle.
    (D) The left main coronary artery supplies blood to right ventricle.

334. Under normal circumstances, which of the following is the correct course of an electrical impulse in the conduction system of the heart?

    (A) atrioventricular (AV) node, sinoatrial (SA) node, bundle of His, internodal atrial pathways, right and left bundle branches, Purkinje fibers, ventricular muscle
    (B) bundle of His, SA node, ventricular muscle, AV node, internodal atrial pathways, right and left bundle branches, Purkinje fibers
    (C) SA node, internodal atrial pathways, AV node, bundle of His, right and left bundle branches, Purkinje fibers, ventricular muscle
    (D) bundle of His, internodal atrial pathways, AV node, SA node, right and left bundle branches, Purkinje fibers, ventricular muscle

335. All of the following are correct statements concerning some of the pacemaker sites in the heart *except*:

    (A) The AV node is normally the dominant pacemaker in the heart.
    (B) If the SA node is damaged or not functioning properly and the AV node becomes the pacemaker for the heart, the heart rate is usually 40–60 beats per minute.
    (C) If the ventricle or Purkinje fibers become the pacemaker for the heart, the heart rate is usually 20–40 beats per minute.
    (D) The SA node paces the heart normally at 60–100 beats per minute.

336. All of the following are stages of cardiac muscle excitation *except*:

    (A) polarization
    (B) depolarization
    (C) repolarization
    (D) reincarnation

337. Electrolytes play a key role in the myocardial action potential. All of the following are such electrolytes, listed with their functions, *except*:

    (A) magnesium (Mg) and chloride (Cl) play a role in the depolarization of the myocardial cells
    (B) sodium (Na): plays a major role in depolarization of the myocardium
    (C) calcium (Ca): plays a role in myocardial depolarization and contraction
    (D) potassium (K): plays a major role in repolarization of the myocardium

338. Starling's law of the heart is defined as

   (A) The pressure in the left ventricle of the heart is proportional to the pressure in the right ventricle.
   (B) The more the myocardium is stretched, up to a limit, the greater its force of contraction.
   (C) The resting pressure in the aorta is inversely related to the pulmonary artery pressure.
   (D) The myocardial resting pressure is directly proportional to the inverse of the systolic blood pressure.

339. All of the following are parts of the autonomic nervous system *except*:

   (A) parasympathetic system
   (B) the sympathetic nervous system
   (C) the gastrointestinal system
   (D) the vagus nerve

340. All of the following are effects of the various parts of the autonomic nervous system on the heart *except*:

   (A) The sympathetic beta-receptor stimulation produces bronchodilation.
   (B) The parasympathetic system slows the heart rate and increases myocardial contractility.
   (C) The sympathetic nervous system increases the heart rate and myocardial contractility.
   (D) The sympathetic alpha-receptor stimulation produces peripheral vasoconstriction.

341. Match the following pathophysiologies with the list of cardiac diseases.

   (A) cardiac arrest _____
   (B) acute pulmonary edema _____
   (C) deep vein thrombosis _____
   (D) acute pulmonary emboli _____
   (E) acute myocardial infarction (MI) _____
   (F) right ventricular heart failure _____
   (G) anginal syndrome _____
   (H) dissecting aortic aneurysm _____

   1. thrombus or clot in an atherosclerotic coronary artery
   2. common causes are left ventricular congestive heart failure, COPD, and pulmonary emboli
   3. most severe form of left ventricular congestive heart failure
   4. believed to be caused by a lethal dysrhythmia
   5. small tear in the inner wall of the aorta
   6. caused by air, fat, amniotic fluid, or blood clots
   7. commonly caused by atherosclerosis and spasm
   8. blood clot in the veins

342. All of the following are signs of cardiovascular disease that can be detected by careful inspection of the patient *except*:

   (A) cool and clammy skin
   (B) barrel chest
   (C) jugular vein distention
   (D) peripheral edema

343. All of the following are physical findings that are detectable by auscultation *except*:

   (A) carotid bruits
   (B) bowel sounds
   (C) abdominal organ enlargement
   (D) heart sounds

344. All of the following are signs of cardiovascular disease that can be detected by palpation *except*:

(A) enlarged lymph nodes
(B) rapid pulse rate
(C) asymmetrical pulses
(D) thready pulse

345. All of the following are correct statements about heart sounds *except*:

(A) The first heart sound, known as S_1, is produced by the closure of the left and right atrial septa.
(B) The second heart sound, known as S_2, is produced by the closure of the aortic and pulmonic valves.
(C) The third heart sound, known as S_3, is associated with congestive heart failure and is a pathologic heart sound.
(D) The fourth heart sound, known as S_4, is produced by left and right atrial contraction.

346. In obtaining a focused history for the patient with a cardiovascular emergency, all of the following are important *except*:

(A) chief complaint
(B) present illness: history of the present event
(C) significant past medical history
(D) history of childhood immunizations

347. The purpose of ECG monitoring is to determine the

(A) myocardial contractile capability
(B) oxygen saturation in the blood
(C) presence and type of electrical activity of the heart
(D) presence of left ventricular hypertrophy

348. Match the following ECG waves with the correct cardiac electrical event.

(A) ST segment _____
(B) RR interval _____
(C) P wave _____
(D) QRS _____
(E) PR interval _____
(F) T wave _____

1. ventricular repolarization
2. time between two ventricular depolarizations
3. atrial depolarization
4. atrial depolarization plus AV junction delay
5. time between ventricular depolarization and repolarization
6. ventricular depolarization

349. Match the following electrical events with the correct time intervals.

(A) ventricular tachycardia _____
(B) atrial fibrillation _____
(C) idioventricular rhythm _____
(D) sinus bradycardia _____
(E) sinus tachycardia _____
(F) supraventricular tachycardia _____
(G) normal sinus rhythm _____
(H) QRS interval _____
(I) junctional rhythm _____
(J) PR interval _____

1. 40–60 beats per minute
2. 60–100 beats per minute
3. 0.12–0.20 seconds
4. 0.08–0.12 seconds
5. 150–250 beats per minute
6. atrial rate 350–600 per minute
7. lower than 60 beats per minute
8. 100–160 beats per minute
9. 20–40 beats per minute
10. 100–250 beats per minute

350. Match the following ECG leads with the correct area of the heart that they represent.

   (A) tall R waves V$_1$ and V$_2$ _____
   (B) 2, 3, and AVF _____
   (C) V$_4$, V$_5$, and V$_6$ _____
   (D) V$_1$, V$_2$, and V$_3$ _____

   1. anteroseptal wall
   2. anterolateral wall
   3. posterior wall
   4. inferior wall

351. The following rhythm strip represents which of the following cardiac rhythms?

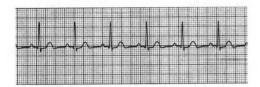

   (A) normal sinus rhythm
   (B) sinus bradycardia
   (C) sinus arrest
   (D) sinus tachycardia

352. The following rhythm strip represents which of the following cardiac rhythms?

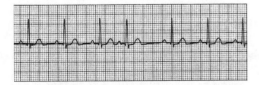

   (A) junctional premature contraction
   (B) ventricular premature contraction
   (C) atrial premature contraction
   (D) sinus bradycardia

353. The following rhythm strip represents which of the following cardiac rhythms?

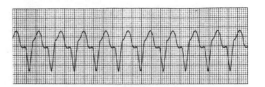

   (A) ventricular tachycardia
   (B) ventricular fibrillation
   (C) junctional rhythm
   (D) supraventricular tachycardia

354. The following rhythm strip represents which of the following cardiac rhythms?

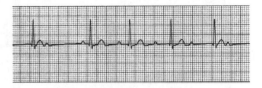

   (A) second-degree AV block, Mobitz type I
   (B) second-degree AV block, Mobitz type II
   (C) first-degree AV block
   (D) third-degree AV block

355. The following rhythm strip represents which of the following cardiac rhythms?

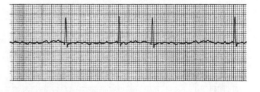

   (A) normal sinus rhythm
   (B) atrial fibrillation
   (C) atrial flutter
   (D) supraventricular tachycardia

356. The following rhythm strip represents which of the following cardiac rhythms?

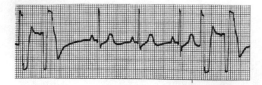

- (A) unifocal premature ventricular contraction (PVC)
- (B) multifocal PVCs
- (C) ventricular bigeminy
- (D) coupled PVCs

357. Match the following ECG rhythm strips with the correct dysrhythmia.

1. premature junctional contractions (PJCs)
2. ventricular tachycardia
3. sinus tachycardia
4. multifocal PVCs

(A) _____

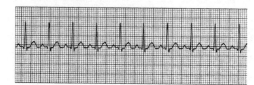

(B) _____

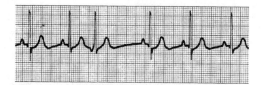

(C) _____

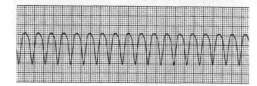

(D) _____

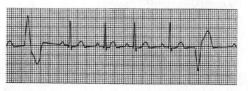

358. Match the following ECG rhythm strips with the correct dysrhythmia.

1. atrial tachycardia
2. sinus arrest
3. junctional rhythm
4. ventricular fibrillation

(A) _____

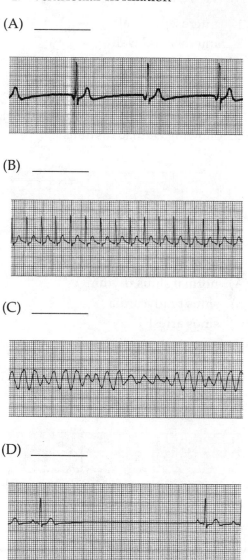

(B) _____

(C) _____

(D) _____

359. Match the following ECG rhythm strips with the correct arrhythmias.

1. second-degree AV block (Mobitz type II), 3:1 AV block
2. unifocal PVCs
3. accelerated junctional rhythm
4. second-degree AV block (Mobitz type I), Wenckebach

(A)  _____

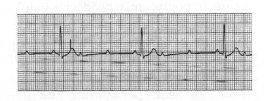

(B) _____

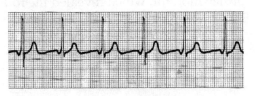

(C) _____

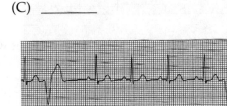

(D)  _____

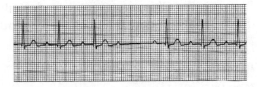

360. Match the following ECG rhythm strips with the correct arrhythmias.

1. third-degree heart block
2. ventricular bigeminy
3. pacemaker rhythm
4. atrial flutter

(A) _____

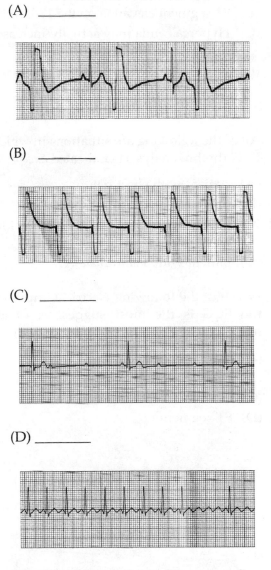

(B) _____

(C) _____

(D) _____

361. All of the following conditions may be associated with pulseless electrical activity (PEA) *except*:

(A) anginal syndrome
(B) cardiogenic shock
(C) cardiac tamponade
(D) acute pulmonary embolism

362. All of the following are correct statements concerning the possible cardiac effects of electrolyte abnormalities *except*:

(A) Hyperkalemia may cause tall, peaked T waves and produce decreased automaticity and cardiac conduction.

(B) Hypernatremia may result in ST-segment elevation on the 12-lead ECG.

(C) Hypercalcemia may actually increase cardiac contractility.

(D) Hypokalemia may produce inverted T waves on the ECG and increase myocardial irritability.

363. All of the following are situations in which an ECG rhythm analysis is indicated *except*:

(A) patient with chest pain

(B) patient in any form of shock

(C) patient with a very fast or a very slow heart rate

(D) patient with a skin rash

364. Which of the following electrical impulses on the ECG is the most suggestive of acute myocardial ischemia and/or infarction?

(A) QRS complex

(B) PR interval

(C) T wave

(D) ST segment

365. You are dispatched to an elderly patient who has passed out at home. On arrival at the patient's home, you find an 86-year-male who is lying on the floor. His neighbor was watching the television with the patient and noticed that the patient attempted to walk to the kitchen and suddenly became unconscious and fell to the floor. The patient was unresponsive for 2–3 minutes on the floor and on awakening denied any memory of the event. The patient and witness denied any signs suggestive of a seizure, hypoglycemia, headache, palpitations, focal weakness, slurred speech, or a drug ingestion. Initial vital signs revealed that the patient had a blood pressure of 110/68, respirations of 14 breaths per minute, and a pulse rate of around 70 beats per minute and irregular. While your partner performed a physical examination, you connected the patient to a cardiac monitor, which revealed the following ECG rhythm strip.

This ECG represents which of the following dysrhythmias?

(A) normal sinus rhythm

(B) sinus tachycardia

(C) sinus arrest

(D) sinus bradycardia

366. Based on the clinical presentation described in question 365, the treatment of choice should be

(A) IV atropine

(B) IV digoxin

(C) IV amiodarone

(D) IV verapamil

367. You are completing your evaluation and initial treatment of a 68-year-old female with chest pain when you notice that she has suddenly stopped breathing. As you quickly confirm that she is pulseless and unconscious, you quickly check the monitor, which reveals the following dysrhythmia.

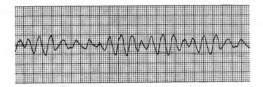

Based on the above dysrhythmia, the treatment of choice is

(A) IV lidocaine
(B) IV bretylium
(C) synchronized cardioversion
(D) immediate defibrillation

368. As you begin to defibrillate the patient with 200 joules, then 300 joules, and finally 360 joules, the patient continues to remain in ventricular fibrillation. All of the following are part of the emergent treatment of the patient who remains in ventricular defibrillation after initially unsuccessful defibrillation *except*:

(A) IV lidocaine and amiodarone
(B) endotracheal intubation
(C) IV epinephrine
(D) IV calcium

369. You are dispatched to a " sick patient." As you arrive at the patient's home, you find a 48-year-old male who admits to having substernal chest pain, shortness of breath, sweating, and nausea for the past 2 hours. On further questioning, the patient admits to smoking two packs of cigarettes per day for the past 30 years, to having been on medication for high blood pressure for the past 5 years, and that his father died of an acute heart attack at age 45. Your partner took the patient's vital signs and found the patient breathing at 26 times per minute, with a blood pressure of 148/72 and a regular pulse rate of 130 beats per minute. The patient's primary assessment is grossly normal. Your partner has hooked the patient up to a cardiac monitor and presents you with the following ECG rhythm strip.

Based on your interpretation of this ECG rhythm strip, the correct initial treatment is

(A) IV diltiazem
(B) sublingual nitroglycerin
(C) IV amiodarone
(D) IV lidocaine

370. As you begin to transport the patient, your patient begins to complain of a funny heartbeat. As you inspect the monitor, you find the patient in the following rhythm.

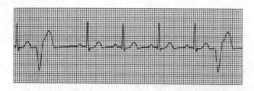

Based on your interpretation of this ECG rhythm strip, after administering oxygen, the treatment of choice is which of the following?

(A) IV lidocaine

(B) IV amiodarone

(C) IV atropine

(D) analgesics for his chest pain

371. You are dispatched to a skilled nursing facility (SNF) to evaluate and transport a 90-year-old female resident who complains of nausea and vomiting associated with dizziness and feeling a little weak. The patient's vital signs are: blood pressure 100/70, respirations 16 breaths per minute, and pulse rate 54 beats per minute. The patient's initial assessment reveals that she is awake, weak, and in no acute distress. As you begin to apply oxygen by nonrebreather face mask, you connect the patient to an ECG monitor, which reveals the following rhythm.

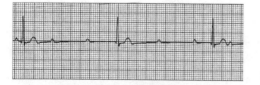

Based on this rhythm, the treatment of choice, with medical control approval, is which of the following?

(A) IV atropine

(B) IV diltiazem

(C) IV amiodarone

(D) transcutaneous pacing

372. As you arrive at the scene of a suspected drug overdose on a Friday night in the back of a schoolyard, you notice a group of nine teenagers. One of the bystanders begins to tell you that this 16-year-old male had been told today that his girlfriend was breaking up with him. He supposedly ran home and gathered up some of his father's medications and swallowed a full bottle of propranolol. As your partner has already begun to assess the patient, he notes that the patient has stopped breathing. Initially, a quick look with the monitor-defibrillator paddles reveals that the patient is in the rhythm below. Since you have confirmed that he is pulseless and apneic, you begin cardiopulmonary resuscitation (CPR), prepare to perform endotracheal intubation with 100% oxygen, connect to a cardiac monitor, and begin an IV line.

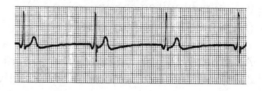

Based on this rhythm and the patient's clinical presentation, the initial treatment of choice is

(A) SQ epinephrine

(B) IV lidocaine

(C) IV atropine 1.0 mg

(D) IV epinephrine 1.0 mg

373. As you continue to treat the patient in cardiac arrest described in question 360, you are becoming frustrated because, despite your best efforts, the patient remains in the same heart rhythm, in PEA. While you have frantically searched for treatable causes of PEA, a friend of the patient has retrieved the empty vial of medications from the patient's home, Cardizem CD 240 mg tablets, dated yesterday, with 90 tablets. Now you immediately begin to package the patient for transport, because you realize that this patient's PEA may be corrected with which of the following medications, which you do not carry in your medication box and is readily available in all EDs?

    (A) IV digoxin
    (B) IV Solumedrol
    (C) IV calcium
    (D) IV Narcan

374. As you arrive at the scene of a motor vehicle accident, you find a 27-year-old female sitting in the back seat of a taxicab who is complaining of being upset but denies any focal pain, headache, whiplash, arm tingling, or numbness. An examination of the vehicle reveals minimal dents on the front bumper and the front left headlight. On initial assessment, the patient appears to show no evidence of any trauma, with vital signs as follows: blood pressure 104/68, respirations 14 breaths per minute, and pulse rate 32 beats per minute. On further questioning, the patient denies taking any medications, drug ingestion, nausea or vomiting, and so on. However, the patient does admit to running 5 miles per day and has been noted to have a slow pulse. As you connect the patient to a cardiac monitor, the patient has the following ECG strip.

    Based on this ECG and clinical presentation, which of the following is the correct course of treatment?

    (A) transcutaneous pacing
    (B) IV isoproterenol
    (C) repeat vital signs and secondary assessment
    (D) IV atropine

375. All of the following are indications for the use of transcutaneous pacing except:

    (A) ventricular fibrillation
    (B) symptomatic atrial fibrillation with a slow ventricular rate
    (C) third-degree heart block with a slow ventricular rate
    (D) symptomatic sinus bradycardia

376. You arrive at the apartment of an 82-year-old male who was found unconscious sitting in his favorite chair, for an unknown period of time. His wife had gone to the store 2 hours ago and left him reading the morning newspaper. As you immediately place the patient on the floor, you realize that he is not breathing and is pulseless. Your partner immediately connects the patient to an ECG monitor, which reveals the following rhythm.

Based on this rhythm, the correct choice of treatment is which of the following?

(A) immediate defibrillation

(B) CPR, intubate, IV access, confirm in more than 1 lead

(C) IV lidocaine

(D) IV amiodarone

377. All of the following are parts of the process of treating a patient with a transcutaneous pacemaker *except*:

(A) Explain the procedure to the patient, place the patient in an upright position, and administer oxygen, IV line, and ECG monitoring.

(B) Confirm the presence of an indication for pacing, such as symptomatic bradycardia, and medical control approval.

(C) Apply the pacing electrodes, connect them to the pacemaker cable, and set the desired pacer rate at 60–80 beats per minute.

(D) Set voltage at 0, turn the pacer on, and slowly increase the voltage until ventricular capture.

378. All of the following are ECG rhythm strip signs of pacemaker malfunction *except*:

(A) slow heart rate, less than 60–70 beats per minute, without pacemaker spike activity

(B) pacemaker spikes without QRS complex following

(C) pacemaker spikes firing on top of or after the QRS complex

(D) heart rate over 88 beats per minute without pacemaker spikes

379. All of the following are possible causes of pacemaker failure *except*:

(A) runaway pacemaker

(B) failure to capture

(C) battery failure

(D) electrolyte imbalance

380. All of the following are risk factors for coronary artery disease with the development of angina pectoris or MI *except*:

(A) cigarette smoking

(B) hypertension

(C) family history of peptic ulcer disease

(D) elevated cholesterol

381. You arrive at the scene of a 68-year-old male who was carrying garbage cans to the street when he suddenly developed substernal chest pain, sweating, difficulty breathing, and nausea, and actually was so weak that he sat down on the grass. As you begin to assess and treat this patient, you think about the pathophysiology of angina pectoris. Which of the following is the best explanation?

(A) Increased myocardial oxygen requirements due to increased exertion and insufficient myocardial oxygen supply due to coronary artery disease.

(B) All coronary arteries are in spasm, resulting in lack of oxygen to the heart.

(C) Complete blockage of all coronary arteries resulting in no coronary artery blood supply to the heart.

(D) Partial blockage of coronary arteries, resulting in increased demands of oxygen.

382. The most common ECG finding in angina pectoris is

   (A) Q waves
   (B) PR-interval prolongation
   (C) tall, peaked T waves
   (D) ST-segment depression

383. In approaching the patient with angina pectoris, which of the following is the correct description of the treatment of this patient?

   (A) Before instituting any treatment, begin to question intensely in order to determine a treatment path for either angina or an acute MI.
   (B) Assume that angina is not a myocardial infarction and treat accordingly.
   (C) With the patient's complaints being consistent with ischemic chest pain, assume that the patient may be having an acute MI and treat accordingly.
   (D) If you are unsure whether the patient is suffering from angina or an acute MI, refrain from any treatment and transport.

384. You are driving back to the ambulance garage when a woman who claims that her sister is having a heart attack frantically waves you down. As you walk up three flights of stairs, you find a 66-year-old female sitting in a chair. She is pale and breathing at 36 times per minute. As the patient informs you about her severe chest pain radiating down her left arm, your partner begins to initiate emergent treatment of the patient. This will include all of the following except:

   (A) as the first intervention, perform a 12-lead ECG
   (B) attach to an ECG monitor
   (C) administer 100% oxygen by nonrebreather face mask
   (D) administer a sublingual nitroglycerin 0.4 mg tablet

385. As you continue to provide emergent prehospital care to the patient described in question 374, you begin to think of the possible complications of an acute MI. All of the following are possible complications of an acute MI except:

   (A) lethal cardiac dysrhythmias
   (B) cardiac rupture
   (C) acute pulmonary edema
   (D) skin rash

386. All of the following are correct statements concerning an acute MI except:

   (A) 4–6% of patients have no chest pain.
   (B) They are responsible for 500,000 deaths per year in the United States.
   (C) They are the leading cause of death in the United States.
   (D) 60–70% occur outside the hospital.

387. All of the following are hemodynamic changes associated with an acute MI except:

   (A) normal blood pressure
   (B) high blood pressure
   (C) increased respiratory rate
   (D) low blood pressure

388. As you arrive at an apartment for a patient with chest pain, you find a 54-year-old male who appears diaphoretic, pale, clammy, and short of breath. On questioning, the patient admits to an acute onset of substernal chest pain, described as a "weight sitting on my chest," which has gradually worsened. The patient was lifting several heavy boxes at the time of the incident. He also admitted to smoking three packs of cigarettes a day, high blood pressure, and an elevated cholesterol level. He also noted that his father had a heart attack at 35 years of age. As you begin to assess and treat this patient with a possible acute MI, you focus on the parameters that you need to assess. All of the following are items to be assessed except:

   (A) skin turgor
   (B) repeat vital signs
   (C) ECG monitoring
   (D) repeat lung sounds

389. All of the following are evolutionary ECG changes associated with an acute MI *except*:

(A) ST-segment depression
(B) T-wave inversion
(C) ST-segment elevation
(D) P-wave inversion

390. All of the following are causes of ST-segment elevations, which are not due to an acute MI and could lead the Paramedic to make a false diagnosis of an acute MI *except*:

(A) acute pericarditis
(B) left bundle branch block (LBBB)
(C) digoxin toxicity
(D) early repolarization

391. You are in the midst of treating a patient at a school fair for a minor allergic reaction when one of the workers asks you to come and evaluate a man with chest pain. The new patient is a 54-year-old male who has been carrying heavy beer barrels into the fairgrounds for the past hour and has suddenly developed substernal chest pain about 20 minutes ago. The patient describes the pain as like "a vice around my chest" and admits that the pain radiates down both arms and is associated with palpitations, weakness, and profuse sweating. He also admits to being under a doctor's care for high blood pressure, diabetes, and poor circulation in his legs. As you begin to assess and treat this patient, you begin to think about him as a possible candidate for thrombolytic therapy. All of the following are inclusion criteria for thrombolytic therapy *except*:

(A) age under 60 years
(C) pain not relieved by nitroglycerin
(C) ST-segment elevation equal to or over 0.5 mm in two adjacent leads
(D) chest pain for longer than 20 minutes and less than 12 hours

392. You are sent to a construction site for a 10-foot fall from a scaffold. As you arrive at the patient's side, the story becomes a little more complicated. The 58-year-old male patient states that he slipped off the scaffold 20 minutes ago. He states that he is having severe pain in his right ankle and midchest. He admits to being treated for angina for 2 years and now complains about the chest pain becoming more intense, despite taking a nitroglycerin tablet about 5 minutes ago. As you begin to complete a primary assessment on this patient, you are contemplating the possibility of this patient's becoming a candidate for thrombolytic therapy. After quickly assessing the patient's chest and confirming that there is no gross evidence of chest trauma, rib fractures, pneumothorax, or chest wounds, you administer another nitroglycerin tablet without relief. A quick examination of his right ankle reveals a grossly deformed, angulated fracture, with a large pool of blood surrounding it. This patient would be excluded from being treated with thrombolytic therapy because of which of the following exclusion criteria?

(A) age
(B) terminal illness
(C) internal bleeding
(D) trauma

393. If the patient in question 392 is excluded from having thrombolytic therapy for an acute MI, the other first-line interventional option available at chest-pain centers used to attempt to reverse the acute MI would be

(A) lithotripsy
(B) percutaneous transluminal coronary angioplasty (PTCA)
(C) laparoscopy
(D) synchronized cardioversion

394. Match the following drugs with the common dose and therapeutic effect.

  (A) atropine sulfate _____
  (B) procainamide _____
  (C) morphine sulfate _____
  (D) dopamine _____
  (E) furosemide _____
  (F) adenosine _____
  (G) amiodarone _____
  (H) lidocaine _____

  1. 1–1.5 mg/kg IV; suppress ventricular dysrhythmias
  2. 6 mg IV bolus; terminate supraventricular tachycardia
  3. 0.5 mg IV bolus; parasympatholytic agent
  4. 3–5 mg slow IV push; pain relief and venodilation
  5. 20–40 mg IV push; venodilation and diuresis
  6. 20–30 mg/kg IV; ventricular dysrhythmias resistant to lidocaine
  7. 2.5–20 μg/kg/min; vasopressor
  8. 150–300 mg slow IV infusion; recurrent ventricular fibrillation or unstable ventricular tachycardia

395. Match the following cardiovascular drugs with the correct side effects.

  (A) nitrates _____
  (B) beta-blockers _____
  (C) amiodarone _____
  (D) isoproterenol _____
  (E) furosemide _____

  1. hypotension
  2. hypokalemia
  3. bradycardia
  4. increased heart rate and myocardial contractility
  5. headache and tingling under the tongue

396. All of the following are causes of left ventricular heart failure *except*:

  (A) acute MI
  (B) advanced COPD
  (C) chronic hypertension
  (D) cardiomyopathy

397. All of the following are symptoms of left ventricular heart failure *except*:

  (A) dyspnea
  (B) headache
  (C) orthopnea
  (D) paroxysmal nocturnal dyspnea

398. You are dispatched to a "difficulty breathing" patient. As you enter the patient's home, you find an 86-year-old female sitting up in bed with three pillows behind her back. The patient tells you that she has had similar episodes in the past because of a very large heart, believed to be due to high blood pressure and two previous heart attacks. As your partner begins to administer oxygen, you begin to perform an initial assessment of this patient with acute pulmonary edema. You would expect to observe all of the following physical findings *except*:

  (A) diffuse, moist rales in the lungs
  (B) neck vein distention
  (C) absent pulses
  (D) pink, frothy sputum

399. All of the following are possible causes of precipitating acute pulmonary edema *except*:

  (A) strep throat
  (B) acute MI
  (C) dysrhythmias
  (D) acute endocarditis

400. You are dispatched to a nearby nursing home because of an elderly resident complaining of acute difficulty breathing. As you arrive at the patient's bedside, you find a 92-year-old female breathing at 46 respirations per minute. The patient's nurse states that the patient has a history of congestive heart failure for the past 2 years and has been maintained on digoxin, lasix, and periodic nasal oxygen. The patient is in the nursing home because of a long-term history of dementia and has been bed bound for the past 3 months. As you begin to examine the patient, you find a blood pressure of 210/114, a pulse rate of 130 beats per minute and regular, and that the patient is afebrile, with jugular neck vein distention and bilateral moist rales throughout the entire chest. All of the following are parts of the treatment of this patient *except*:

(A) 100% oxygen by nonrebreather face mask
(B) nitroglycerin 0.4 mg tablet or spray
(C) morphine sulfate 2–mg slow IV
(D) furosemide 5 mg IV bolus

401. The main therapeutic action of morphine sulfate, which results in improvement in the pulmonary edema patient, is which of the following?

(A) alleviates anxiety
(B) slows respiratory rate
(C) lowers blood pressure
(D) decreases venous return (preload)

402. Which of the following is the best definition of *cardiac tamponade*?

(A) As blood fills the pericardial sac, the coronary arteries become occluded.
(B) As blood fills the pericardium, the heart's function is progressively compromised.
(C) As blood fills the pericardium, the blood pressure elevates dramatically.
(D) As blood fills the pericardium, the aortic and mitral valves become narrowed.

403. You are dispatched to a shooting at the scene of a robbery. As you pull up to the store, you find a 28-year-old male lying unconscious on the floor. As you begin to assess the patient, you notice that he has a bloodstained shirt. His airway is patent, and he is breathing at 22 breaths per minute, has a pulse rate of 140 beats per minute, and has a blood pressure only palpable at 50 systolic. On further examination, the patient's lung sounds are clear and symmetrical, he has distended neck veins and cyanosis, and auscultation of the heart reveals crisp heart sounds. All of the following are clinical signs of cardiac tamponade *except*:

(A) distended neck veins
(B) crisp heart sounds
(C) hypotension
(D) tachycardia

404. While hypertension is a medical condition that affects over 60 million Americans, the definition of a hypertensive emergency includes an acute elevation of blood pressure along with evidence of end-organ damage. All of the following are examples of end-organ damage, which is caused by uncontrolled hypertension, *except*:

(A) hypertensive encephalopathy
(B) acute pulmonary edema
(C) dissecting aortic aneurysm
(D) diabetes

405. You arrive at the home of a 56-year-old male whose wife states that he had initially been acting confused since lunch but now has become increasingly sleepy and difficult to arouse. She states that he does not drink alcohol and does not take any medications. He had been told that he had high blood pressure, and his physician had started him on blood pressure medications a year ago, but he did not continue to take them and has not seen his physician again. He had been complaining of a headache on and off for the past 2 weeks and was taking more aspirin and tylenol than usual. On examining the patient, you notice that he is breathing at 20 respirations per minute, with a pulse rate of 84 beats per minute, and a blood pressure of 240/130 bilaterally. The patient's entire physical assessment is grossly normal, without any signs of focal weakness. As you contemplate an approach to treatment of this patient with a hypertensive emergency, you consider administering all of the following treatment options, with medical control approval, *except*:

(A) labetalol 20 mg slowly IV push
(B) dilantin 500 mg IV push
(C) nitroglycerin 0.4 mg sublingual tablet or spray
(D) furosemide 20–40 mg IV push

406. All of the following are signs of cardiogenic shock *except*:

(A) cool, clammy skin
(B) tachycardia
(C) hypertension
(D) tachypnea

407. You arrive at the scene of a chest-pain patient and find a 68-year-old male patient lying on the floor, diaphoretic, and breathing at 40 breaths per minute. He is cool and clammy, has a pulse rate of 130 beats per minute, and appears very weak and lethargic. The patient is unable to give a history, and his blood pressure is only 40 systolic palpable bilaterally. As your partner begins to apply oxygen, connect to an ECG monitor, and initiate an IV line, the patient's wife states that he has had two previous MIs, suffers from congestive heart failure, and complained of substernal chest pain this morning for 25 minutes prior to the call to 911. As you complete your assessment of the patient, you contemplate treatment options. Which of the following would appear to be the best initial treatment of this patient?

(A) norepinephrine (Levophed) 0.5–30 µg/min
(B) labetalol 20 mg IV push slowly
(C) dopamine (Intropin), initially 2–5 µg/kg/min
(D) pneumatic antishock trousers

408. All of the following are possible past medical histories leading to cardiogenic shock *except*:

(A) acute pericarditis
(B) advanced cardiomyopathy
(C) massive anterior wall acute MI
(D) pericardial tamponade

409. All of the following are acute emergencies that may progress to cardiac arrest *except*:

(A) acute MI
(B) viral flu syndrome
(C) foreign-body airway obstruction
(D) gunshot wound

410. All of the following are the most common conditions associated with the cardiac arrest patient *except*:

(A) asystole
(B) ventricular fibrillation
(C) first-degree heart block
(D) PEA

411. You are dispatched to a hardware store for a 50-year-old unconscious patient. However, when you arrive and begin to examine the patient, you note that she is unresponsive, pulseless, and apneic. You immediately reach for which of the following piece of equipment?

    (A) oxygen mask
    (B) IV line
    (C) IV dextrose
    (D) quick-look monitor-defibrillator paddles

412. As you respond to a cardiac arrest call, you find a 68-year-old female lying in the hallway of an apartment building. The patient is unresponsive, pulseless, and apneic. As you begin to perform a quick-look with the ECG monitor paddles, you find that the patient is in a junctional tachycardia. Rechecking, you find that the patient is truly without a pulse. As you begin to perform CPR, you try to reflect on the possible correctable causes of PEA. All of the following are possible correctable causes of PEA *except*:

    (A) cardiac tamponade
    (B) tension pneumothorax
    (C) bronchitis
    (D) severe hypovolemia

413. Match each of the following medications, which are used in treating cardiac arrest patients, with the correct desired therapeutic effect.

    (A) IV lidocaine _____
    (B) IV epinephrine _____
    (C) IV amiodarone _____
    (D) IV magnesium sulfate _____
    (E) IV sodium bicarbonate _____
    (F) IV atropine _____

    1. corrects metabolic acidosis
    2. increases cerebral and coronary blood flow
    3. prevents recurrence of ventricular fibrillation
    4. corrects magnesium deficiency
    5. prevents recurrence of ventricular tachycardia
    6. may stimulate activity in asystole

414. All of the following are critical actions required for treating patients in nontraumatic cardiac arrest *except*:

    (A) establishing IV access
    (B) applying quick-look ECG monitor-defibrillator
    (C) administering IV calcium
    (D) endotracheal intubation

415. All of the following are criteria for termination of resuscitation *except*:

    (A) patient's family is upset with resuscitative actions
    (B) no restoration of spontaneous circulation
    (C) absence of recurring or refractory ventricular fibrillation or ventricular tachycardia or continued neurologic activity
    (D) standard advanced life support for 25 minutes

416. You are sent to a 74-year-old male with acute nontraumatic leg pain. As you arrive at the patient's bedside, you find the patient grimacing in pain, pointing to his left leg. The patient admits to smoking three packs of cigarettes per day for over 50 years and has a history of mild diabetes but again denies any recent trauma. On examination, you find the patient's left leg to be pale, cool, cyanotic, and pulseless, and the patient has decreased ability to move his left foot. This patient's presentation is consistent with which of the following diagnoses?

    (A) acute arterial occlusion
    (B) acute phlebitis
    (C) acute cellulitis
    (D) acute arthritis

417. Which of the following cardiac dysrhythmias would be one of the possible causes of the patient's emergent problem in question 405?

    (A) ventricular fibrillation
    (B) atrial fibrillation
    (C) junctional rhythm
    (D) junctional tachycardia

418. Which of the following is the correct definition of *aneurysm*?

(A) blockage of an artery
(B) weakening and dilation of a vessel wall
(C) congenital defect of a vein
(D) increased curvature of an artery

419. *Claudication* is defined as

(A) cramp-like pain in the calf
(B) intermittent heat and redness of a leg
(C) abdominal cramps
(D) focal headache

420. All of the following are types of aneurysms *except*:

(A) embolic
(B) congenital
(C) traumatic
(D) atherosclerotic

421. You are dispatched to a chest-pain patient. As you walk into the office, you find a 68-year-old male lying on the office floor. He states that he has substernal chest pain, which began 1 hour ago and has a ripping quality. He states that the pain was very severe at onset and remains the same but now is moving from the substernal location to the epigastric area. In taking the patient's vital signs, your partner is confused because he found the blood pressure to be 178/68 in the right arm and 120/52 in the left arm, even with repeating the readings twice. This patient's presentation is most suggestive of

(A) acute gallbladder attack
(B) acute MI
(C) acute arterial occlusion
(D) dissecting aortic aneurysm

422. While on your way for gas, a bystander, who states that her father is having severe stomach pains that spread to his back, flags you down. As you gather your equipment, you have found out that the patient is a 66-year-old male who has had acute abdominal pain for only 30 minutes, and it was not associated with vomiting, diarrhea, or fever. As you arrive at the patient's bedside, you find an acutely ill, pale patient who appears to be writhing in pain. As you begin to examine the patient, you find that the patient has a blood pressure of 50 palpable bilaterally, no bowel sounds, and a pulsating abdominal mass. This patient appears to have which of the following acute emergencies?

(A) acute appendicitis
(B) acute gastroenteritis
(C) acute urinary retention
(D) acute abdominal aortic aneurysm

423. All of the following are parts of the prehospital emergency medical care for a patient with an abdominal aortic aneurysm *except*:

(A) high-concentration oxygen
(B) ECG monitoring
(C) on-scene stabilization if the patient is hypotensive
(D) IV access

424. As you transport a 64-year-old female patient with possibly her third acute MI, her emotionally upset daughter asks you if there is anything that she may do in order to prevent heart disease for herself and her children. Before you answer, you begin to think of the risk factors for cardiovascular disease that can be modified. All of the following are modifiable risk factors *except*:

(A) family history of premature cardiovascular disease
(B) hypertension
(C) smoking
(D) hypercholesterolemia

425. Match the following areas of the heart with the correct coronary artery which is responsible for its blood supply (must use more than one answer twice):

(A) right ventricle _____

(B) anterior wall of the left ventricle _____

(C) inferior wall of the left ventricle _____

(D) lateral wall of the left ventricle _____

(E) septum of the left ventricle _____

  1. right coronary artery
  2. LAD
  3. left circumflex artery

426. You are assigned to an 88-year-old male patient in a SNF for difficulty breathing. As you come off the elevator on the third floor, a nurse approaches you and states that the patient had arrived from the local hospital after having undergone repair of a fractured left hip about 2 weeks ago. The patient had a prolonged hospital stay because of pneumonia, which developed 3 days after surgery and required bed rest, oxygen, and IV antibiotics. The patient was coming to the nursing home for short-term rehab but he still had only been out of bed in a chair. This morning the patient's nurse noticed that his left leg was red and swollen and planned to have the doctor examine the patient on afternoon rounds; however, the patient developed acute shortness of breath and acute pleuritic chest pain about 30 minutes ago and even coughed up some blood. This clinical presentation is most likely caused by which of the following?

(A) acute left-leg arterial occlusion

(B) congestive heart failure

(C) acute pulmonary embolism

(D) acute gouty arthritis

427. You are dispatched to a patient with "stomach upset and doesn't feel well." As you arrive at an office building, you are directed to a 14th floor office. You find a 48-year-old female lying on the couch who admits to epigastric stomach upset, nausea, and just not feeling well. She quickly mentions that she has high blood pressure and smokes two packs of cigarettes per day for 30 years. Reluctantly, she also mentions that her father died at age 42 of a heart attack. On examination, her vital signs were as follows: blood pressure 178/102, pulse rate 94 beats per minute and regular, afebrile, and respiratory rate 14 breaths per minute. She appears diaphoretic, pale, and anxious. Her lungs are clear bilaterally; heart is 102 beats per minute and regular without murmurs; her abdomen is soft and nontender; her extremities are symmetrical without edema. While you obtained the patient's history and examined the patient, your partner performed a 12-lead ECG and hands it to you. Based on the ECG on the following page, your initial impression is

(A) acute anterior wall MI

(B) acute anterolateral wall MI

(C) old inferior wall MI

(D) acute pulmonary embolism

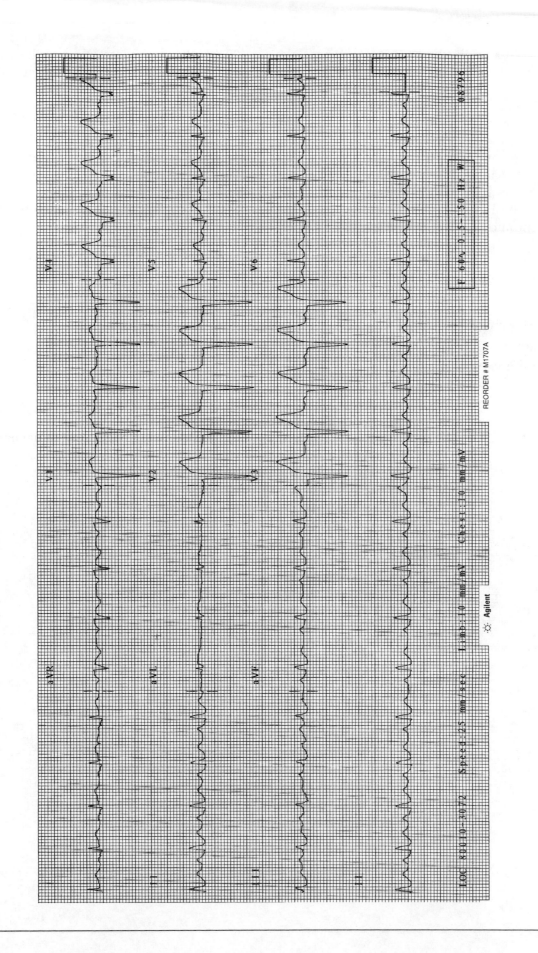

428. You arrive at the bedside of a 58-year-old female, two packs per day smoker, diabetic, who called 911 because of 2 hours of substernal chest pain. As you begin to question the patient, she admits to having the same mild chest pain with long walks and exercising in the gym for the past 2–3 months. She also admits to having shortness of breath and a little nausea. As your partner begins to start an IV, attach the ECG monitor to administer high-concentration oxygen, you take a 12-lead ECG. Based on the 12-lead ECG below, which additional part of the heart (not visible on the 12-lead ECG) may be infarcting at the same time?

(A) base of the aorta

(B) mitral valve

(C) aortic valve

(D) right ventricle

429. Match the 12-lead ECGs on the next two pages with the correct interpretation.

1. LBBB
2. acute anterior-lateral wall MI
3. RBBB (right bundle branch block)
4. acute inferior-lateral wall MI

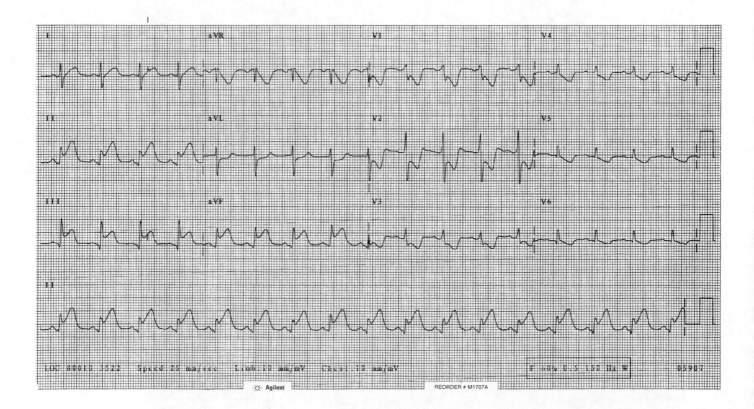

(A)

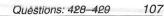

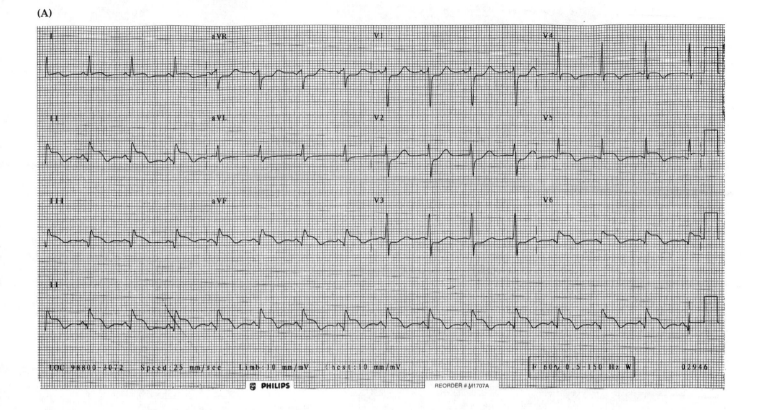

(B)

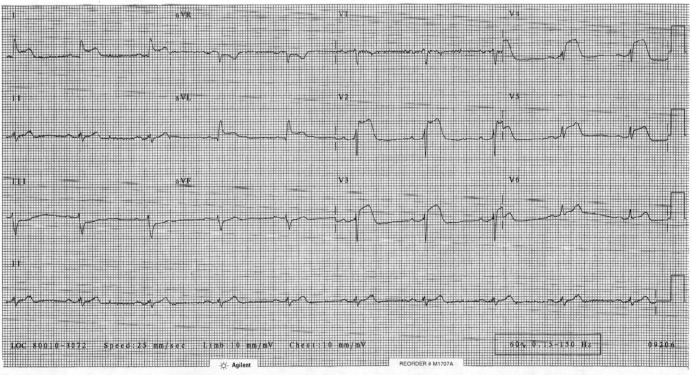

(C)

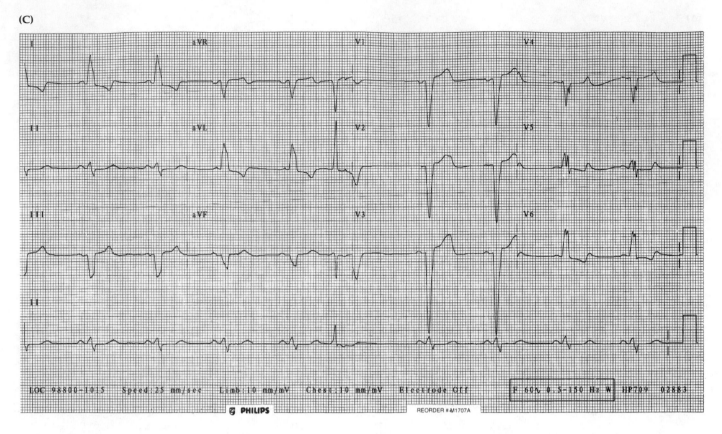

(D)

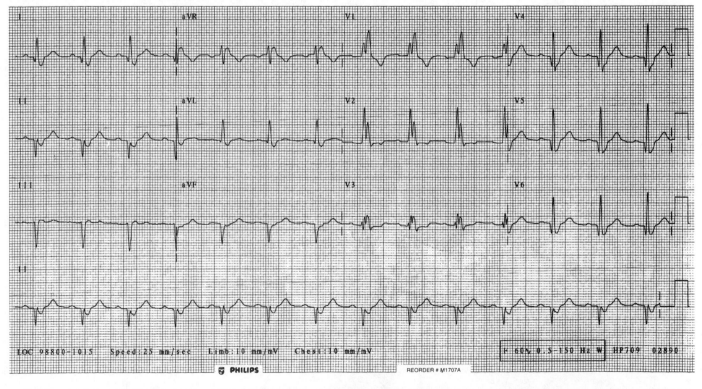

430. Match the following 12-lead ECGs with the correct interpretation.

1. pacemaker rhythm with ventricular rate 72 per minute
2. supraventricular tachycardia with ventricular rate 200 per minute
3. third-degree heart block
4. atrial flutter with variable AV block

(A)

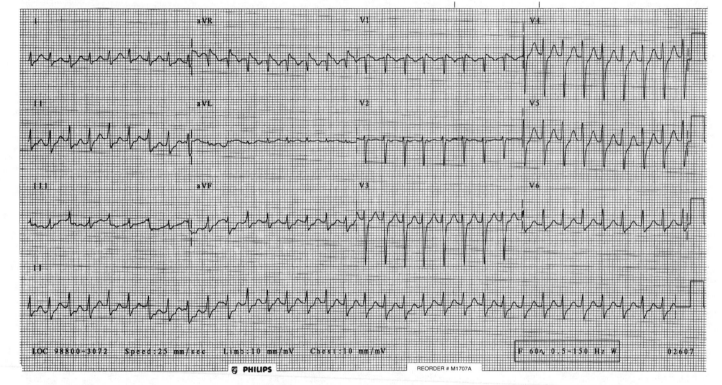

(B)

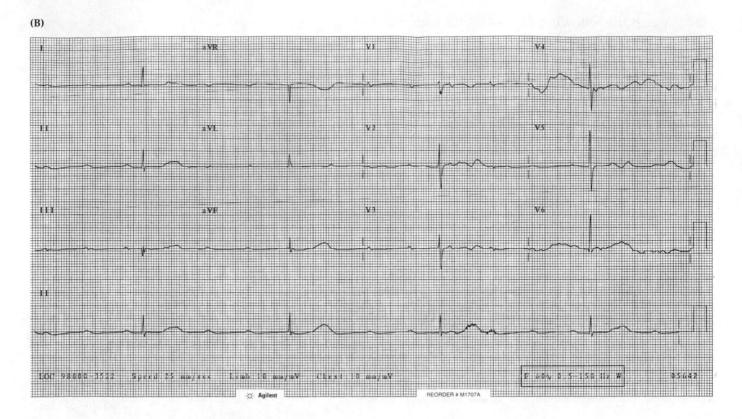

(C)

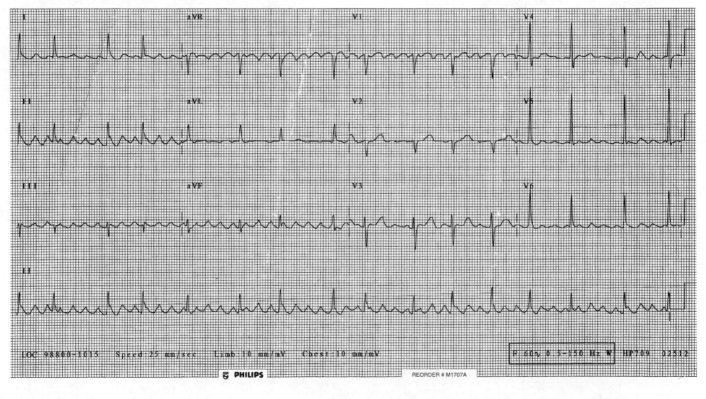

(D)

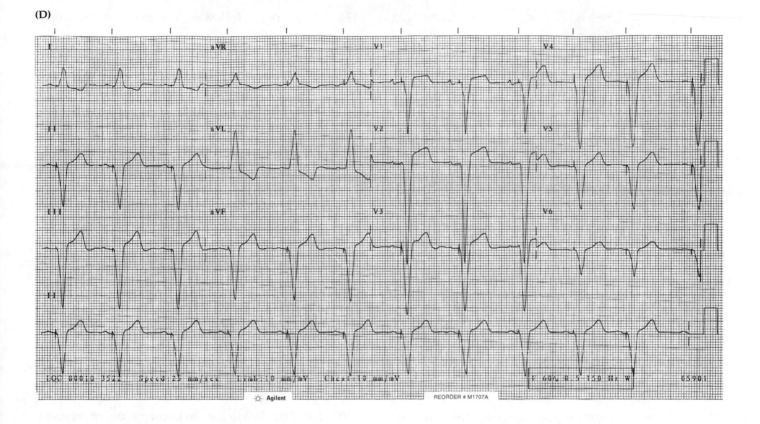

MEDICAL NEUROLOGY

DIRECTIONS: Each item below contains four suggested responses. Select the one best response to each item.

431. Neurologic emergencies are often a consequence of all of the following *except*:

  (A) intravascular protein concentration changes
  (B) intracranial pressure changes
  (C) circulatory changes
  (D) head trauma

432. The main reason an increase in intracranial volume results in a significant increase in intracranial pressure is

  (A) because the skull is a rigid, closed space
  (B) a change in the brain's oncotic pressure
  (C) the cerebral collateral blood supply
  (D) the volume of cerebrospinal fluid

433. After evaluating a patient with any type of non-traumatic neurologic emergency, the primary survey includes all of the following *except*:

  (A) drawing baseline blood work
  (B) circulation: check for a pulse
  (C) breathing: make sure depth and rate are adequate
  (D) establish and maintain an airway

434. All of the following are examples of patients with altered mental status *except*:

  (A) narcotic overdose
  (B) syncope
  (C) seizures
  (D) speaking in a foreign language

435. All of the following are possible causes of coma *except*:

  (A) head trauma
  (B) antibiotics
  (C) drug overdose
  (D) hypoglycemia

436. You are dispatched to the home of a 52-year-old male who is unresponsive. As you arrive in the patient's bedroom, the patient's wife states that he failed to awaken in the morning and she thought that he was sleeping late. However, after an hour, she decided to awaken him but was unable to do so. She states that he was known to have hypertension and that he drank socially but went to bed normally last night. The patient's wife denies all questions related to other possible causes of coma. As you begin to examine the patient, you begin by establishing an airway, initiating breathing without a problem, and noting that the patient's pulse and blood pressure are normal. All of the following are important next steps in examining the comatose patient *except*:

    (A) check the response to pain
    (B) check for nasal discharge
    (C) check for pupillary response
    (D) check for eye response.

437. You are dispatched to a warehouse for an unconscious 52-year-old male. This patient delivers supplies to this company, but no one is aware of his medical history. A search of his wallet and clothing fails to reveal any additional information. The patient's assessment reveals stable vital signs and that he is not responsive to any stimuli. After cervical spine immobilization, securing a stable airway, and confirming adequate breathing and circulation, all of the following are parts of the emergent management of this patient *except*:

    (A) Perform a finger-stick glucose test or draw a blood glucose sample, and then administer 50 mL (25 g) of 50% dextrose IV push and repeat as necessary.
    (B) If a narcotic overdose is suspected, administer 1–2 mg IV, endotracheally, intramuscularly, or SC, and repeat at 2- to 3-minute intervals.
    (C) If increased intracranial pressure is suspected, hypoventilate the patient at 10 breaths per minute
    (D) If the patient is an alcoholic, administer 100 mg of thiamine IV

438. Which of the following is the correct definition of a *seizure*?

    (A) A permanent alteration in behavior due to an electrical discharge of a neuron or group of neurons.
    (B) A temporary alteration of behavior due to an electrical discharge of a neuron or group of neurons.
    (C) A complete loss of consciousness due to an emotional upset.
    (D) A temporary alteration of behavior due to a cardiac dysrhythmia.

439. Which of the following is considered the most common cause of seizures?

    (A) brain tumor
    (B) head trauma
    (C) meningitis
    (D) epileptic patient's failure to take prescribed medications

440. All of the following are known types of seizures *except*:

    (A) absence seizures
    (B) generalized seizures
    (C) simple partial seizures
    (D) allergic seizures

441. Your ambulance is flagged down outside a bar, and a customer states that the patient appeared to have a seizure. The patient had been drinking all afternoon and had stated that he was having problems at home and at work. As a result, the patient stated that he was binge drinking and not taking his medications. The patient was noted to fall abruptly to the floor and began to have dramatic movements of all four extremities. A physical examination revealed that the patient had become incontinent of urine and was now unconscious yet had an adequate airway, was breathing adequately, and had a strong pulse with a blood pressure of 112/76. All of the following are additional priorities for the physical examination of this patient *except*:

(A) examine for any evidence of head trauma

(B) examine for any leg swelling

(C) examine for pupillary size and reaction to light

(D) examine for any signs of additional trauma secondary to the seizure activity

442. All of the following are phases of a generalized, grand mal seizure *except*:

(A) hypotonic phase

(B) aura

(C) clonic phase

(D) postictal phase

443. You are dispatched to the scene of a seizing patient. As you arrive at an office building, another employee states that this patient has had a long history of seizures. Today, he was found on the floor of his office actively seizing. The patient was noted to have tonic-clonic contractions of his arms and legs for about 10 minutes, which stopped about 2 minutes ago. As you begin to examine the patient, you note that he is unresponsive and yet his airway appears open and he does not accept an oropharyngeal airway. While placing the patient on a stretcher, he begins again to have another generalized seizure. Treatment of this seizure may include all of the following *except*:

(A) Administer IV 100 g of 50% dextrose.

(B) Administer IV 100 mg of thiamine.

(C) Continue to maintain the airway.

(D) Administer IV slowly up to 10 mg of diazepam (Valium).

444. You are dispatched to a bingo game where an 80-year-old female has passed out. As you arrive at the patient's side, a neighbor states that she had become very excited and admitted to feeling a little dizzy because she had just won the grand prize. On yelling out "bingo" and jumping up, she passed out and landed on the floor. After about a minute, she woke up. As you begin to obtain a history from the patient, she notes that she has just had a yearly physical examination and has not had any significant medical problems. She had her appendix out 40 years ago and a total knee replacement 30 years ago. She does not take any medications. She does admit to passing out several years ago at a funeral and having a similar lightheaded feeling before passing out. You next begin to examine the patient in order to determine the cause of the syncopal episode. All of the following areas of physical examination would help to determine the cause of the syncope *except*:

(A) focal weakness

(B) pulse rate

(C) blood pressure, supine and erect

(D) checking for thickening of her toe nails

445. Match the following symptoms or physical findings with the list of causes of syncope.

(A) postural increase in pulse rate of 20 beats per minute, decrease in systolic blood pressure of 20 mmHg

(B) finger-stick glucose level of 32

(C) pulse rate 180 beats per minute, blood pressure 62/46

(D) pulse rate 30 beats per minute, blood pressure 60 palpable

(E) unconsciousness, urinary incontinence, and confusion on awakening

1. Stokes-Adams syncope due to tachy- or bradydysrhythmia
2. seizure disorder
3. acute gastrointestinal bleeding
4. vasovagal syncope
5. hypoglycemia

446. As you await the end of a busy day, you are dispatched to a 92-year-old male who has just "passed out" at home. On your arrival, you find the patient lying on the floor. He apologizes for his wife's calling the ambulance because he truly feels fine now. The patient's wife interrupts by stating that he was simply walking across the room and suddenly fainted and hit the floor without any warning. His wife stated that he was unconscious for about 2 minutes but then awakened without any signs of confusion, weakness, slurred speech, or headache. As you examine the patient, you note that he has normal vital signs without orthostatic changes, and an initial survey reveals only abrasions of both knees. The patient also is alert; oriented to person, place, and time; and has grossly symmetrical neurologic findings. The appropriate prehospital management of this patient includes all of the following except:

(A) cardiac monitoring

(B) high-flow oxygen

(C) IV to keep vein open (KVO)

(D) encouraging the patient to sign to be released against medical advice

447. You are dispatched to a patient with a severe headache who is frightened. As you arrive at the patient's home, you find a 42-year-old male who is grimacing with his head in his hands, stating that about 25 minutes ago, he experienced the worst headache in his life. He noted that his day began as usual, with breakfast and dressing to go to work, when he experienced an acute left-sided headache. On further questioning, he admitted to rarely having mild to moderate headaches, one to two times a year, which immediately resolved with aspirin or Tylenol. Today, the headache was so intense that the Tylenol did nothing, and the severity of the headache persisted. Your initial physical examination reveals that the patient is afebrile to touch and has a blood pressure of 124/78, a regular pulse rate of 88 beats per minute, respirations of 20 breathsper minute, pupils that are equal and reactive to light, and normal gross neurologic findings. All of the following are signs or symptoms that would heighten your concerns of a possibly serious or potentially life-threatening cause of a headache except:

(A) Patient complains of a fever and a stiff neck.

(B) Patient has a bleeding disorder or is taking blood-thinning medications.

(C) Patient demonstrates focal neurologic abnormality.

(D) Patient complains of congestion, postnasal drip, with facial pain and tenderness.

448. Match the following types of headache with the appropriate pathophysiologic or identifying characteristic.

(A) toxic exposure

(B) migraine

(C) hypertensive

(D) meningitis

(E) sinus

(F) subarachnoid hemorrhage

(G) tension

1. throbbing headache, often with nausea and vomiting

2. fever and stiff neck

3. stress-related, in the front of the head to the occipital area

4. sudden onset of worse headache, vomiting, and stiff neck

5. associated with confusion, chest tightness, and fumes

6. associated with diastolic blood pressure above 120 mmHg

7. nasal congestion, forehead or cheek tenderness

449. Which of the following is the most accurate description of the most likely clinical presentation of a patient with a brain tumor?

(A) sudden onset of headache associated with coma

(B) fever, chills, and stiff neck

(C) memory difficulty and personality change over a long period of time

(D) nasal congestion with facial pain into the upper teeth

450. You are stopped at an intersection when a teenage boy runs out in front of the ambulance to ask for your help. His mother was told 6 months ago that she has a malignant brain tumor on the right side of her brain. This morning she had difficulty climbing out of bed and needed assistance because of weakness. As you enter the patient's bedroom, you find the patient lying in bed with a blank stare on her face. As you begin to examine the patient, you find focal weakness. With this presentation, you would expect to find the weakness in which of the following areas?

(A) bilateral lower extremities

(B) right upper and/or lower extremity

(C) bilateral upper extremities

(D) left upper and/or lower extremity

451. All of the following are examples of critical signs of a probable neurologic or medical emergency *except*:

(A) a single dilated, unreactive pupil

(B) unresponsiveness with elevated blood pressure

(C) decreasing level of responsiveness

(D) memory deficit

452. All of the following are mechanisms of strokes *except*:

(A) metastatic

(B) embolic

(C) thrombotic

(D) hemorrhagic

453. A stroke leads to weakness, paralysis, speech disorders, confusion, coma, and other acute neurologic deficits that are due to which of the following?

(A) syncope

(B) acute increase in intracranial pressure

(C) brain metastasis

(D) sudden vascular catastrophe

454. You are dispatched to a nursing home for a 78-year-old male with an acute onset of confusion and left-sided weakness. The nurse on the floor notes that the patient has a history of hypertension and an old left-sided cerebrovascular accident, resulting in right-leg weakness. On review of last evening's nurse's notes, it is found that the patient did complain of a mild headache, which responded to two aspirins. At present, the patient is too confused to answer any of your questions concerning this episode. All of the following are physical findings due to an acute stroke *except*:

(A) focal hemiparesis or hemiplegia (opposite to the side of the brain damage)

(B) skin rash

(C) hypertension and bradycardia

(D) loss of gag reflex

455. All of the following are correct statements concerning an acute hemorrhagic stroke *except*:

(A) The two types are intracerebral hemorrhage and subarachnoid hemorrhage.

(B) The mortality rate is 50–80%

(C) The average age is fifties to early sixties.

(D) Patients frequently have a history of cancer.

456. You are dispatched to a business office for a 62-year-old female complaining of a severe headache. On your arrival, you find the patient lying on a couch in the lobby. The patient notes that she has been under the care of an internist for hypertension. Today, she awoke and went to work and felt normal. Then, about an hour ago, she felt an acute onset of the worst headache of her entire life. She also notes that she feels pain in her neck and then down her back, associated with feeling very nauseous. As you begin to assess the patient and your partner begins to take the patient's vital signs, you note that the patient is acting confused and becoming more somnolent. Since the only abnormality on physical examination is elevated blood pressure of 178/124 bilaterally and the patient has grossly symmetrical neurologic findings, you suspect that the cause of the patient's symptoms is which of the following events?

(A) a ruptured cerebral aneurysm

(B) brain tumor

(C) thrombosed cerebral vessel

(D) a syncopal episode

457. You are called to respond to a possible stroke patient. When you arrive at the patient's apartment, you find a 92-year-old male who awoke feeling weak. On attempting to walk to the bathroom, the patient noted that his right leg was dragging, and his friend could not understand him on the telephone. On examining the patient, you note that his blood pressure is 186/120 bilaterally, his speech is truly slurred, and he has 2 out of 4 strength in his right arm and 1 out of 4 strength in his right leg. All of the following are appropriate treatment options for this patient *except*:

(A) Establish and maintain the airway.

(B) Administer oxygen and attach the patient to an ECG monitor.

(C) Protect the paretic limbs in order to prevent injury during transport.

(D) Request permission to open and administer a sublingual nifedipine capsule to lower the blood pressure.

458. As you proceed to an 88-year-old female with a stroke at the Sunshine Nursing Home, you jest with your partner as to what the true nature of this call could be. Yet, as you arrive at the patient's bedside, you note that several members of the staff are very upset with the patient's condition. Evidently, the patient awoke complaining of a headache and then gradually became more confused, with left-sided upper- and lower-extremity paralysis. After the staff called 911, the patient became barely responsive to verbal stimuli and responsive to painful stimuli. Your assessment of this very lethargic patient revealed that she had a blood pressure of 168/104 bilaterally, symmetrical pupils that reacted to light, an absent gag reflex, and insignificant findings on the remainder of the physical examination. However, the patient's neurologic examination documented that the patient had left-sided flaccid paralysis. All of the following are parts of the emergency care rendered to this patient *except*:

(A) Perform a finger-stick glucose determination, and treat hypoglycemia if present.

(B) Hyperventilate the patient.

(C) Immediately perform endotracheal intubation.

(D) Transport in the stable side position.

459. Transient ischemic attacks are episodes of focal neurologic deficits, similar to cerebrovascular accidents, that totally resolve within

(A) 4 hours

(B) 8–10 hours

(C) 24 hours

(D) 24–48 hours

460. A transient ischemic attack is clinically most important because it is a reliable sign of an impending

(A) stroke

(B) sudden death

(C) gastrointestinal bleed

(D) status epilepticus

461. You arrive at a senior-citizen center to find a 78-year-old male who complains that, at lunch about an hour ago, he noticed that his left hand became numb and weak and he spilled his coffee. He is embarrassed because the supervisor of the center called for the ambulance. He notes that his hand has come back to normal in the past 5 minutes, and he desires to simply go home. On your examination, the patient has a blood pressure of 156/102, a regular pulse rate of 86 beats per minute, and respirations at 18 breaths per minute. His physical examination findings are grossly normal, and his neurologic assessment reveals symmetrical motor and sensory findings, with orientation to person, place, and time. While the patient is playing down his complaints and wants to sign out against medical advice, you and the center's supervisor are successful in convincing the patient to go to the hospital. During transport, the patient again notes that he is feeling numbness and weakness in his left hand. Your assessment confirms that the patient's strength in the hand is 2 out of 4, and his blood pressure is now 156/100 bilaterally. All of the following are part of the emergency care rendered to this patient *except*:

(A) Establish and maintain the airway.

(B) Administer sublingual nifedipine to lower the blood pressure.

(C) Administer oxygen.

(D) Start an IV with normal saline solution or lactated Ringer's solution.

462. All of the following are symptoms or signs of transient ischemic attacks *except*:

(A) monocular blindness

(B) staggering gait

(C) numbness and/or paresthesias

(D) dysuria

463. You are dispatched to a "possible stroke" and arrive to find an 86-year-old female with her family. The patient's daughter called because her mother had just awoken from a nap and was found to have a half-paralyzed face. The patient's family was afraid that she had a stroke and called the ambulance. The patient was noted to have had a bad cold with a temperature for 2 days. As you question the patient, you note that she denies any headaches, weakened arm or leg, or loss of consciousness. On physical examination, you note that the patient has a one-sided facial droop with loss of forehead wrinkling and some saliva drooling out of the corner of the mouth on the affected side. Which of the following is the correct definition of this patient's presentation?

    (A) acute stroke
    (B) transient ischemic attack
    (C) Bell's palsy
    (D) sciatica

ENDOCRINOLOGY

DIRECTIONS: Each item below contains four suggested responses. Select the one best response to each item.

464. Diabetes mellitus is a disease characterized by a lack of

    (A) insulin
    (B) potassium
    (C) epinephrine
    (D) testosterone

465. Type I diabetes mellitus is characterized by all of the following *except*:

    (A) inadequate production of insulin
    (B) total body edema
    (C) accumulation of organic acids and ketones
    (D) metabolic acidosis

466. Which of the following is the correct explanation of the manner in which osmotic diuresis produces dehydration in the type I diabetes mellitus patient?

    (A) The elevation of the blood sugar level results in a comatose state and the patient is unable to drink so that the patient becomes dehydrated.
    (B) As the blood sugar level rises in the blood, it spills into the urine and pulls water with it. This increased urination, known as polyuria, results in dehydration.
    (C) Type I diabetes mellitus frequently results in acute kidney damage, which results in dehydration.
    (D) As the blood sugar level rises in the urine, this always results in a urinary tract infection, which produces urinary frequency, which results in dehydration.

467. You are dispatched to a "sick" patient and find a 38-year-old male who admits to having diabetes. He complains of having the flu for the past week and has not had much of an appetite. As a result, he has not taken his insulin for 3 days. He now feels very weak and tired and yet has been urinating more than usual. Your assessment reveals a hot-to-touch patient with a blood pressure of 82/52, a pulse rate of 124 beats per minute, and respirations of 32 breaths per minute, with a patent airway and adequate ventilation. After performing a finger-stick glucose test or obtaining a blood sugar level, the next most important treatment is

    (A) 20 units IV neutral protamine Hagedorn (NPH) insulin
    (B) 25 g of $D_{50}W$
    (C) 1–2 L IV 0.9% normal saline solution
    (D) 10 meq potassium chloride

468. You are dispatched to an 18-year-old female who was found unconscious in her college bedroom. Her roommate states that the patient appeared sick and refused to go to the student infirmary. She also states that she has only known the girl for the past 4 weeks but truly believes that the patient showed no signs of alcohol or drug use. Your assessment reveals that this patient is warm to touch and unresponsive to all stimuli. The vital signs are: blood pressure of 80 palpable, pulse rate of 120 beats per minute, and respirations of 22 breaths per minute. As you begin to perform a rapid physical examination, you find a bracelet that states that the patient is a diabetic. Based on this presentation, after checking the airway, breathing, and circulation (ABCs), the first priority in the management of this patient should consist of which of the following?

(A) immediate administration of 0.9% normal saline solution IV

(B) 10 units regular insulin IV

(C) IV epinephrine 1.0 mg of 1:10,000 solution

(D) 50 mL of 50% dextrose

469. All of the following are correct statements concerning type II diabetes mellitus *except*:

(A) It usually occurs in later life, not childhood.

(B) Obesity causes an increase in blood sugar by converting protein to sugar.

(C) Most patients are treated with diet and oral agents.

(D) It usually occurs in obese patients.

470. All of the following are signs and symptoms of a hypoglycemic reaction *except*:

(A) frequent urination, increased thirst, and increased appetite

(B) confusion, irritability, and combative behavior

(C) rapid pulse, and cold and clammy skin

(D) nervousness, drowsiness, and coma

471. All of the following are possible long-term complications of diabetes mellitus *except*:

(A) kidney failure

(B) heart disease and strokes

(C) emphysema

(D) blindness

472. You are dispatched to an unresponsive diabetic at work. As you arrive in the factory, you find a 24-year-old male, unresponsive to all stimuli. His coworkers state that the patient was acting strange and arguing vehemently, when he went to the bathroom and did not return for 10 minutes. As his coworkers opened the bathroom door, they found the unresponsive patient lying on the bathroom floor. All of the following are causes of hypoglycemia in diabetic patients *except*:

(A) increased dose of insulin or oral hypoglycemic agents

(B) increased physical activity or exercise

(C) increased intake of carbohydrates in the diet

(D) decreased dietary intake

473. You are dispatched to the home of a 26-year-old female who has been complaining for 2 weeks of gradual weakness associated with increased desire to urinate, drink fluids, and eat. Since she is obese, her family had become suspicious that she had some form of eating disorder and had made an appointment with a special eating disorder center in about 4 weeks. However, in the last 2 days she has simply felt weaker and has been sleeping more, even during most of the day. Finally, she asked for help to go to the bathroom and had to be caught before passing out on walking. The patient's mother did note that her husband's family had a history of diabetes, with his brother dying at an early age with complications related to it. As you begin to assess this patient, you might expect to find all of the following signs of diabetic ketoacidosis *except*:

    (A) bradypnea, with a respiratory rate of 8 breaths per minute
    (B) warm, dry skin, with dry parched mucous membranes
    (C) hypotension and tachycardia
    (D) fruity breath odor

474. All of the following are symptoms of patients in diabetic ketoacidosis *except*:

    (A) polyuria, polydipsia, and polyphagia
    (B) skin moles
    (C) nausea, vomiting, and severe abdominal pain
    (D) weakness, tiredness, and lethargy

475. All of the following are known causes of diabetic ketoacidosis in known diabetics *except*:

    (A) infection
    (B) taking too much insulin
    (C) increased stress from surgery or trauma
    (D) failing to take insulin

476. All of the following are frequent causes of hypoglycemia in insulin-dependent diabetics *except*:

    (A) an error in insulin or oral hypoglycemic agent dosage
    (B) decreased dietary intake in a patient taking insulin
    (C) insomnia
    (D) a combination of A and B

477. Hypoglycemia is an acute medical emergency because the failure to recognize and correct it may result in which of the following?

    (A) kidney failure
    (B) permanent brain damage
    (C) peripheral neuropathy
    (D) acute MI

478. You are dispatched to an unconscious male found in an alley. As you arrive at the patient's side, a local bartender identifies the patient as a regular customer at his bar for the past several years. The bartender states that the patient has told him his life's story several times over the years and notes that the patient has high blood pressure and arthritis, and had his appendix removed 2 years ago and fractured his hip 5 years ago. He is adamant that the patient has never had diabetes, nor has anyone in his family. After your partner reveals an overall normal physical and neurologic assessment, an argument ensues between the well-meaning bartender and your partner over the need for IV dextrose, since the patient is not a diabetic and has never taken insulin or oral hypoglycemic medications. Acute hypoglycemia may occur in patients with all of the following diseases *except*:

    (A) certain drug overdoses
    (B) prostatism
    (C) alcoholics
    (D) certain cancers

479. You are completing the assessment and initial management of a 32-year-old homeless diabetic with classic diabetic ketoacidosis and are making final preparations to transport the patient. Suddenly, the Paramedic student riding with you notes that the ECG rhythm strip looks funny. As you and your partner review it, you note that the gross abnormality appears to be very tall, peaked T waves. You quickly change leads and note that it is truly present in each lead checked. In diabetic ketoacidosis, the tall, peaked T waves are due to which of the following abnormalities?

   (A) hyperkalemia
   (B) dehydration
   (C) hyperglycemia
   (D) hypernatremia

480. You are called to respond to an emotionally disturbed man. As you pull up to the scene, a police officer tells you to be careful with this emotionally charged patient. A bystander notes that a car was weaving in and out of traffic with an emotionally upset driver. As the police stopped the car, the driver appeared very upset but was making little sense. While you begin to slowly approach the patient, another bystander comes by to tell you that this patient is his neighbor and he believes that he is a diabetic. He recalls a similar episode, when the patient's wife called 911 because he was acting bizarre about 2 years ago. On approaching the patient, you note that he is sweating. His vital signs are: blood pressure of 126/86, respirations of 18 breaths per minute, and a regular pulse rate of 156 beats per minute. Your findings on initial assessment are grossly normal, but you did discover a wrist bracelet that confirms that he is a diabetic on insulin. While the patient will not allow you to perform a finger-stick glucose test or draw blood, he will allow you to treat him to make him feel better. Which of the following is the correct first step in treating this patient?

   (A) immediate 50–100 mL 50% dextrose IV push
   (B) oral glucose administration with orange juice, soda, or some form of glucose paste
   (C) adenosine 6 mg IV push
   (D) arm and leg restraints

481. All of the following are correct statements about hyperosmolar hyperglycemic nonketotic coma *except*:

   (A) Hyperventilating the patient is helpful in correcting the ketoacidosis.
   (B) A 0.9% saline solution IV is a priority.
   (C) It usually occurs in elderly patients.
   (D) It is sometimes precipitated by certain medications, such as thiazide diuretics or steroids, and sometimes by enteral or parenteral feedings.

482. Hyperthyroidism is a condition consisting of an overactive thyroid gland. All of the following are signs or symptoms of hyperthyroidism *except*:

    (A) weight loss
    (B) hypertension
    (C) tachycardia
    (D) cold intolerance

483. All of the following are signs or symptoms of hypothyroidism *except*:

    (A) cold intolerance
    (B) dry skin and brittle hair
    (C) altered mental status
    (D) lethargy

484. All of the following are a part of the prehospital emergent treatment of hyper- or hypothyroidism *except*:

    (A) ABCs
    (B) cardiac monitoring
    (C) IV access
    (D) IV lidocaine

485. Cushing's disease, which is another name for hyperadrenalism, may consist of all of the following *except*:

    (A) unusual fat distribution, buffalo hump, moon facies
    (B) rapid mood swings, depression
    (C) hyperkalemia, weight loss
    (D) increased blood sugar

486. Hypoadrenalism, also known as Addison's disease, may present with all of the following signs and symptoms *except*:

    (A) hypoglycemia
    (B) nausea and vomiting
    (C) hypertension
    (D) weakness and fatigue

ALLERGIES AND ANAPHYLAXIS

DIRECTIONS: Each item below contains four suggested responses. Select the one best response to each item.

487. A hypersensitivity response to an allergen to which an organism has previously been exposed and to which the organism has developed antibodies is the definition of

    (A) an allergic reaction
    (B) asthma
    (C) a panic attack
    (D) immune deficiency

488. An acute, generalized, and violent antigen-antibody reaction, the most severe allergic reaction, which may be rapidly fatal, even with prompt and appropriate emergency medical care, is the definition of

    (A) immune deficiency
    (B) urticaria
    (C) anaphylaxis
    (D) status epilepticus

489. An allergic reaction and/or an anaphylactic reaction is usually initiated after the body is exposed to

    (A) an antigen
    (B) a medication
    (C) a bacteria
    (D) an antibody

490. During an allergic and/or anaphylactic reaction, the mast cells and basophils produce a number of chemical mediators. The principal chemical mediator released is

    (A) epinephrine
    (B) histamine
    (C) norepinephrine
    (D) insulin

491. During an anaphylactic reaction, histamine produces all of the following effects *except*:

    (A) vascular permeability, causing dilation of capillaries and venules
    (B) contraction of smooth muscle, especially in the gastrointestinal tract and bronchi
    (C) contraction of the coronary arteries
    (D) increase in gastric, nasal, and lacrimal secretions

492. All of the following are agents that may cause anaphylaxis *except*:

    (A) water, vasoline, and air
    (B) nuts, eggs, and seafood
    (C) nonsteroidal anti-inflammatory agents, aspirin, and x-ray contrast material
    (D) antibiotics, bee stings, and aspirin

493. You are called to a holiday party to evaluate a 44-year-old female who is complaining of having eaten some fish with a fine gravy that contained some crushed almond nuts. Within 30 seconds, the patient complained of itching, hives, hoarseness, wheezing, dizziness, headache, nausea, vomiting, and diarrhea. In performing your assessment of this patient, all of the following are consistent with an allergic reaction or anaphylaxis *except*:

    (A) hoarseness and wheezing
    (B) hives
    (C) nausea, vomiting, and diarrhea
    (D) a pulse rate of 34 beats per minute

494. As you and your partner are cruising along a road by the beach, a frantic teenage boy is waving you down. He is screaming that a friend of his just got stung by a bee and is having difficulty breathing. As you approach this patient, you would expect all of the following possibilities *except*:

    (A) patient's stating that he feels as if he is going to die
    (B) swelling of the lips, tongue, and eyelids
    (C) nosebleeding
    (D) chest tightness and wheezing

495. Which of the following is a less common manner in which an allergen gains access to the body and causes an anaphylactic reaction?

    (A) injection by a needle or bee sting
    (B) ingestion
    (C) inhalation
    (D) absorption across the skin

496. All of the following are signs or symptoms of anaphylaxis, rather than an allergic reaction, *except*:

    (A) hoarseness and stridor
    (B) confusion and headache
    (C) hypotension
    (D) hives and itching

497. You arrive at a private physician's office in your community for a 24-year-old male who has had an allergic reaction to an injection of penicillin. On your arrival, the nurse tells you that the patient had a strep throat and was given an intramuscular injection of penicillin about 15 minutes ago. Then, about 5 minutes ago, he began to complain about itchiness of the throat and swelling of the tongue. The doctor gave the patient an intramuscular injection of 50 mg Benadryl, but the patient then began to complain of hoarseness and having difficulty taking in air. As you walk into the examining room, you see a young man who is stridorous and in acute respiratory distress, breathing at 40 respirations per minute. His physical assessment revealed blood pressure of 124/78; pulse rate of 124 beats per minute; a large, swollen tongue; loud wheezing on lung examination; and several widespread hives. Which of the following is the first priority in the emergent treatment of this patient?

    (A) establish and maintain an airway
    (B) pulse oximetry
    (C) 2 L of Ringer's lactate solution wide open
    (D) ECG monitoring

498. In the patient presented in question 497, which would be the correct way to establish and maintain an airway?

(A) immediate cricothyrotomy

(B) blind insertion of an oropharyngeal airway

(C) oral tongue blade-guided insertion of an oropharyngeal airway

(D) oral endotracheal intubation

499. You are dispatched to a 75-year-old female who has taken a neighbor's prescription for a pain medication for arthritis. The patient admits to having two very dangerous reactions to ibuprofen and has been told to avoid medications in the same category. However, her neighbor's pain medication is naproxen, another nonsteroidal medication, like ibuprofen. After taking the medication, the patient noticed within 20 minutes that she became very itchy, with hives and an upset stomach. Over the past hour, the patient complains of weakness, dizziness, and inability to walk for fear of falling. Your assessment reveals a flushed female who appears very weak, with a blood pressure of 70/46 supine and only palpable with sitting up. The patient otherwise shows diffuse hives, facial flushing, with clear lungs and a clear oral airway. After ensuring an open airway, all of the following are a part of the emergency care of this patient *except*:

(A) 0.3–0.5 mg of 1:1000 epinephrine IV push

(B) administration of 100% oxygen by nonrebreather mask

(C) large-bore IV line, with Ringer's lactate, to run wide open

(D) slow IV infusion of 5–10 mL of 1:10,000 epinephrine

500. In addition to the emergency care outlined in the questions 497–499, all of the following are additional treatment options for a patient with anaphylaxis *except*:

(A) diphenhydramine (Benadryl) 25–50 mg intramuscular or slow IV push

(B) IV steroids (Solumedrol or hydrocortisone)

(C) IV beta-blockers

(D) inhaled beta agonists

501. Match all of the following medications used in the treatment of anaphylaxis with the correct dosage.

(A) epinephrine SC

(B) epinephrine IV

(C) Benadryl

(D) Solumedrol

(E) aminophylline

(F) beta-agonist inhaler

1. 25–50 mg

2. 0.3–0.5 mg of 1:10,000

3. 125–250 mg

4. 2.5 mg in 3.0 mL normal saline solution

5. 5.0 mg/kg loading dose

6. 0.3–0.5 mg of 1:1000

502. You are dispatched to a 52-year-old male at an outpatient radiology center who has been injected with IV iodine in order to undergo an intravenous pyelogram to diagnose a possible kidney stone. The nursing staff notes that the patient was given an injection of iodine and, within 30 seconds, broke out in hives and complained of difficulty breathing. As you go into the examining room, you note that the patient is lying down. He is breathing at 26 breaths per minute and is able to speak clearly. His other vital signs are: a normal temperature of 98°F, a blood pressure of 106/74, a regular pulse rate of 102 beats per minute, and a pulse oximetric measurement of 96%. Your assessment reveals a frightened male with bilateral diffuse wheezes, normal heart sounds, a soft abdomen with normal bowel sounds, grossly normal neurologic findings, and diffuse hives on the skin. After confirming a patent airway and initiating oxygen by nonrebreather mask, which is the first medication you should administer?

   (A) IV Solumedrol 125 mg
   (B) Benadryl 25–50 mg
   (C) SC epinephrine 0.3–0.5 mg 1:1000 solution
   (D) albuterol 2.5 mg in 3.0 mL of normal saline solution

GASTROENTEROLOGY

DIRECTIONS: Each item below contains four suggested responses. Select the one best response to each item.

503. The intrathoracic abdomen includes all of the following except:

   (A) spleen
   (B) stomach
   (C) liver
   (D) kidneys

504. All of the following are classified as hollow abdominal organs except:

   (A) stomach
   (B) urinary bladder
   (C) spleen
   (D) gallbladder

505. The stretching of the autonomic nerve fibers that surround abdominal organs is known as

   (A) visceral pain
   (B) hypochondriacal pain
   (C) referred pain
   (D) cephalic pain

506. Irritation of the nerve fibers in the peritoneum by chemical or bacterial inflammation is known as

   (A) somatic pain
   (B) visceral pain
   (C) cephalic pain
   (D) referred pain

507. Pain that is felt in an area that is removed from the diseased organ is known as

   (A) visceral pain
   (B) referred pain
   (C) distant pain
   (D) cervical pain

508. In obtaining a history from a patient with abdominal pain, the key points to be defined are represented by the letters PQRST. All of the following are matched with the correct definition except:

   (A) P = provocative
   (B) Q = quantity
   (C) R = region
   (D) T = timing

509. In the prehospital setting, all of the following are parts of the abdominal examination of the patient complaining of abdominal pain *except*:

(A) determination of vital signs
(B) auscultation for bowel sounds
(C) palpation
(D) inspection

510. You are dispatched to a 68-year-old female with acute abdominal pain. As you arrive at this patient's home, the patient admits to having a long-standing history of arthritis, which she self-medicates with Advil and aspirin. She notes that the arthritis has been particularly painful for the past 4 weeks, and she states that she has increased the use of both of these medications. The patient notes that her pain has been in the epigastric area for the past 5 days and that it is a burning pain associated with belching and vomiting. Your physical assessment reveals vital signs as follows: blood pressure 146/82, pulse rate 110 beats per minute, respirations 20 breaths per minute. The patient is pale and diaphoretic and appears to be in mild distress. The abdominal examination reveals a nondistended abdomen, active bowel sounds, and epigastric tenderness without guarding or rebound. This presentation best represents which of the following diagnoses?

(A) acute appendicitis
(B) acute gastrointestinal bleeding
(C) acute kidney stone
(D) acute gastritis

511. As you drive to get gas, you are waved down by a frantic child, who states that his mother is having terrible stomach pains and needs help right away. As you run up the stairs to the patient's apartment, you find a 38-year-old female moaning in bed. She slowly explains that the pain started early this morning, with pain around the umbilicus associated with a lack of appetite, nausea, and constipation. During the day, the pain began to localize in the right lower quadrant. On assessment, the vital signs are: blood pressure 100/72, pulse rate 112 beats per minute, and respirations 16 breaths per minute. Your abdominal examination reveals absent bowel sounds and marked right lower quadrant tenderness. The patient grabs your hand on examination (guarding), and there is rebound tenderness as well. This acute abdominal emergency best represents which of the following diagnoses?

(A) acute duodenal ulcer
(B) acute dysentery
(C) acute appendicitis
(D) acute cholecystitis

512. In the questions 510 and 511, the prehospital management of the acute abdomen includes all of the following *except*:

(A) high-concentration oxygen
(B) repeat abdominal examinations prior to transport
(C) IV saline solution or Ringer's lactate
(D) immediate transport

513. As you arrive at the home of an 88-year-old male with abdominal pain, you request a history from the patient. He states that he has had left lower quadrant abdominal pain for over a week. However, only this morning the patient had the sudden onset of intense generalized abdominal pain, which intensifies with deep inspirations. Your assessment reveals the following vital signs: blood pressure 90/50, pulse rate 120 beats per minute, respiration rate 14 breaths per minute, and hot to touch. The abdominal examination reveals a distended abdomen without bowel sounds that is rigid and boardlike to palpation, with diffuse guarding and rebound. This case presentation best represents which of the following diagnoses?

(A) perforated abdominal viscus
(B) acute appendicitis
(C) acute hepatitis
(D) acute upper gastrointestinal bleed

514. All of the following are signs or symptoms of acute upper gastrointestinal bleeding *except*:

(A) hematemesis
(B) pain in the epigastric or upper quadrants, if present
(C) dark stools or melena
(D) bleeding only with defecation

515. Match the following causes of upper gastrointestinal bleeding with the correct pathophysiology.

(A) esophagitis
(B) bleeding esophageal varices
(C) duodenal ulcer
(D) Mallory-Weiss tear
(E) gastric ulcer
(F) gastritis

1. eroding ulcer in the stomach
2. esophageal inflammation and erosions
3. diffuse inflammation in the stomach
4. eroding ulcer in the duodenum
5. bleeding, swollen esophageal veins
6. esophageal injury due to recurrent vomiting

516. You are dispatched to a 76-year-old female who is vomiting blood. On your arrival at the patient's home, you notice four large pans filled with blood and mucus. The patient states that she has arthritis and has been getting progressively worse. Under her doctor's direction, she has been taking increasing amounts of Advil and aspirin. In the past week, she has taken two tablets of 200-mg Advil five times per day and two aspirins two to three times a day as well. She has been having stomach pains, nausea, and anorexia over this same period of time but just this morning began to vomit. Initially, the vomit was only blood streaked; however, since noon it has been almost entirely bright-red blood. Your initial assessment reveals that the patient is afebrile and has the following vital signs: respiratory rate 16 breaths per minute, pulse rate 132 beats per minute lying supine and 160 beats per minute sitting upright, and blood pressure 90/62 lying supine and 60 palpable sitting upright. All of the following are part of the prehospital emergency care of the patient suffering from acute upper gastrointestinal bleeding *except*:

(A) two large-bore IVs and beginning to administer Ringer's lactate or normal saline solution
(B) securing a patent airway
(C) initiating blood transfusions
(D) 100% oxygen

517. Which of the following is the best definition of lower gastrointestinal bleeding?

(A) left lower abdominal pain
(B) urinating bright-red blood
(C) vomiting blood with lower abdominal pain
(D) bright-red blood or wine-colored bleeding per rectum

518. Match the following causes of lower gastrointestinal hemorrhage with the correct pathophysiology.

(A) anal fissures
(B) arteriovenous malformations
(C) hemorrhoids
(D) diverticulosis
(E) colon carcinoma (cancer) or tumor
(F) inflammatory bowel disease

1. external and/or internal bleeding rectal veins
2. vascular abnormalities, frequently in right colon
3. ulcerations and erythema of colon and/or small bowel
4. bleeding diverticulum of the colon
5. cracks in the anal tissue
6. abnormal growths in colon

519. You are assigned to an 86-year-old male with rectal bleeding. As you enter the patient's bedroom, you find the patient appearing weak and pale, with blood and clots in the sheets. The patient denies having previous episodes of rectal bleeding. As you begin to assess the patient, you find that the patient's vital signs are: respiratory rate 16 breaths per minute, pulse rate 110 beats per minute supine and 140 beats per minute sitting up, and blood pressure 94 supine and 70 palpable sitting up. The abdominal examination reveals a nondistended abdomen that is soft, and nontender, with active bowel sounds. The prehospital treatment of a lower gastrointestinal hemorrhage includes all of the following *except*:

(A) 100% oxygen
(B) ECG monitoring
(C) IV line with saline lock KVO
(D) rapid transport

520. You are assigned to a 76-year-old female nursing home resident for stomach upset. As you arrive at the patient's bedside, she admits to a 3-day history of feeling sick with nausea, vomiting, and occasional watery diarrhea associated with mild abdominal cramps. The patient felt sick but was still able to ambulate and take care of her needs. The patient stated that everyone at the nursing home was worried about her inability to keep food down. Your physical assessment reveals that the patient's vital signs are: blood pressure 118/74 without postural changes, pulse rate 86 beats per minute, and respirations 16 breaths per minute. The patient's abdomen is soft and nontender, with active bowel sounds. Which of the following best represents the cause of this patient's problem?

(A) acute gastrointestinal hemorrhage
(B) acute gastroenteritis
(C) acute appendicitis
(D) ulcerative colitis

521. Match each of the following conditions with the correct pathophysiology.

(A) pancreatitis
(B) peptic ulcer disease
(C) intestinal obstruction
(D) diverticulitis
(E) appendicitis
(F) Crohn's disease

1. inflammation of tissue at tip of the cecum
2. inflammation of an epigastric organ caused by trauma, alcohol, drugs, and so on
3. ulceration, edema, and erythema of the small intestine and colon
4. ulceration, edema, and erythema of stomach and/or duodenum
5. blockage of the movement of intestinal contents due to adhesions, tumor, hernia, fecal impaction, and other conditions
6. inflammation of pockets off the colon

522. You are dispatched to a nursing home for a "sick and jaundiced" 76-year-old male. As you arrive at the home, the nurse in charge rushes to tell you that this is the third patient in the past week with the same type of illness. This patient complains of 4–5 days of feeling very tired, with darkening of urine; light, clay-colored stools; dull, right upper quadrant pain; and loss of appetite. Your physical examination reveals a blood pressure of 128/72, respirations of 14 breaths per minute, a pulse rate of 74 beats per minute, yellow sclera, yellow skin, clear lungs, and a nondistended, soft abdomen with active bowel sounds and mild right upper quadrant tenderness without guarding and without rebound tenderness. As you discuss the approach to treating this patient with your partner, which of the following is most important in preventing any possible spread of this condition?

(A) Use of body-substance isolation precautions.

(B) Draw blood work to specifically define the type of disease.

(C) Vaccinating all of the nursing home residents.

(D) Carefully collect all vomitus and stool-stained sheets and clothing.

523. You are assigned to a 38-year-old female with abdominal pain. You arrive at the patient's home and find the patient lying in bed in acute pain. The patient notes that, for the past 12 hours, she has had recurrent episodes of severe epigastric and right upper quadrant pain that is severe and associated with nausea, vomiting, and shaking chills. Your assessment reveals a blood pressure of 112/72, respirations of 12 breaths per minute, a pulse rate of 90 beats per minute, and a slightly distended abdomen with active bowel sounds and marked right upper quadrant tenderness without guarding or rebound. All of the following are correct statements concerning this patient's illness *except*:

(A) The pain is often precipitated by fatty foods.

(B) It should be treated with IV fluids.

(C) Prehospital treatment may include IV narcotics for pain control.

(D) There is often a patient and/or family history of gallstones.

524. You are dispatched to a "sick call" at a very well-known "crack house" in your city. As you enter the poorly lit, run-down building, a young man comes up to you to tell you that the patient has been sick for about a week. In the beginning he had a fever, was tired, didn't want to eat, and even lost his taste for cigarettes. Now he has begun to complain of pain on the right side of his stomach and is frightened because his eyes and skin are yellow, his urine is brown, and his stools are very light. All of the following are correct statements concerning this patient's illness *except*:

(A) He is contagious.

(B) Increased risk of spread occurs in crowded, poor sanitary living conditions.

(C) There are types A, B, C, D, and E.

(D) There is no need for any precautions in treating this patient.

RENAL AND UROLOGY

DIRECTIONS: Each item below contains four suggested responses. Select the one best response to each item.

525. Which of the following is the best definition of *acute renal failure*?

    (A) rapid and potentially reversible deterioration in kidney function
    (B) patient on renal dialysis machine with difficulty breathing
    (C) acute urinating of blood
    (D) acute urinary tract infection with difficulty urinating

526. Which of the following is the correct sequence for the flow of urine through the renal and urinary system?

    (A) ureters, bladder, kidneys, urethra
    (B) bladder, kidneys, urethra, ureters
    (C) kidneys, ureters, bladder, urethra
    (D) ureters, kidneys, bladder, urethra

527. All of the following are various presentations of common acute urinary disorders *except*:

    (A) urinary tract infection
    (B) urinary alkalosis
    (C) urinary retention
    (D) urinary stones

528. All of the following are mechanisms for the development of acute renal failure *except*:

    (A) urinary tract infection
    (B) renal: trauma, nephrotoxic drugs, or kidney infection
    (C) postrenal: obstruction of the urinary flow
    (D) prerenal: shock and dehydration

529. You are dispatched to an 86-year-old "sick" male. On questioning the patient and his family, you are told that he has a long-standing history of difficulty urinating and getting up to urinate several times at night. However, in the past 3–4 days, the patient's wife noted that he developed a high fever but strangely was not going to the bathroom and yet was not incontinent of urine on his clothes or in the bed. Now, in the past 3 hours, he has been moaning and is less coherent. Your physical assessment reveals a blood pressure of 98/72, respirations of 20 breaths per minute, a pulse rate of 112 beats per minute, clear lungs, normal heart sounds, and a distended abdomen, active bowel sounds, and a palpable fullness in the lower abdomen. The most likely cause of this patient's problem is

    (A) acute renal failure due to the ingestion of renal toxic medications
    (B) acute renal failure due to a urinary tract obstruction due to an enlarged prostate with a secondary infection
    (C) acute renal failure due to a kidney stone
    (D) acute renal failure due to cancer of the kidney

530. You arrive at the home of an 84-year-old female who has a history of "kidney problems" and is complaining of decreased urinary output, fatigue, loss of appetite, nausea, vomiting, and generalized swelling of her legs and abdomen. Your initial assessment reveals a blood pressure of 192/124, a pulse rate of 88 beats per minute, respirations of 28 breaths per minute, and pasty yellow skin and 4+ pitting leg edema. This patient's case best represents which of the following diagnoses?

    (A) acute renal failure
    (B) prostate cancer
    (C) acute urinary tract infection
    (D) chronic renal failure

531. Based on the case presentation in question 530, which of the following are the most probable blood work results in this patient with chronic renal failure?

  (A) hyperkalemia and metabolic acidosis

  (B) hypokalemia and metabolic alkalosis

  (C) hypernatremia and normal serum creatinine

  (D) hypernatremia and hypokalemia

532. All of the following are possible nervous system presentations of chronic renal failure *except*:

  (A) delirium

  (B) seizures

  (C) tinnitus

  (D) muscle twitching

533. Which of the following is the best definition of *renal dialysis*?

  (A) Process of exchanging biochemical substances across a semipermeable membrane to remove toxic substances.

  (B) Process of passing a nasogastric tube in order to remove toxic ingestions.

  (C) Process of providing antibiotics to an infected kidney(s) by way of an arterial catheter.

  (D) Process of using a programmable machine to assist in the urinating process.

534. All of the following are known complications of dialysis *except*:

  (A) stomach ulcers

  (B) hypotension

  (C) chest pain or dysrhythmia

  (D) disequilibrium syndrome

535. Which of the following is the best definition of *renal calculi*?

  (A) Kidney stones, the result of crystal aggregation in the kidney's collecting system.

  (B) A kidney dialysis machine's calculator.

  (C) The formula used to calculate whether a patient is in kidney failure.

  (D) Stones that form in other organs and result in damaging kidney function.

536. You are dispatched to a 34-year-old male complaining of the acute onset, 1 hour ago, of severe pain in his right side. The patient states that he went to work this morning feeling fine and then suddenly felt an intense pain, which he rated as a 10 in severity. He stated that the pain was associated with nausea, and he even vomited once. After about 20 minutes, the pain suddenly resolved and he was joking with his coworkers that he must have had gas. Then, about 15 minutes later, the pain returned but was a little lower in his right side and seemed to spread into his right testicle. He noted that his testicle appeared normal and was not tender to touch. He again noted that the pain was very intense and was as painful as when he fractured his leg in a football game. Your physical assessment reveals a blood pressure of 146/88, a pulse rate of 94 beats per minute, respirations of 18 breaths per minute, active bowel sounds, a nondistended and nontender abdomen, and no guarding or rebound tenderness. Based on this patient's presentation, the key part of his emergent prehospital treatment would include which of the following?

  (A) request for only IV morphine from medical control

  (B) IV fluids

  (C) only nasal oxygen and ECG monitoring

  (D) syrup of ipecac

TOXICOLOGY

DIRECTIONS: Each item below contains four suggested responses. Select the one best response to each item.

537. All of the following are routes of exposure for toxicologic emergencies *except*:

    (A) ingestion
    (B) surface absorption
    (C) aspiration
    (D) inhalation

538. Regional poison control centers are available for assisting in the treatment of toxicologic emergencies in all of the following manners *except*:

    (A) They will always dispatch personnel to the scene to assist with the emergent treatment of each acutely poisoned patient.
    (B) With their assistance, definitive care can often be initiated in the prehospital setting for over 8% of toxicologic emergencies.
    (C) Emergency medical services (EMS) professionals are often able to contact them directly.
    (D) They can help coordinate the treatment of the poisoned patient by calling ahead and notifying the receiving hospital while the ambulance is en route.

539. The total number of reported poisonings in the United States each year is approximately

    (A) 150,000 patients
    (B) 250,000 patients
    (C) 975,000 patients
    (D) over 4,000,000 patients

540. Of the total annual poisonings, which is the correct percentage of cases occurring in children less than 6 years of age?

    (A) 10–15%
    (B) 25–30%
    (C) 50–70%
    (D) 90–95%

541. All of the following are contraindications to inducing vomiting in the poisoned patient *except*:

    (A) a patient with an acetaminophen (Tylenol) overdose
    (B) a patient actively seizing
    (C) a stuporous patient
    (D) a pregnant patient

542. You are dispatched to the home of a 3-year-old boy who was found lying on the floor next to an empty bottle of adult acetaminophen (Tylenol) tablets. The patient's mother is very upset and states that she just bought the bottle of 100 tablets of 500-mg acetaminophen 4 days ago. She herself had taken 10 tablets in the past few days and had just taken two tablets a few hours ago and left the top off of the bottle when the telephone rang. On returning to the bedroom, she found her child chewing on a few tablets, with only 60 tablets remaining in the bottle. The child appears alert, is in no distress, and has stable vital signs and normal physical examination findings. When you call medical control, the telemetry physician wants you to begin to prevent the child from absorbing the acetaminophen. All of the following are prehospital emergency care treatment options for preventing absorption of an ingested poison *except*:

    (A) Administer syrup of ipecac.
    (B) Administer activated charcoal.
    (C) Perform colon lavage.
    (D) Pass an orogastric tube to perform gastric lavage.

543. You are dispatched to a 4-year-old child who is having difficulty breathing. As you arrive at the house, the child's tearful father calls you into the kitchen. His son is sitting on the floor, complaining of a very sore throat. The child's father notes that he left him eating his cereal, while he took a shower and shaved, about 45 minutes ago. On returning, he found the child sitting on the floor with an open Drano container. The child readily admits swallowing three handfuls of the contents and is complaining of increasing throat pain. The patient's vital signs are: blood pressure 96/62, pulse rate 110 beats per minute and regular, and respiratory rate 32 breaths per minute. The child is becoming hoarse, and his respiratory rate is continuing to rise to 40 breaths per minute. His mouth reveals small Drano particles and some redness and swelling. His chest is clear, but he is beginning to use his accessory muscles and has some nasal flaring. Which of the following is the top priority in caring for this child with a caustic ingestion?

(A) Administer syrup of ipecac.

(B) Perform gastric lavage.

(C) Try to administer lemon juice or vinegar to neutralize this alkali ingestion.

(D) Immediately transport to the hospital with 100% oxygen and focusing on airway management with possible airway obstruction.

544. The dispatcher sounds frantic in trying to get you to respond to a seizing 6-year-old boy in his next-door neighbor's garage. As you pull up to the scene, there are two women crying and a man trying to comfort the child who is actively seizing. Evidently their son and a few of his friends were playing in the garage before he became acutely ill. The patient was lying next to an open container of insecticide. Initially the child was sweating, drooling, crying, and having a lot of difficulty breathing but then suddenly began to seize. Which of the following is a similar presentation with a substance which causes the same symptoms and signs and requires the same treatment medications?

(A) hypoglycemia and IV dextrose

(B) asthma and albuterol inhaler

(C) anaphylaxis and IM epinephrine

(D) sarin gas and parenteral atropine and pralidoxime

545. You arrive at the apartment of an elderly female who states that she was babysitting her 3-year-old granddaughter today. About 15 minutes ago, she found the child crying in the dining room with an opened bottle of furniture polish. The child appears to have taken half of the bottle and is having obvious difficulty breathing, with a respiratory rate of 50 breaths per minute. At present, the child's airway is open, yet she is beginning to have increasing use of accessory muscles and central cyanosis. On physical examination, the child has diffuse rales and rhonchi. Which of the following is the first priority in providing emergency care to this child?

(A) administering nasal oxygen at 3–4 L/min

(B) calling medical control to discuss options for inducing vomiting

(C) endotracheal intubation followed by administration of 100% oxygen

(D) administering IV morphine sulfate

546. All of the following are true statements concerning toxic inhalations *except*:

(A) Often there is more than one victim.

(B) Removal of the patient from the toxic environment is crucial.

(C) The Paramedic should not enter the toxic environment without protective breathing apparatus.

(D) Carbon monoxide poisoning is a part of every toxic inhalation.

547. All of the following are causes of inhalation poisoning *except*:

(A) cyanide

(B) chlorine gas

(C) carbon monoxide

(D) alcohol

548. In the middle of winter, you are called to evaluate a 68-year-old man because he was found "acting bizarre." As you arrive at the patient's home, his wife hurriedly waves you into the house. She tells you that they have recently purchased this winter home, which had not been used for over 2 years. Her husband went into the basement to start up a small fireplace about 40 minutes ago. He had come up about 10 minutes ago, complaining of a headache. He was nauseous and actually vomited on the floor. On questioning him, she found that he was confused and did not make sense. Right after she called 911 for an ambulance, she returned to find her husband having a seizure, and then he became unresponsive. All of the following are parts of the emergency treatment options for this patient *except*:

(A) immediately removing the patient from the home

(B) assessing the ABCs and beginning to administer 100% oxygen

(C) contacting poison control or medical control to discuss the quickest means of transfer to a hyperbaric chamber

(D) immediately proceeding down to the basement to personally investigate the possible source of the problem in order to prevent additional victims

549. You are called to a home of a 14-year-old boy who is exhibiting bizarre behavior. As you arrive at the scene, you find the patient being surrounded by his family and acting upset and scared because of frightening hallucinations. As you are trying to calmly talk with and assess this emotionally disturbed patient, his 12-year-old brother states that the patient has sniffed glue in the past few weeks. All of the following are possible signs of inhalant abuse *except*:

(A) smell of a chemical solvent on the patient's breath

(B) evidence of product containers or huffing or bagging paraphernalia

(C) diffuse red skin rash

(D) glue or paint on the patient's hands, face, or clothes

550. All of the following are causes of injected poisoning *except*:

(A) wasp bite

(B) bee sting

(C) spider bite

(D) dog bite

551. You are dispatched to the county fair for a 6-year-old boy who has been stung by a bee. As you approach the crying child in his mother's arms, you notice that his right forearm is red and swollen at the site of the witnessed sting. You have determined that the child has only a localized reaction to the sting, with stable vital signs and no signs of anaphylaxis. As you begin to treat the bite site, you notice that the stinger is still present at the site. Which of the following is the correct way to remove the stinger?

(A) Gently squeeze two sides of the sting site and pull the stinger out.

(B) Use a forceps or tweezers to pull it out.

(C) Use a scalpel blade to cut out the piece of skin containing the stinger.

(D) Use a scalpel or knife blade, carefully scrape the stinger and its sac from the wound.

552. You are dispatched to a 20-year-old with a spider bite. As you walk up to the patient, he explains that he went outside to the woodshed to get a few pieces of firewood. He initially thought that he saw a spider near the woodpile, but then it was gone. In proceeding to pick up a few logs, he felt a bite on his lower leg. When he looked down, he recognized a large black widow spider. As you begin to examine the patient, you think of the possible physical findings that may be caused by a black widow spider bite. All of the following are such findings *except*:

(A) immediate localized redness and swelling at the site of the bite

(B) gross hematuria

(C) severe abdominal pain with lower-extremity bite

(D) progressive severe muscle spasms

553. Which of the following is the best definition of *drug overdose*?

(A) taking prescription medications too rapidly

(B) poisoning from a pharmacologic substance, either legal or illegal

(C) a combination of normal doses of prescribed medications and a moderate amount of alcohol

(D) refers only to taking "street" drugs

554. You are dispatched to a nearby college dormitory for an unresponsive 18-year-old male. As you arrive at his room, two students approach you and ask that you please keep the story they are about to tell confidential. Evidently, last night was initiation into their fraternity and the patient was one of the new pledges. As part of the ritual, he was made to drink several glasses of straight liquor, including scotch, bourbon, gin, and others. As the night progressed, this young man became increasingly drunk, and so they simply escorted him to a bed in the fraternity house. However, when the fire alarm went off this morning, about 4 hours after he went to bed, he did not respond and was found unresponsive in bed. As you examine the patient, you note that he is truly unresponsive to painful stimuli, with midsize reactive pupils. His vital signs are a blood pressure of 88/64, a pulse rate of 114 beats per minute and regular, and respirations of 8 breaths per minute. In assessing his airway, you note the presence of alcoholic-smelling vomit in his mouth and on his face, gurgling respirations, and absence of a gag reflex. As a Paramedic, your emergency medical care should include all of the following *except*:

(A) oral suctioning

(B) syrup of ipecac

(C) IV thiamine, naloxone (Narcan), and $D_{50}W$

(D) endotracheal intubation

555. You respond to an "overdosed" 24-year-old female. As you enter the patient's apartment and approach the patient, you notice that the patient and her mother are crying. The patient's mother states that about a week ago, her daughter's boyfriend was returning home from law school to see her, when he had a fatal car accident. She has been distraught ever since and, according to her mother, very depressed. Today, after being out all day with some friends, the mother found the patient in her bedroom with an empty bottle of her pheno-barbital (30 mg tablets), which she takes for a seizure disorder. Her mother states that she usually takes one tablet three times a day and just yesterday had received a new month's supply of 90 tablets. As you approach the patient, you notice that she appears to be in a drunken state, with slurred speech, and is falling asleep. The patient's initial vital signs include a pulse rate of 120 beats per minute, respirations of 18 breaths per minute, and a blood pressure of 90/64. She also has dilated pupils, clammy skin, and an intact gag reflex. All of the following are part of the Paramedic's emergency care for this patient except:

(A) IV thiamine, naloxone (Narcan), and $D_{50}W$
(B) IV fluids and ECG monitoring
(C) activated charcoal
(D) syrup of ipecac

556. In treating a patient with a cocaine overdose, all of the following medications may be given, if indicated, except:

(A) nitroglycerin for chest pain
(B) benzodiazepines, such as midazolam (Versed) or lorazepam (Ativan), for seizures
(C) IV flumazenil (Mazecon) for a concurrent diazepam (Valium) overdose
(D) IV lidocaine for ventricular tachycardia with a pulse

557. You are waved down at the site of one of the city's well-known crack houses by an upset 20-year-old female. She states that she and her boyfriend went inside to look for a friend, and then her boyfriend proceeded to try "a little" crack. Now she is very upset because he is inside acting very strange and appears very sick. As you enter the house accompanied by a police escort, you find a 24-year-old male sitting on an old couch, excited and appearing bizarre. All of the following are possible physical findings in a patient with a cocaine overdose except:

(A) twitching, anxiety, psychosis
(B) euphoria, dilated pupils, and bradycardia
(C) tachycardia, somnolence, and hypertension
(D) hyperactivity, rapid and irregular pulse, and seizures

558. Match the following drugs with their "street" names.

(A) barbiturates _____
(B) phencyclidine _____
(C) marijuana _____
(D) methadone _____
(E) heroin _____
(F) methaqualone (Quaalude) _____
(G) amphetamines _____
(H) cocaine _____

1. bennies, black beauties, uppers
2. angel dust, loveboat, hog
3. lude, quay, soaps
4. snow, blow, white powder
5. horse, smack, antifreeze
6. dollies, dolls
7. blues, downs, downers
8. pot, reefer, weed

559. You are dispatched to a small, old hotel for a 52-year-old male who is "acting crazy." As you climb up the stairs to the third floor, you find the manager of the hotel next to the patient. The manager states that the patient was a long-time heavy drinker who had begun to attend nearby church meetings and decided 3 days ago to just stop drinking. Not seeing the patient for the past 3 days, the manager called the police to break down the door of his apartment. On entering the apartment, you find the patient lying in his bed, tremulous, weak, sweating, and arousable but very irritable. Your partner recorded the following set of vital signs: blood pressure 180/104, respirations 20 breaths per minute, and pulse rate 124 beats per minute. As you contact medical control and present the case, the telemetry physician may ask you to administer which of the following medications?

(A) IV diazepam (Valium)

(B) IV lidocaine

(C) IV diphenylhydantoin (Dilantin)

(D) IV flumazenil (Mazecon)

560. You receive a dispatch to a farm on the north side of town. As you pull up to the house, you are met by a young girl, who states that her father is out behind the house and is very sick. As you approach the patient, his wife states that her husband was working out in the fields for the past 5 hours, on an unusually hot spring day, with his shirt off. She also notes that she found a letter this afternoon, under the kitchen table, notifying farmers that all fields were going to be sprayed with insecticides by airplane today. She did not think that her husband was aware of it. About 10 minutes ago, she looked out her kitchen window and saw her husband staggering out of the fields and then suddenly collapsing. As you begin to examine this 40-year-old, muscular man, you notice that he appears unconscious, with tearing eyes and profuse salivation. He has been vomiting and has been incontinent of urine and diarrhea. The patient's vital signs are: blood pressure 102/68, pulse rate 108 beats per minute, and respirations 28 breaths per minute. He is gurgling and has constricted pupils. As you begin to establish an airway, your partner contacts medical control. All of the following are appropriate telemetry physician requests to assist you with the care of this patient *except*:

(A) Suction vigorously.

(B) Perform endotracheal intubation if you cannot ventilate adequately.

(C) Remove all of the patient's clothes and immediately wash him off with copious amounts of soap and water.

(D) Administer 0.5 mg IV atropine.

561. You arrive at the home of a 35-year-old female who states that she must have eaten something bad because, after going out to eat with her boyfriend about 3–4 hours ago, she has felt sicker and sicker. She noticed that she began to have stomach cramps about 2 hours ago and then began to have some vomiting and severe diarrhea, which has not abated. Her vital signs are: blood pressure 112/74 supine and 88/62 sitting up, pulse rate 94 beats per minute supine and 132 beats per minute sitting up, and respirations 18 breaths per minute. On the basis of this presentation, all of the following would be appropriate parts of the Paramedic's emergency care *except*:

(A) IV fluids

(B) endotracheal intubation

(C) obtaining samples of any contaminated food brought home

(D) high-flow oxygen

562. As you cruise by the wildest fraternity at your local college on Friday night, you notice that they appear to be having another loud party with some obviously intoxicated students. Later that night about 4 a.m., you are sent to the college's gymnasium, which is only a few buildings away from the fraternity party, because the night watchman has found a female unconscious and naked in the trainer's room. As you begin to examine the patient, two of her roommates arrive. As you began to inquire about the patient's history of alcohol and/or substance abuse, the two girls become very angry with you and state that the patient has a well-known social history of being very straight and never has had more than a single beer at any college party for the past 3 years. When they saw her tonight at the fraternity party, they did notice that a couple of the most notorious "ladies' men" were giving her their undivided attention toward the middle of the night. Then they noticed that suddenly she was gone. They both figured that she had left the party to either go back to their room or hang out in some other girls' room. When one of the girls went to the bathroom an hour ago and saw that she had not returned to her bed, they both were very frightened and began to search the campus for her. Despite your own experience with these fraternity parties, you did notice that there is no scent of alcohol around the patient. Which of the following is the most likely cause of this patient's presentation?

(A) simple alcohol overdose

(B) Rohypnol ingestion

(C) hypoglycemia

(D) aspirin overdose

HEMATOLOGY

DIRECTIONS: Each item below contains four suggested responses. Select the one best response to each item.

563. All of the following are parts of the hematopoietic (blood-cell-producing) system *except*:

    (A) liver
    (B) yellow bone marrow
    (C) red bone marrow
    (D) spleen

564. All of the following are correct statements concerning red blood cells (RBCs) *except*:

    (A) Myoglobin is the key molecule in RBCs, which enables the blood to efficiently transport oxygen.
    (B) RBCs are the most abundant blood cells and are responsible for tissue oxygenation.
    (C) When RBCs become old or damaged, they are removed from the blood by the spleen.
    (D) RBC production is increased in response to anemia, hypoxia, high altitudes, or pulmonary disease.

565. All of the following are true statements about anemia *except*:

    (A) Some physical findings of anemia are tachypnea, tachycardia, and orthostatic hypotension.
    (B) Anemia is defined as a reduction in the level of circulating RBCs.
    (C) Some symptoms of anemia include weakness, fatigue, headache, tiredness, and syncope.
    (D) In the adult, the most common cause of anemia is abnormal RBC production.

566. You are dispatched to the home of a 41-year-old female for weakness and difficulty breathing. As you enter the patient's living room, you see that the patient is lying on the couch and appears very weak. She states that she has been told of being anemic due to very heavy menstrual periods due to uterine fibroids. She is a single parent of three small children and has been unable to find the time to have the fibroids removed, as recommended by her gynecologist. Her vital signs are: blood pressure 104/68 supine and 60 palpable sitting up, pulse rate 110 beats per minute supine and 148 beats per minute sitting up, and respiration rate 28 breaths per minute. All of the following are parts of the prehospital emergency care for suspected anemia *except*:

    (A) IV fluids
    (B) nasal oxygen 2–3 L/min
    (C) ECG monitoring
    (D) frequently repeated measurement of vital signs

567. All of the following are correct statements about white blood cells (WBCs) *except*:

    (A) WBCs act in the spleen and are transported by the bone marrow.
    (B) WBCs are produced in the red bone marrow in adults and are destroyed in the spleen.
    (C) WBCs are part of the body's immunologic system, which defends against infection.
    (D) Measurement of the WBC count is helpful in determining the presence of infection or disease.

568. All of the following are leukocyte (WBC) disorders *except*:

    (A) acute leukemia
    (B) chronic leukemia
    (C) anemia
    (D) leukopenia

569. You are sent to a 21-year-old Black male who is complaining of "pain all over." As you enter the patient's home and begin to take a history, the patient tells you that he has sickle cell anemia. He usually has one or two attacks per year. Two days ago, he developed a cold with sneezing, a cough, and generalized achiness. However, last night he began to feel severe pain in his arms and legs, both sides of his chest, and his abdomen. He took some Advil and Tylenol, with no relief. He also complains of feeling a little short of breath. The patient's vital signs are: blood pressure 130/80, pulse rate 100 beats per minute, and respiration rate 24 breaths per minute. On physical examination, the patient appears to be uncomfortable and in pain, and has a few rhonchi and no rales on lung examination. The heart examination reveals a heart rate of 110 beats per minute. The abdominal examination shows active bowel sounds, and the abdomen is soft and diffusely tender. The extremities all demonstrate muscular tenderness and are without edema or cyanosis. The prehospital emergency medical care by a Paramedic includes all of the following *except*:

(A) high-concentration oxygen with a nonrebreather mask

(B) morphine sulfate 2–3 mg IV

(C) IV fluids

(D) rapid transport

570. You are dispatched to a dentist's office for a 14-year-old boy with persistent, heavy bleeding after a routine tooth extraction. As you enter the dentist's office, you immediately are escorted to the patient, in the dentist's chair, with the dentist applying direct pressure to the bleeding site in the boy's mouth. The dentist states that he had no difficulty extracting the tooth, but he cannot stop the bleeding. As you begin to approach the patient, his mother tells you that the patient had a minor injury to his left knee about 2 months ago and had a large amount of bleeding into the joint. Since then, an occasional squeeze of his arm results in bruising. He also had a spontaneous nosebleed one night last week. He does not take any medications. His vital signs are: blood pressure 102/78 lying down and 88 systolic sitting up, pulse rate 100 beats per minute lying down and 128 beats per minute sitting up, and respiration rate of 18 breaths per minute. All of the following are possible causes of this patient's bleeding episodes *except*:

(A) anemia

(B) acute leukemia

(C) warfarin (Coumadin) overdose

(D) hemophilia

571. All of the following are correct statements about platelets *except*:

(A) They are essential for blood coagulation and control of bleeding.

(B) They live about 10 days.

(C) Like RBCs and WBCs, they are the third line of cells in the blood.

(D) They are produced in the bone marrow and are removed from the circulation in the spleen.

572. On a bright Sunday morning, you arrive at the home of a 15-year-old boy who has been sick for over a month. Initially the patient's family brought him to their family doctor but they were told that he probably had a viral flu and needed time to get better. As you begin to question and listen to the patient he complains of feeling very weak, losing weight, continuous fever, with very sore bones. As you examine the patient, you notice that he has several large swollen glands in the front and back of his neck and then he points out more under his armpits and in his groin as well. You also note that he has several bruises and patches of purple dots in various places over his skin and also that his gums are bleeding. Which of the following is the most likely cause of this patient's condition?

(A) acute leukemia
(B) the viral flu
(C) the bird flu
(D) pneumonia

ENVIRONMENTAL EMERGENCIES

DIRECTIONS: Each item below contains four suggested responses. Select the one best response to each item.

573. Which of the following is the best definition of an *environmental emergency*?

(A) an emergency occurring to another person who is physically near to you
(B) a medical emergency occurring in a foreign country
(C) a patient's garden and/or lawn being dried up from the summer heat
(D) a medical emergency related to environmental conditions

574. All of the following are environmental factors that may affect the care of an emergently ill patient *except*:

(A) ionizing radiation
(B) heat
(C) alcohol
(D) cold

575. You arrive at the apartment of a 90-year-old female in the middle of a hot summer day. As you enter, you notice that it feels very hot, all of the windows are closed, and the patient is lying on the bed dressed with a sweater and winter coat. As you begin to examine the patient, you notice that her skin is hot and dry and she is very confused and disoriented as to place and time. Her vital signs are: blood pressure 70 systolic, a regular pulse rate of 140 beats per minute, and shallow respirations at a rate of 42 breaths per minute. As you begin to remove her clothing, the patient begins to have a generalized seizure. Which of the following best describes this patient's condition?

(A) viral flu syndrome
(B) heat cramps
(C) heat exhaustion
(D) heat stroke

576. All of the following are parts of the prehospital emergency care of the patient suffering from heat stroke *except*:

(A) rapid cooling of the patient using ice water–soaked sheets, ice packs, and fans
(B) ECG monitoring
(C) rapid administration of IV fluids
(D) nasal oxygen at 2–3 L/min

577. All of the following are correct statements concerning body temperatures *except*:

    (A) Heat stroke is usually associated with a temperature of at least 105°F.
    (B) Lethal hypothermia is associated with a temperature of less than 80°F.
    (C) Severe hypothermia is associated with a temperature less than 86°F.
    (D) Mild hypothermia is associated with a temperature between 94 and 97°F.

578. All of the following are predisposing factors for heat (hyperthermia) and cold (hypothermia) disorders *except*:

    (A) pediatric and geriatric patients
    (B) health of the patient
    (C) patient's religious affiliation
    (D) medications

579. Which of the following is a correct definition of *hypothermia*?

    (A) a generalized cooling of the body due to exposure to low temperature
    (B) a clinically dead person with a pulse
    (C) a condition in which a patient is shivering
    (D) a clinical state occurring only during the winter

580. On a freezing winter's night, you are dispatched to a park for a 68-year-old male reported to be cold and confused. As you approach the patient, you notice that he is shivering, confused, and ambulating with a stumbling gait. Which of the following is the best categorization of this patient's condition?

    (A) frostbite
    (B) severe hypothermia
    (C) mild to moderate hypothermia
    (D) alcohol intoxication

581. Which of the following is the best definition of *frostbite*?

    (A) a localized injury due to freezing of body tissues
    (B) hypothermia induced by prolonged exposure to frosty snow
    (C) a rare insect bite occurring in frosty snow
    (D) a bite-like injury occurring in frosty snow

582. Which of the following is the best explanation of the difference between superficial and deep frostbite?

    (A) Superficial frostbite produces only pale skin, while deep frostbite produces black skin.
    (B) In superficial frostbite, after several days, blackened tissue peels away, revealing shiny, red skin beneath, while in deep frostbite eventually black eschar mummifies and sloughs away from viable tissue.
    (C) In superficial frostbite, rewarming is painless, with blisters forming within 24 hours, while in deep frostbite blisters never form.
    (D) Superficial frostbite initially is painless, while in deep frostbite the tissue becomes pink and warm after rewarming.

583. All of the following are parts of the emergency care of a patient with frostbite *except*:

    (A) elevation and protection of the involved extremity
    (B) rapid transport to the hospital
    (C) not allowing the patient to walk if the patient's lower extremity is affected by frostbite
    (D) vigorous rubbing of the involved extremity

584. *Near-drowning* is best defined as

(A) The patient suffers submersion, but death either does not occur or occurs in more than 24 hours.

(B) The patient suffers submersion near another patient who has just drowned.

(C) The patient suffers submersion and becomes depressed from a nearby drowning.

(D) Death occurs within 24 hours of submersion.

585. While in a "wet" drowning patient a significant amount of water enters the lungs, in a "dry" drowning patient a significant amount of water does not enter the lungs, because of

(A) laryngospasm

(B) drowning in very shallow water

(C) the patient's actually dying of respiratory arrest prior to falling into the water and then drowning

(D) hot, humid weather

586. You are dispatched to the town beach for a man drowning. As you drive up to the ocean, you find a 48-year-old man lying on the wet sand, with the lifeguards performing two-person CPR. The patient's wife stated that he appeared to be taken out by the undertow. All of the following are parts of the emergency care of the near-drowning patient *except*:

(A) If there is any possibility of a neck injury, maintain the neck in a neutral position on a wooden backboard.

(B) Perform endotracheal intubation and ventilate with 100% oxygen.

(C) Since the airway is obstructed by water, administer the Heimlich maneuver.

(D) If possible, try to administer positive end-expiratory pressure (PEEP) to keep the alveoli from collapsing.

587. Which of the following is the best definition of *scuba diving*?

(A) self-confined usable breathing abnormality

(B) self-contained underwater breathing apparatus

(C) sorted containable unused breathing airway

(D) sudden-contained underwater breathing access

588. You are dispatched to a summer cabin for a 24-year-old man who had been scuba diving in the local springs about 2 hours ago. Since arriving back at the cabin, he has complained of itchy skin, joint aches, diffuse numbness, and weakness of all of his extremities. When the patient began to stagger and actually fell, his roommates called 911. As you begin to assess the patient, you find the following vital signs: blood pressure 120/70, respiration rate 18 breaths per minute, and a regular pulse rate of 90 beats per minute. On examination, the patient is now found to be paraplegic. Which of the following is the best explanation for this patient's problems?

(A) air embolism

(B) acute cerebrovascular accident

(C) seizure disorder

(D) decompression sickness

589. Which of the following is the most important part of the emergency care for a patient with decompression sickness?

(A) IV fluids

(B) administration of 100% oxygen with PEEP

(C) transportation to a hyperbaric center

(D) IV naloxone (Narcan)

V: Patient Presentations: Medical

590. You are assigned to a "sick diver" at a local ocean beach. The patient was diving several miles out in the ocean for over an hour. On resurfacing, the patient immediately complained to friends of a rapid onset of an acute tearing chest pain accompanied by right-sided paralysis. The patient was driven quickly by motorboat to the shore. As you approach the patient, you note that he is weak, confused, tachypneic, and not moving his right upper and lower extremities. The patient's vital signs are: blood pressure 158/52, pulse rate 114 beats per minute, and a respiratory rate of 32 breaths per minute. All of the following are parts of the emergency care of this patient *except*:

(A) Sit upright on the stretcher.
(B) Administer 100% oxygen by nonrebreather mask.
(C) Monitor vital signs frequently.
(D) Transport to a hyperbaric center.

591. Which of the following is the best definition of *high-altitude sickness*?

(A) On exposure to reduced atmospheric pressures, the patient begins to feel nervous.
(B) On walking up a mountain, the patient becomes anxious.
(C) On flying in an airplane, on ascent, the patient feels his or her ears pop.
(D) On exposure to reduced atmospheric pressures, hypobaric hypoxia occurs.

592. All of the following are true statements concerning acute mountain sickness *except*:

(A) Symptoms occur because of decreased oxygen saturation in the blood.
(B) It usually occurs after rapid ascent to elevations of 5000 feet.
(C) Symptoms may include headache, dizziness, nausea, vomiting, and irritability.
(D) The most important part of the treatment is descent to a lower altitude.

593. You are dispatched to a ski lodge for a 40-year-old man with difficulty breathing. As you arrive at the patient's bedside, you are told that the patient had taken a hike up to the top of a nearby mountain 2 days ago and was in the middle of carrying all of his family's skiing equipment and suitcases into the car when he acutely complained of difficulty breathing. The patient's family note that he has never been sick before and has been in excellent health. As you approach the patient, you note that he is extremely short of breath, cyanotic, and coughing up pink frothy sputum. His vital signs reveal a blood pressure of 174/102, a pulse rate of 124 beats per minute, and a respiratory rate of 42 breaths per minute. The patient is very lethargic and confused. On listening to the patient's chest, you note that he has diffuse crackles. All of the following are parts of the emergency care of this patient *except*:

(A) 100% oxygen by nonrebreather
(B) IV furosemide and morphine used with caution
(C) oral or intramuscular dexamethasone (Decadron) every 6 hours
(D) stabilization before any transport is undertaken

594. All of the following are correct statements concerning high-altitude cerebral edema *except*:

(A) There is progression of global cerebral symptoms of acute mountain sickness.
(B) It is probably caused by increased intracranial pressure.
(C) The patient may progress to stupor and coma.
(D) Immediate oxygen is the most important part of the treatment.

INFECTIOUS AND COMMUNICABLE DISEASES

DIRECTIONS: Each item below contains four suggested responses. Select the one best response to each item.

595. All of the following are possible causes of infectious and/or communicable diseases *except*:

    (A) bacteria
    (B) parasites
    (C) carcinoma
    (D) viruses

596. All of the following are parts of the human body's host defense mechanism against infections *except*:

    (A) the lymphatic system
    (B) the circulatory system
    (C) T lymphocytes
    (D) B lymphocytes

597. All of the following are routes of exposure for the potential transmission of infectious diseases *except*:

    (A) airborne
    (B) bloodborne
    (C) fecal-oral
    (D) talking to an exposed individual

598. All of the following are included in universal precautions *except*:

    (A) hand washing
    (B) wearing gloves and other barrier precautions
    (C) immediate vaccinations
    (D) use of sharp containers to discard needles, syringes, scalpels, sponges, and the like

599. HIV infection may be transmitted by all of the following body secretions *except*:

    (A) blood
    (B) vaginal secretions
    (C) feces
    (D) semen

600. You arrive at the apartment of a 41-year-old male with AIDS who is complaining of fever, chills, and shortness of breath with any activity. He admits to previously being diagnosed with hepatitis B, amebiasis, and Kaposi's sarcoma of the skin. All of the following are parts of the universal precautions, which need to be instituted before beginning to examine and treat this patient, *except*:

    (A) carefully recapping each used needle before putting it in a sharps container
    (B) wearing gloves
    (C) placing all soiled bandages in a puncture-resistant container
    (D) considering use of masks, protective eye wear, or face shields if any procedure to be performed may cause blood droplets or body fluids

601. As you clean up after starting an IV on the patient mentioned in question 600, you are trying to hustle a little at the end of a long night shift. As you gather the used drapes, you inadvertently stick yourself with the recently used bloodstained needle. As you examine your own punctured bleeding finger, you realize the potential consequences of this injury and become very upset. You and your partner begin to care for your injury and then begin to transport the patient to the hospital. On arrival at the hospital, which of the following individuals must be contacted to insure that your present exposure is properly documented and cared for?

    (A) the hospital lawyer
    (B) your supervisor
    (C) the infection disease control officer (IDCO)
    (D) the medical director for the Centers for Disease Control (CDC)

602. You are dispatched to a 78-year-old male who is having fever and just feels very sick. As you arrive at the patient's home, the patient's wife tells you that he has had a high fever for 6–7 days, along with a productive cough, occasionally mixed with blood. The patient also complains of night sweats and a 10-pound weight loss. The wife states that her husband has been volunteering at a local hospital with patients dying from a myriad of illnesses and infections. Your examination reveals a blood pressure of 110/68, respirations of 22 breaths per minute, and a pulse rate of 110 beats per minute. The patient is hot to touch. His chest reveals a few rhonchi, and his heart rate is 100 beats per minute and regular, without any murmurs. All of the following are important precautions to be taken in treating this patient *except*:

(A) Ask the patient to wear a disposable mask.
(B) Avoid contact with the patient's sputum.
(C) Wear disposable gloves.
(D) Paramedics do not need to wear masks.

603. You arrive at a local grammar school and are escorted to the nurse's office. You are informed that there have been two cases of meningitis in the past week. Both of the children are still hospitalized, and one remains in a coma. The nurse states that a 6-year-old boy was taken out of class after feeling sick. The child tells you that he feels hot, has a headache, and just wants to go to sleep. The nurse also notes that the child had vomited in the toilet. All of the following need to be done before assessing this child *except*:

(A) putting on disposable gloves
(B) putting a disposable mask on the patient
(C) having each Paramedic put on a disposable mask
(D) placing all linen in bags and labeling them for the protection of laundry personnel

604. At 12 noon, you are dispatched to a summer camp for an animal bite. As you walk to the playground, one of the teenage counselors directs you to a 4-year-old girl. Evidently, about an hour ago, a group of five small children approached a large "cat" that was licking its paws. The patient was scratched deeply in her right arm and was bleeding and crying. Another counselor, who observed the episode, noticed that the "cat" was actually a raccoon. As you approach the patient, you can see the raccoon walking around on the side of the playground slowly, with a staggering gait. All of the following are important parts of the emergency care of this patient *except*:

(A) Encourage the counselors to calmly remove all of the children near the raccoon.
(B) Disposable gloves are not necessary in this case.
(C) Contact local police and an animal control agency for immediate assistance.
(D) Make sure to notify the ED staff of the nature of the child's wound so that they can safely take care of the child and dispose of all soiled bandages.

605. Match each of the following communicable diseases with the correct medical name.

(A) whooping cough _____
(B) German measles _____
(C) chickenpox _____
(D) measles _____
(E) mumps _____

1. pertussis
2. rubeola
3. rubella
4. varicella
5. mumps

606. Match each of the following communicable diseases with the correct statement.

(A) herpes simplex type II _____

(B) mumps _____

(C) chickenpox _____

(D) gastroenteritis _____

(E) herpes simplex type I _____

(F) pertussis _____

(G) measles _____

(H) rubella _____

(I) influenza _____

(J) mononucleosis _____

1. causes the common cold and the flu
2. causes cold sores around the mouth and nose
3. German measles, red rash
4. produces vesicles on the genitalia
5. infection of the stomach and intestines
6. red rash first on face and then on trunk
7. red rash first on trunk and then on extremities
8. swelling of salivary glands and cheeks
9. swollen glands, fever, and enlarged spleen
10. whooping cough

607. You arrive at the home of a 5-year-old girl, whose parents state that they found her in bed this morning with a high fever, appearing sick, and with red spots all over her skin. Two weeks ago, the child slept over her cousins' house, and one of the children had become sick the next day. As you begin to examine the child, you note that she is alert and uncomfortable, with the following vital signs: blood pressure 100/68, pulse rate 110 beats per minute, and respiratory rate 24 breaths per minute. The patient has discrete red spots, some of them fluid filled, on her chest, stomach, and back. All of the following are appropriate steps for the Paramedic to take in order to prevent acquiring and spreading this disease *except*:

(A) Unlike major trauma, it is not necessary to call ahead and notify the ED of this patient's diagnosis and arrival.

(B) Wear a face mask.

(C) Place all linens and trash in separate bags for the protection of others.

(D) Wear disposable gloves.

608. Which of the following illnesses are prevented by the use of the MMR vaccine?

(A) measles, meningitis, and rabies

(B) measles, mumps, and rubella

(C) measles, mumps, and rubeola

(D) measles, meningitis, and rubeola

609. You are stationed at a county fair when a teenage girl runs up to tell you that her pregnant girlfriend is going into labor. As you approach the 18-year-old patient, you notice that she is crying and appears to be very upset. She has had regular contractions for several hours, but now they are much stronger and only 3 minutes apart. Her vital signs are stable, and her water breaks on the stretcher sheets. In the back of the ambulance, the patient tells you that she is very upset because she has a flare-up of genital herpes. Which of the following is the correct reason for calling ahead and notifying the ED of this patient's condition and arrival?

(A) Women in labor with active herpes genitalis are delivered by cesarean section.

(B) The ED staff can put on masks and gowns prior to this patient's arrival.

(C) Women in labor with active herpes genitalis are only delivered with forceps.

(D) Secure an isolation room for this patient.

610. You are dispatched to a 46-year-old homeless male in an alleyway complaining of severe itching. As you approach the patient, you notice that his hair is covered with white specks and his skin actually has small, white, moving organisms. All of the following are important parts of the treatment of this patient *except*:

(A) wearing disposable gloves

(B) hand washing after contact with this patient

(C) calling ahead to the ED to request an isolation bed for this patient

(D) bagging and labeling all linen

611. You are sent to a 64-year-old male, who is "very sick." The patient states that he began to feel sick 2 days ago and complains of abdominal cramps, nausea, and vomiting. As he began to feel a little better, he developed diarrhea. He noted that he had 15 bowel movements yesterday and now over 7 today. He is becoming concerned because he is gradually becoming weaker and has no appetite. He denies any blood in the stool, present abdominal pain, or any previous gastrointestinal diseases. The patient's vital signs are: blood pressure 108/70 supine and 80 systolic palpable sitting up, pulse rate 90 beats per minute supine and 120 beats per minute sitting up, and respirations of 18 breaths per minute. The patient appears weak and has a dry tongue and dry mucous membranes. The patient's abdomen is soft, nondistended, and nontender with active bowel sounds and no masses. This patient's presentation is most consistent with which of the following?

(A) viral gastroenteritis with dehydration

(B) peptic ulcer disease with dehydration

(C) acute appendicitis with dehydration

(D) acute diverticulitis with dehydration

612. You arrive at the home of a 56-year-old female who says that she saw her doctor 2 weeks ago because of severe joint pains and a rash. The patient was worried because she regularly works in her garden and has frequently removed deer ticks. However, currently she complains of severe headaches, tiredness, and difficulty concentrating. The patient's vital signs are a blood pressure of 138/80, a regular pulse rate of 72 beats per minute, and respirations of 16 breaths per minute. Results of the patient's examination, including a neurologic assessment, are normal. However, the patient has a large, 5-cm, red, circular rash on her back, with clearing in the middle. All of the following are complications of Lyme disease *except*:

(A) arthritis

(B) first-degree heart block

(C) cranial nerve paralysis

(D) kidney stones

613. As you walk into the patient's apartment, the family immediately informs you that the patient is a 24-year-old male who has just returned from a 3-week visit with his family in China. He actually lived with relatives on a farm in the country. The patient said that he initially felt like he was coming down with the flu because of severe muscle aches, fever, chills, and a headache but over the past 6–7 days he has developed a dry cough with worsening shortness of breath, even at bed rest. All of the following are important parts of the personal protective equipment (PPE) to be used by you and your partner *except*:

(A) disposable gloves
(B) disposable fluid-resistant gowns
(C) N-95 or greater respirators
(D) neoprene rubber boots

BEHAVIORAL AND PSYCHIATRIC DISORDERS

DIRECTIONS: Each item below contains four suggested responses. Select the one best response to each item.

614. Which of the following is the best definition of a *psychiatric* or *behavioral emergency*?

(A) The patient presents with strange attire and verbalizes concerns with the country's political direction.
(B) The patient's family calls because the patient has been verbally argumentative for the past several years.
(C) The patient has been crying on and off after a spouse died from cancer 3 weeks ago.
(D) The patient presents with a disorder of mood, thought, or behavior that is dangerous to him- or herself or to others.

615. Match the following terms with the correct definition or description.

(A) mental status _____
(B) posture _____
(C) anger _____
(D) anxiety _____
(E) affect _____
(F) depression _____

1. sad expression, crying, and apathetic behavior
2. sometimes caused by feelings of helplessness
3. dominant mood of fear and apprehension
4. means of establishing mental vital signs
5. outward expression of a person's mood
6. sitting at the edge of a chair or gripping the armrest

616. You are dispatched to the home of a 47-year-old hostile male who is acting "crazy." As you enter the patient's apartment, you notice the patient sitting on a kitchen chair with his arms tightly crossed and appearing very angry. As you slowly approach the patient, you notice that his friends are actually raising their voices with the patient. Which of the following is one of the best reasons for having friends, relatives, or bystanders removed from the scene of a psychiatric or behavioral emergency?

(A) They truly appear to be making the situation worse and escalating any violence.
(B) You want to quickly restrain the patient because your shift is almost over.
(C) They are supportive and quiet.
(D) You personally do not like their answers to your questions.

617. All of the following are useful interviewing skills in managing the emotionally disturbed patient *except*:

(A) listening to the patient in a concerned and receptive manner

(B) admonishing the patient for demonstrating any feelings

(C) offering realistic reassurance and support

(D) providing information about aspects of the upcoming treatment at the hospital

618. Which of the following is the best category for situations in which a Paramedic would be expected to transport a patient forcibly against his or her will?

(A) a troubled senior citizen worried about the country's future

(B) an anxiety reaction with panic attacks

(C) a grieving widow with a number of friends present

(D) when the patient appears to be a danger to him- or herself or to others

619. All of the following are methods of restraint that may be necessary in managing an emotionally disturbed patient *except*:

(A) verbal restraint

(B) mouth-gagging devices

(C) leather restraints

(D) small towels, cravats, and roll bandages

620. All of the following are risk factors for suicide *except*:

(A) financial setback or job loss

(B) previous suicide attempt

(C) depressed or sudden improvement in depression

(D) female sex, age under 40

621. You are dispatched to a 20-year-old emotionally disturbed male. As you arrive at the patient's home, the patient is lying on the couch. The patient appears withdrawn and states that he feels "useless" after just being let go from his job. He admits to having thoughts of killing himself and even goes on to describe his plan to go to a nearby, quiet subway station and jump in front of a train. Which of the following is the correct approach to this patient?

(A) Calmly interview the patient and encourage him to be transported to the hospital in order to be evaluated and treated.

(B) Call medical control and request permission to administer 10 mg IV diazepam (Valium) in order to sedate the patient.

(C) Calmly talk with the patient and encourage him to see a psychiatrist in the morning.

(D) Leave the patient alone, proceed down to the ambulance, and call medical control to discuss the case.

622. All of the following are factors which help to determine the potential for a violent episode *except*:

(A) the patient has a past history of previous violent behavior

(B) the location of the call

(C) the patient's posture

(D) the patient's physical activity

GYNECOLOGY

DIRECTIONS: Each item below contains four suggested responses. Select the one best response to each item.

623. Match the following female reproductive organs with the correct function.

   (A) vagina _____
   (B) cervix _____
   (C) endometrium _____
   (D) fallopian tubes _____
   (E) ovaries _____
   (F) uterus _____
   (G) urethra _____
   (H) labia _____

   1. two sets of organs that protect the vagina and urethra
   2. produces a menstrual period by its monthly sloughing
   3. produces eggs and hormones
   4. organ in which a developing fetus grows
   5. dilates during labor, allowing passage of the baby
   6. opening of the urinary system for draining of the bladder
   7. connects the uterus with the outside of the body
   8. transports eggs from the ovary to the uterus

624. All of the following are common symptoms of gynecologic emergencies *except*:

   (A) excessive vaginal bleeding
   (B) pregnancy with lower abdominal pain
   (C) fever and lower abdominal pain
   (D) dysuria and increased urinary frequency

625. You are dispatched to a 48-year-old female who called because of excess vaginal bleeding and extreme weakness. As you arrive at the patient's bedside, you note that there is a large amount of blood on the bed sheets. As you begin to interview the patient, she notes that she has a long-standing history of fibroids. However, in the past few months, she has been having increasingly heavy vaginal bleeding with her periods and even in between. On physical examination, you note the following vital signs: blood pressure 96/64 supine and 60 palpable systolic sitting up, pulse rate 110 beats per minute supine and 140 beats per minute sitting up, and respirations 18 breaths per minute. All of the following are part of the emergency care of the patient with a gynecologic emergency *except*:

   (A) keeping the patient supine
   (B) remaining on the scene and contacting medical control for additional options for stabilization at the scene
   (C) monitoring ECG and repeat vital signs
   (D) administering oxygen and IV fluids

626. You arrive at one of the local college's dormitories to evaluate a 19-year-old female who is complaining of abdominal pain. As you approach the patient, she admits to having had left lower quadrant abdominal pain for the past 24 hours. She hesitantly adds that she missed her last menstrual period 3 weeks ago and has noticed some slight vaginal bleeding with the onset of the pain. She does admit to being sexually active with her boyfriend and rarely without birth control protection. On examination, the patient's vital signs are: blood pressure 104/72 supine and 84 palpable systolic sitting up, pulse rate 96 beats per minute supine and 132 beats per minute sitting up, and respiratory rate 18 breaths per minute. The abdominal examination reveals a very tender left lower quadrant with guarding and rebound tenderness. All of the following are possible gynecologic emergencies occurring in this patient *except*:

(A) acute peptic ulcer disease

(B) ectopic pregnancy

(C) ruptured ovarian cyst

(D) ruptured tubo-ovarian abscess

627. You are dispatched to a possible sexual assault victim in her apartment. As you enter the room, the patient states that she was raped 4 hours ago. She lives alone and is very upset. After establishing that the patient does not have any life-threatening traumatic injuries, you proceed to document that her vital signs are all normal. All of the following are part of the care rendered to the sexual assault victim *except*:

(A) trying to question the victim about the details of the incident

(B) allowing a female to accompany the victim to the hospital

(C) psychologic and emotional support

(D) providing a safe environment as possible for the patient

628. In continuing to care for the sexual assault victim mentioned in question 627, in addition to the above, all of the following are important in preserving potential evidence from the crime scene *except*:

(A) do not allow the patient to change clothes, shower, douche, or clean under her finger nails before going to the hospital

(B) try not to clean any wounds

(C) do not allow the patient to drink or brush teeth

(D) use only plastic bags to transport for bloodstained articles

OBSTETRICS

DIRECTIONS: Each item below contains four suggested responses. Select the one best response to each item.

629. All of the following are correct statements concerning pregnancy *except*:

(A) At 20 weeks, the fetus has a good chance of surviving if born prematurely.

(B) The first trimester is the first 90 days of pregnancy and is crucial for fetal development.

(C) In the second trimester, the fetus develops bone structure, and the uterus is palpable.

(D) In the third trimester, the uterus reaches its maximal size.

630. All of the following are important approaches to assessing the obstetric patient *except*:

(A) obtaining key historical information, such as the mother's previous number of pregnancies and deliveries, the length of this pregnancy, and the expected delivery date

(B) history of vaginal bleeding, vaginal discharge, and ruptured membranes

(C) abdominal examination for gross deformity, presence of masses, distended bladder, intestinal distention, or enlarged organs

(D) evaluating routine vital signs but not orthostatic vital signs

631. All of the following are predelivery emergencies *except*:

(A) breech delivery

(B) ectopic pregnancy

(C) eclampsia

(D) spontaneous abortion

632. You are called to see a 21-year-old female who is 33 weeks pregnant and has vaginal bleeding. On questioning, the patient admits to having had 10 hours of vaginal bleeding associated with acute abdominal pain. The patient's vital signs are: blood pressure 124/84 supine and 80/50 sitting up, pulse rate 106 beats per minute supine and 136 beats per minute sitting up, and respirations 16 breaths per minute. The most likely cause of this presentation is

(A) eclampsia

(B) placenta previa

(C) postpartum hemorrhage

(D) abruptio placenta

633. All of the following are correct statements concerning the three stages of labor *except*:

(A) In the first stage of labor, uterine contractions begin to increase in frequency, force, and duration, in association with progressive dilation of the cervix.

(B) In the first stage of labor, the average duration of uterine contractions is 8–12 hours and includes the rupture of the membranes.

(C) The second stage of labor is defined as the time from the full dilation of the cervix to the delivery of the baby.

(D) The third stage of labor is defined as the time from the delivery of the baby to the termination of uterine contractions.

634. You are dispatched to the home of a 36-year-old pregnant female in labor. As you walk up the stairs, the patient's husband tells you that his wife is pregnant for the fourth time. As you enter the bedroom, the patient makes eye contact with you and starts to yell, "The baby is coming." As you glance at the patient's perineal area, you see that the baby's head is crowning. All of the following are parts of the preparation for a prehospital imminent delivery *except*:

(A) Open the sterile obstetrics kit.

(B) Position the patient in a prone position, with her legs apart.

(C) Place sterile towels under the mother's buttocks, on the bed between the mother's legs, on the mother's abdomen and on each leg.

(D) Wash your hands thoroughly and put on sterile gloves.

635. You are flagged down on a street corner by a teenage girl stating that her aunt is about to have her seventh child in her bedroom. As you enter the bedroom, the patient, a 36-year-old female, is beginning to push, and the baby's head is about to deliver. As you quickly put on a pair of sterile gloves, you immediately prepare to assist this mother with the delivery of her child. All of the following are parts of the emergency care to be rendered for this prehospital delivery *except*:

(A) Put on sterile gloves.
(B) After delivery of the head, check to make sure the cord is not looped around the neck.
(C) As the entire body delivers, be careful to grasp and support it because the baby is very slippery.
(D) Suction the infant's mouth and nose for the first time only after the entire delivery is completed.

636. You are called to a college student health service for a 17-year-old student who is about to deliver. A fellow student, who is a nurse, is trying to assist the patient in doing special breathing exercises, and you take a look at the patient's perineum. You note that the baby's head is crowning, and the patient tells you that it feels like the baby is coming. As you prepare the patient with drapes, the nurse tells you that the patient broke her water about 2 hours ago and shows you a sheet that is stained with yellow-green fluid. As you realize that the patient's amniotic fluid is meconium stained, you immediately ask your partner to prepare for all of the following *except*:

(A) Assemble a pediatric intubation kit.
(B) As soon as the baby's head delivers, wipe the nostrils and mouth with sterile gauze and use the bulb aspirator to suction the nose and mouth.
(C) Next use the DeLee suction trap to suction the mouth gently.
(D) With the delivery of the complete baby, if you note heavy meconium staining, you should contact medical control to request permission to perform intubation and to connect a meconium aspirator and begin to suction while removing the endotracheal tube. This may need to be repeated.

637. Which of the following is the correct location for clamping the umbilical cord?

(A) about 12–15 inches from the placenta
(B) about 12–15 inches from the baby
(C) about 6–9 inches from the infant
(D) about 6–9 inches from the placenta

638. All of the following are parts of providing neonatal resuscitation *except*:

(A) oxygen, ideally warm and humidified
(B) fluid boluses administered at 20 mL/kg
(C) epinephrine and naloxone by endotracheal tube if there is no IV access
(D) chest compressions with a 3:1 ratio at a rate of 120 per minute

639. All of the following are abnormal deliveries for which the patient must be rapidly transported to the hospital for cesarean section delivery *except*:

(A) footling breech delivery
(B) buttocks breech delivery
(C) transverse-lie presentation
(D) face presentation

640. You are dispatched to a birthing center for a 39-year-old female who has just delivered her sixth child after an uneventful pregnancy. However, the nurse-midwife became concerned when the patient continued to have a large amount of vaginal hemorrhaging even after delivering the placenta. As you approach the patient, you note that she appears weak and pale. The patient's vital signs are: blood pressure 122/72 supine and 80 systolic palpable sitting up, pulse rate 112 beats per minute supine and 138 beats per minute sitting up, and respirations 18 breaths per minute. All of the following are parts of the emergency care of the postpartum hemorrhaging patient *except*:

(A) Continue gentle uterine massage.
(B) Gently pack the patient's vagina with sterile dressings.
(C) Add 10 units of oxytocin to the IV fluid bag and administer at 20–30 mL/min.
(D) Start a large-bore IV.

641. You arrive at the scene of a motor vehicle accident with a Honda Civic wrapped around a tree. You quickly grab your equipment and hustle to the scene just as you see the fire fighters extricating an obviously third trimester pregnant female. The patient has a large volume of blood loss on her clothing and in the car and has angulated fractures to both lower extremities. The resuscitation of the mother is the key to the survival of the mother and fetus. All of the following are priorities in assessing and managing the pregnant trauma patient *except*:

(A) airway, ventilation, and circulatory support
(B) spinal precautions
(C) hemorrhage control
(D) repeat serial vital signs and full secondary assessment on-scene prior to transport

Answers and Explanations

311. **The answer is C.** (A), (B), (D), pursed lips, inability to speak, altered mental status, a pulse rate above 130 beats per minute or below 60 beats per minute in an adult, respirations greater than 30 breaths per minute, absent breath sounds, and one- to two-word dyspnea are all signs of impending respiratory failure. (C) is incorrect. (*Brady, Paramedic Care 2e, Principles and Practice, Volume 3—Pulmonary. Mosby, Paramedic Textbook 3e, Pulmonary Emergencies.*)

312. **The answer is A.** (A) is correct because markedly decreased air movement, a silent chest, and decreasing oxygen saturation are ominous signs of respiratory failure. In such cases, the Paramedics must be prepared to support the patient's ventilation. (B) is incorrect because severe inspiratory and expiratory wheezing is a sign of mild to moderate asthma. (C) is incorrect because mild expiratory wheezing is a common finding in the mild to moderately symptomatic asthmatic patient. (D) is incorrect because rhonchi are usually a sign of mucous in the airways and along with fever are present in bronchitis or pneumonia. (*Brady, Paramedic Care 2e, Principles and Practice, Volume 3—Pulmonary. Mosby, Paramedic Textbook 3e, Pulmonary Emergencies.*)

313. **The answer is A.** (B), (C), (D), high-concentration (100%) oxygen, and IV aminophylline and IV magnesium sulfate are all emergency care treatments available to you. (A) is not appropriate because asthmatics complaining of difficulty breathing should be treated with high-concentration, 100% oxygen by nonrebreather mask. (*Brady, Paramedic Care 2e, Principles and Practice, Volume 3—Pulmonary. Mosby, Paramedic Textbook 3e, Pulmonary Emergencies.*)

314. **The answer is D.** (D) is correct because a foreign body in the bronchus may produce unilateral wheezing, but it is not part of the pathology of asthma. (A), (B), and (C) are all part of the pathology of the asthmatics' airways. (*Brady, Paramedic Care 2e, Principles and Practice, Volume 3—Pulmonary. Mosby, Paramedic Textbook 3e, Pulmonary Emergencies.*)

315. **The answer is C.** (A), (B), and (D) are all common medications prescribed for long-term management of the asthmatic patient. (C) is the exception because there is no role for oral ibuprofen in the treatment of asthma. Some asthmatic patients with a known allergy to aspirin may actually be allergic to oral ibuprofen, and it may worsen the patient's asthma. (*Brady, Paramedic Care 2e, Principles and Practice, Volume 3—Pulmonary. Mosby, Paramedic Textbook 3e, Pulmonary Emergencies.*)

316. **The answer is A.** (A) is correct because the PEFR measures the airflow rate during maximal exhalation and is used to repetitively measure the severity of the asthmatic attack. It is also used to measure the response to treatment. (B), (C), and (D) are all important adjuncts that help to evaluate and monitor all emergently ill patients. However, the PEFR is specifically most helpful for the acutely ill asthmatic patients. (*Brady, Paramedic Care 2e, Principles and Practice, Volume 3—Pulmonary. Mosby, Paramedic Textbook 3e, Pulmonary Emergencies.*)

317. **The answer is B.** (A) and (C) are two chronic pulmonary conditions, which may, over a long period of time, cause pulmonary hypertension. Pulmonary hypertension may lead to the development of right heart failure, known as cor pulmonale (D). (B) is the exception because renal failure has no association with COPD. (*Brady, Paramedic Care 2e, Principles and Practice, Volume 3—Pulmonary. Mosby, Paramedic Textbook 3e, Pulmonary Emergencies.*)

318. **The answer is B.** (A), (C), and (D) are all part of the emergency treatment of the patient with decompensated COPD. (B) is not appropriate because SC epinephrine is given for the treatment of asthma, not COPD. (*Brady, Paramedic Care 2e, Principles and Practice, Volume 3—Pulmonary. Mosby, Paramedic Textbook 3e, Pulmonary Emergencies.*)

319. **The answer is D.** (D) is correct because this patient's presentation is consistent with a spontaneous pneumothorax, and 100% oxygen, frequent checking of vital signs, and watching for the development of a tension pneumothorax are important treatment options. (A) is incorrect because this is the treatment of a confirmed tension pneumothorax, not a simple pneumothorax. (B) and (C) have no place in the treatment of a simple pneumothorax. (*Brady, Paramedic Care 2e, Principles and Practice, Volume 3—Pulmonary. Mosby, Paramedic Textbook 3e, Pulmonary Emergencies.*)

320. **The answers are:** (A) 1, (B) 5, (C) 4, (D) 3, (E) 2. (*Brady, Paramedic Care 2e, Principles and Practice, Volume 3—Pulmonary. Mosby, Paramedic Textbook 3e, Pulmonary Emergencies.*)

321. **The answer is D.** (D) is correct and is caused as a complication of various disorders, such as trauma, infections, drug overdose, toxic gas inhalation, aspiration of gastric contents, hematologic disorders, and certain toxic metabolic disorders. Treatment involves the aggressive administration of oxygen using endotracheal intubation with the administration of PEEP, which helps to keep alveoli open by pushing fluid out of the alveoli back into the interstitium or capillaries. (A), (B), and (C) are incorrect. (*Brady, Paramedic Care 2e, Principles and Practice,*

Volume 3—Pulmonary. Mosby, Paramedic Textbook 3e, Pulmonary Emergencies.)

322. **The answer is B.** (B) is correct because this patient demonstrates the hyperventilation syndrome. However, hyperventilation may be a part of the presentation of a number of emergent conditions, such as an acute MI, acute pulmonary embolism, and diabetic ketoacidosis. As a result, the patient needs to be given supplemental oxygen. (A) and (C) have no place in the treatment of the hyperventilation syndrome. (D) Allowing the patient to rebreathe in a paper bag will permit the patient to raise his CO_2 levels by rebreathing his own CO_2 but may actually worsen the patient's condition by lowering his blood oxygen level. As the patient rebreathes his own exhaled air, the oxygen content of the paper bag continues to drop to very low levels. (*Brady, Paramedic Care 2e, Principles and Practice, Volume 3—Pulmonary. Mosby, Paramedic Textbook 3e, Pulmonary Emergencies.*)

323. **The answer is C.** The medications in (C) are used primarily to treat gastrointestinal problems, such as peptic ulcer disease and gastroesophageal reflux disease (GERD). The medications in (A) are used for myriad pulmonary diseases, which often produce difficulty breathing, especially asthma and COPD. The medications in (B) are used to treat patients with congestive heart failure. The medications in (D) are antibiotics used to treat pulmonary infections such as acute bronchitis and pneumonia. (*Brady, Paramedic Care 2e, Principles and Practice, Volume 3—Pulmonary. Mosby, Paramedic Textbook 3e, Pulmonary Emergencies.*)

324. **The answer is D.** (D) is correct because the administration of IV antibiotics is truly a hospital-based, nonemergent treatment. (A), (B), (C), and transportation to the ED are all parts of the prehospital emergent care of the patient with pneumonia. (*Brady, Paramedic Care 2e, Principles and Practice, Volume 3—Pulmonary. Mosby, Paramedic Textbook 3e, Pulmonary Emergencies.*)

325. **The answer is A.** (A) is incorrect because AIDS stands for the acquired immune deficiency syndrome which may result in various types of infections, including pneumonia, but none of them are called AIDS pneumonia. (B), (C), (D), viral, bacterial, and legionnaires' disease are all types of pneumonia. *(Brady, Paramedic Care 2e, Principles and Practice, Volume 3—Pulmonary. Mosby, Paramedic Textbook 3e, Pulmonary Emergencies.)*

326. **The answer is C.** (C) is incorrect because while smoking is a predisposing factor for the development of various pulmonary disorders, such as COPD, it is not a predisposing factor for developing aspiration pneumonia. (A), (B), (D), seizures, shock, infections are all capable of causing an alteration of the patient's mental status and decreasing ability to protect his/her airway which may result in aspiration. *(Brady, Paramedic Care 2e, Principles and Practice, Volume 3—Pulmonary. Mosby, Paramedic Textbook 3e, Pulmonary Emergencies.)*

327. **The answer is C.** (A), (B), and (D) are correct. (C) is incorrect because decreased $ETCO_2$ levels are seen in patients suffering with cardiac arrest, shock, pulmonary emboli, bronchospasm, and incomplete airway obstruction. *(Brady, Paramedic Care 2e, Principles and Practice, Volume 3—Pulmonary. Mosby, Paramedic Textbook 3e, Airway Management and Ventilation.)*

MEDICAL CARDIOLOGY

328. **The answer is C.** (A), (B), and (D) are correct statements. (C) is an incorrect statement because a family history of premature coronary artery disease is a risk factor for coronary artery disease; however, your sister is correct because it is not reversible. *(Brady, Paramedic Care 2e, Principles and Practice, Volume 3—Cardiology.)*

329. **The answer is B.** (A), (C), (D), obesity, male sex, and a family history of premature coronary artery disease are all major risk factors for coronary artery disease. (B) is incorrect because, while cocaine use is a risk factor, marijuana use is not. *(Brady, Paramedic Care 2e, Principles and Practice, Volume 3—Cardiology. Mosby, Paramedic Textbook 3e, Cardiology.)*

330. **The answer is D.** (A), (B), and (C) are correct statements. (D) is an incorrect statement because

the four heart valves are the tricuspid, pulmonic, mitral, and the aortic, not the ventricular. *(Brady, Paramedic Care 2e, Principles and Practice, Volume 3—Cardiology. Mosby, Paramedic Textbook 3e, Cardiology.)*

331. **The answer is D.** (D) is the correct sequence in following the flow of blood from the left ventricle to all of the body by way of the arterial system and then returning by way of the venous system. (A), (B), and (C) are all incorrect. *(Brady, Paramedic Care 2e, Principles and Practice, Volume 3—Cardiology. Mosby, Paramedic Textbook 3e, Cardiology.)*

332. **The answer is A.** (A) is the correct formula used to determine cardiac output. (B) is Einstein's famous formula for determining energy. (C) and (D) are incorrect. *(Brady, Paramedic Care 2e, Principles and Practice, Volume 3—Cardiology. Mosby, Paramedic Textbook 3e, Cardiology.)*

333. **The answer is D.** (A), (B), and (C) are all correct examples. (D) is an incorrect example because the left main coronary artery supplies blood to its branches, the LAD artery, and the left circumflex artery. While the left main coronary artery normally supplies all of the coronary artery blood supply to its two branches, it is usually not associated with supplying blood to any particular geographic area of the left ventricle. *(Brady, Paramedic Care 2e, Principles and Practice, Volume 3—Cardiology. Mosby,. Paramedic Textbook 3e, Cardiology.)*

334. **The answer is C.** (C) is the correct sequence for an electrical impulse to follow in the normal heart. (A), (B), and (D) are incorrect. *(Brady, Paramedic Care 2e, Principles and Practice, Volume 3—Cardiology. Mosby, Paramedic Textbook 3e, Cardiology.)*

335. **The answer is A.** (B), (C), and (D) are correct statements. (A) is not a correct statement because the SA node is normally the dominant pacemaker in the heart. *(Brady, Paramedic Care 2e, Principles and Practice, Volume 3—Cardiology. Mosby, Paramedic Textbook 3e, Cardiology.)*

336. **The answer is D.** (A), (B), and (C) are all stages of cardiac muscle excitation. (D) is unrelated to cardiac muscle excitation. It refers to being brought back to life again. *(Brady, Paramedic*

Care 2e, Principles and Practice, Volume 3—Cardiology. Mosby, Paramedic Textbook 3e, Cardiology.)

337. **The answer is A.** (B), (C), and (D) are all involved in the myocardial action potential. (A) is the exception because while magnesium (Mg) and chloride (Cl) are believed to be involved in the electrical activity of the cardiac cycle, their roles are still unknown. *(Brady, Paramedic Care 2e, Principles and Practice, Volume 3—Cardiology. Mosby, Paramedic Textbook 3e, Cardiology.)*

338. **The answer is B.** (A), (C), and (D) are incorrect. (B) is correct because the greater the volume of blood filling the chamber, the more forceful the myocardial contraction. Therefore, the greater the venous return, the greater the preload and stroke volume. *(Brady, Paramedic Care 2e, Principles and Practice, Volume 3—Cardiology. Mosby, Paramedic Textbook 3e, Cardiology.)*

339. **The answer is C.** (A), (B), and (D) are all parts of the autonomic nervous system. (C) is the exception because, while the gastrointestinal system may be affected by the autonomic nervous system, it contains the esophagus, stomach, small intestine, and colon. *(Brady, Paramedic Care 2e, Principles and Practice, Volume 3—Cardiology. Mosby, Paramedic Textbook 3e, Cardiology.)*

340. **The answer is B.** (A), (C), and (D) are correct statements. (B) is an incorrect statement because, while the parasympathetic nervous system slows the heart rate, it also decreases myocardial contractility. *(Brady, Paramedic Care 2e, Principles and Practice, Volume 3—Cardiology. Mosby, Paramedic Textbook 3e, Cardiology.)*

341. **The answers are:** (A) 4, (B) 3, (C) 8, (D) 6, (E) 1, (F) 2, (G) 7, (H) 5. *(Brady, Paramedic Care 2e, Principles and Practice, Volume 3—Cardiology. Mosby, Paramedic Textbook 3e, Cardiology.)*

342. **The answer is B.** (A), (C), and (D) may all be signs of cardiovascular disease. (B) is the exception because a barrel chest is usually a sign of pulmonary emphysema, not cardiovascular disease. *(Brady, Paramedic Care 2e, Principles and Practice, Volume 3—Cardiology. Mosby, Paramedic Textbook 3e, Cardiology.)*

343. **The answer is C.** (A), (B), and (D) are all findings detectable by auscultation. (C) is the exception because abdominal organ enlargement is detected by palpation of the abdomen, not auscultation. *(Brady, Paramedic Care 2e, Principles and Practice, Volume 3—Cardiology. Mosby, Paramedic Textbook 3e, Cardiology.)*

344. **The answer is A.** (B), (C), and (D) are correct. (A) is incorrect because, even though enlarged lymph nodes are detected by palpation, they are not a sign of cardiovascular disease. Enlarged lymph nodes are usually due to a nearby infection or blood disorder. *(Brady, Paramedic Care 2e, Principles and Practice, Volume 3—Cardiology. Mosby, Paramedic Textbook 3e, Cardiology.)*

345. **The answer is A.** (B), (C), and (D) are correct. (A) is incorrect because the first heart sound is produced by the closure of the tricuspid and mitral AV valves. *(Brady, Paramedic Care 2e, Principles and Practice, Volume 3—Cardiology. Mosby, Paramedic Textbook 3e, Cardiology.)*

346. **The answer is D.** (A), (B), and (C) are correct. (D) is incorrect because the history of childhood immunizations is not pertinent to a cardiovascular emergency evaluation and treatment in the prehospital and ED setting. *(Brady, Paramedic Care 2e, Principles and Practice, Volume 3—Cardiology. Mosby, Paramedic Textbook 3e, Cardiology.)*

347. **The answer is D.** (C) is correct. (A) is incorrect because the ECG does not give any information about the myocardial muscle contracting capability; an echocardiogram would determine myocardial muscle contractility. Pulse oximetry, not ECG monitoring, determines the oxygen saturation (B). Left and right ventricular hypertrophy (D) is determined by a 12-lead ECG or by an echocardiogram, not by ECG monitoring. *(Brady, Paramedic Care 2e, Principles and Practice, Volume 3—Cardiology. Mosby, Paramedic Textbook 3e, Cardiology.)*

348. **The answers are:** (A) 5, (B) 2, (C) 3, (D) 6, (E) 4, (F) 1. *(Brady, Paramedic Care 2e, Principles and Practice, Volume 3—Cardiology. Mosby, Paramedic Textbook 3e, Cardiology.)*

349. The answers are: (A) 10, **(B)** 6, **(C)** 9, **(D)** 7, **(E)** 8, **(F)** 5, **(G)** 2, **(H)** 4, **(I)** 1, **(J)** 3. *(Brady, Paramedic Care 2e, Principles and Practice, Volume 3—Cardiology. Mosby, Paramedic Textbook 3e, Cardiology.)*

350. The answers are: (A) 3, **(B)** 4, **(C)** 2, **(D)** 1. *(Brady, Paramedic Care 2e, Principles and Practice, Volume 3— Cardiology. Mosby, Paramedic Textbook 3e, Cardiology.)*

351. The answer is A. (A) Normal sinus rhythm is a regular rhythm, with P waves before every QRS complex, at a rate of 60–100 beats per minute. (B) is incorrect because sinus brady-cardia has a rate of less than 60 beats per minute. (C) is incorrect because sinus arrest has a period of no electrical activity (pause), which is not demonstrated here. (D) is incorrect because sinus tachycardia has a rate of 100–160 beats per minute. *(Brady, Paramedic Care 2e, Principles and Practice, Volume 3—Cardiology. Mosby, Paramedic Textbook 3e, Cardiology.)*

352. The answer is C. (C) is correct because there is a premature P wave, which is different from the normal P wave. (A) is incorrect because, with junctional premature contraction, there is a premature QRS complex, which may have no P wave. If a P wave is present, it comes either shortly before (less than 0.12 seconds) or after the QRS. (B) is incorrect because, with a ventricular premature contraction, the premature QRS is wide (greater than 0.12 seconds), with a T wave of polarity opposite to that of the QRS. (D) is incorrect because it is a regular rhythm with a rate less than 60 beats per minute. *(Brady, Paramedic Care 2e, Principles and Practice, Volume 3— Cardiology. Mosby, Paramedic Textbook 3e, Cardiology.)*

353. The answer is A. (A) is correct because, with ventricular tachycardia, the rhythm is regular or slightly irregular, with wide QRS complexes (greater than 0.12 seconds), with a rate of 100–250 beats per minute. (B) is incorrect because ventricular fibrillation is a chaotic, irreg-ular rhythm with no QRS complexes, only fib-rillatory waves. (C) is incorrect because a junctional rhythm is a regular rhythm, with narrow QRS complexes and a rate of 40–60 beats per minute. (D) is incorrect because supraven-tricular tachycardia usually has narrow QRS complexes (less than 0.12 seconds) with a regu-lar rhythm and a rate of 150–250 beats per minute. *(Brady, Paramedic Care 2e, Principles and Practice, Volume 3—Cardiology. Mosby, Paramedic Textbook 3e, Cardiology.)*

354. The answer is A. (A) is correct because in second-degree AV block, Mobitz type I, also known as Wenckebach, the rhythm is charac-terized by progressive widening of the PR inter-val until an atrial beat is blocked (not followed by a QRS complex). (B) is incorrect, because second-degree AV block, Mobitz type II, is a regular rhythm characterized by P waves not always followed by QRS complexes, with an atrial to ventricular ratio of 2:1, 3:1, 4:1, and so on. (C) is incorrect because first-degree AV block is a rhythm characterized by a regular rhythm with a prolonged PR interval greater than 0.20 seconds. (D) is incorrect because third-degree AV block is a regular rhythm character-ized by no relationship between the atrial and ventricular complexes, with different rates as well. *(Brady, Paramedic Care 2e, Principles and Practice, Volume 3—Cardiology. Mosby, Paramedic Textbook 3e, Cardiology.)*

355. The answer is B. (B) is correct because atrial fibrillation is characterized by a rhythm that is irregular, with atrial fibrillatory waves and no P waves. The atrial rate is between 350 and 600 beats per minute, and the ventricular rate is usually between 100 and 160 beats per minute. (A) is incorrect because normal sinus rhythm is characterized by a regular rhythm, with P waves before every QRS, with a rate of 60–100 beats per minute. (C) is incorrect because atrial flutter is a regular rhythm with an atrial rate of 250–350 beats per minute, with P waves that have the flutter wave, sawtooth pattern. (D) is incorrect because supraventricular tachycardia is regular and characterized by a regular rhythm with a ventricular rate of 150–250 beats per minute. *(Brady, Paramedic Care 2e, Principles and Practice, Volume 3—Cardiology. Mosby, Paramedic Textbook 3e, Cardiology.)*

356. The answer is D. (D) is correct because coupled PVCs are characterized by premature, wide QRS (greater than 0.12 seconds), which are repetitive (next to each other). (A) is incorrect because unifocal PVCs are characterized by premature, wide QRS (greater than 0.12 seconds) from the same focus (appearing the same). (B) is incorrect because multifocal PVCs are characterized by premature, QRS (greater than 0.12 seconds), which originate in different foci (different appearances). (C) is incorrect because ventricular bigeminy is characterized by a rhythm in which every other beat is a PVC. *(Brady, Paramedic Care 2e, Principles and Practice, Volume 3—Cardiology. Mosby, Paramedic Textbook 3e, Cardiology.)*

357. **The answers are: (A)** 3, **(B)** 1, **(C)** 2, **(D)** 4. *(Brady, Paramedic Care 2e, Principles and Practice, Volume 3—Cardiology. Mosby, Paramedic Textbook 3e, Cardiology.)*

358. **The answers are: (A)** 3, **(B)** 1, **(C)** 4, **(D)** 2. *(Brady, Paramedic Care 2e, Principles and Practice, Volume 3—Cardiology. Mosby, Paramedic Textbook 3e, Cardiology.)*

359. **The answers are: (A)** 1, **(B)** 3, **(C)** 2, **(D)** 4. *(Brady, Paramedic Care 2e, Principles and Practice, Volume 3—Cardiology. Mosby, Paramedic Textbook 3e, Cardiology.)*

360. **The answers are: (A)** 2, **(B)** 3, **(C)** 1, **(D)** 4. *(Brady, Paramedic Care 2e, Principles and Practice, Volume 3—Cardiology. Mosby, Paramedic Textbook 3e, Cardiology.)*

361. **The answer is A.** (B), (C), (D), hypovolemia, tension pneumothorax, hypoxemia, acidosis, hyperkalemia, hypothermia, certain drug overdoses (e.g., beta-blockers, calcium blockers, tricyclic antidepressants, and digoxin), and any type of shock are all conditions that may be associated with PEA. Ideally, the detection and correction of one of these associated critical conditions may result in the reversal of PEA. (A) is incorrect because patients with anginal syndromes usually have stable vital signs, with a strong pulse. In PEA, the patient is in cardiac arrest, pulseless, with an electrical rhythm. *(Brady, Paramedic Care 2e, Principles and Practice, Volume 3—Cardiology. Mosby, Paramedic Textbook 3e, Cardiology.)*

362. **The answer is B.** (A), (C), and (D) are correct. Hyperkalemia, an increase in the blood potassium level, is sometimes caused by kidney failure, patients missing dialysis treatments, metabolic acidosis (e.g., diabetic ketoacidosis), and potassium-sparing diuretics (e.g., spironolactone). Severe hyperkalemia may cause life-threatening dysrhythmias. Hypercalcemia, an increase in the blood calcium level, is sometimes caused by an excessive intake of calcium tablets, an overactive parathyroid gland, and occasionally with certain types of cancers. Hypokalemia, a decrease in the blood potassium level, is frequently caused by recurrent vomiting and/or diarrhea, and certain potassium wasting diuretics (e.g., furosemide). (B) is incorrect because hypernatremia, an increase in the blood sodium level, does not produce ECG changes. It is most commonly caused by dehydration. *(Brady, Paramedic Care 2e, Principles and Practice, Volume 3—Cardiology. Mosby, Paramedic Textbook 3e, Cardiology.)*

363. **The answer is D.** (A), (B), (C), and patients suffering from myriad critical and/or potentially unstable conditions, such as cardiac arrest, drug overdose, difficulty breathing, heart failure, major trauma, syncope, coma, anaphylaxis, and so on, are all situations in which an ECG analysis is indicated. (D) is incorrect because a skin rash by itself is not an indication for ECG rhythm analysis. *(Brady, Paramedic Care 2e, Principles and Practice, Volume 3—Cardiology. Mosby, Paramedic Textbook 3e, Cardiology.)*

364. **The answer is D.** (D) is correct because elevation or depression of the ST segment is the most suggestive ECG finding in the patient who may be having acute myocardial ischemia and/or infarction. A series of Q waves in certain parts of the ECG may be evidence of old MI(s). (A) is incorrect because the development of a new Q wave in the QRS complex may be a sign of an old MI but not acute one. (B) is incorrect even though, in some acute MI patients, one can see prolongation of the PR interval, known as first-degree heart block. (C) is incorrect even though, in many patients with acute myocardial ischemia and/or infarction, there may be elevation and/or inversion of the T wave. However, a number of abnormalities may affect the T wave, such as an increase or decrease of blood potassium levels, patients taking digoxin, left ventricular hypertrophy, and bundle branch blocks. *(Brady,*

Paramedic Care 2e, Principles and Practice, Volume 3—Cardiology. Mosby, Paramedic Textbook 3e, Cardiology.)

365. **The answer is C.** (A), (B), and (D) are incorrect. (C) is correct because there is a long pause of electrical activity before any P-wave activity appears. Significant electrical pauses may be related to a period of loss of consciousness. *(Brady, Paramedic Care 2e, Principles and Practice, Volume 3—Cardiology. Mosby, Paramedic Textbook 3e, Cardiology.)*

366. **The answer is A.** (A) is correct, with the realization that, if the patient's heart rate fails to respond to the maximal dose of atropine, then the Paramedic should consider applying a transcutaneous pacemaker. (B), (C), and (D) are incorrect. *(Brady, Paramedic Care 2e, Principles and Practice, Volume 3—Cardiology. Mosby, Paramedic Textbook 3e, Cardiology.)*

367. **The answer is D.** (D) is the correct immediate treatment for ventricular fibrillation and pulseless ventricular tachycardia. However, in monitored patients who go into ventricular fibrillation or pulseless ventricular tachycardia, performing a precordial thump is also an option. (A), (B), and (C) are incorrect. *(Brady, Paramedic Care 2e, Principles and Practice, Volume 3—Cardiology. Mosby, Paramedic Textbook 3e, Cardiology.)*

368. **The answer is D.** (A), (B), (C), repeat defibrillation, and possibly sodium bicarbonate are all part of the emergent treatment options available. *(Brady, Paramedic Care 2e, Principles and Practice, Volume 3—Cardiology. Mosby, Paramedic Textbook 3e, Cardiology.)*

369. **The answer is B.** (B) is correct. Since the ECG rhythm strip is sinus tachycardia with a rate of 130 per minute, there is no treatment for this. The first priority is to treat the patient's chest pain, with medical control approval, with sublingual nitroglycerin. (A), (C), and (D) are all incorrect treatments for sinus tachycardia. *(Brady, Paramedic Care 2e, Principles and Practice, Volume 3—Cardiology. Mosby, Paramedic Textbook 3e, Cardiology.)*

370. **The answer is A.** (A) is correct because the patient is symptomatic with chest pain and malignant PVCs. (B) is incorrect because it is used for more serious ventricular dysrhythmias, such as ventricular fibrillation and ventricular tachycardia, but not for PVCs alone. (C) and (D) are incorrect because neither is the treatment of choice for this patient. *(Brady, Paramedic Care 2e, Principles and Practice, Volume 3—Cardiology. Mosby, Paramedic Textbook 3e, Cardiology.)*

371. **The answer is D.** (D) is correct because, in patients with high-grade heart blocks, atropine (A) should be used with caution, as it may accelerate the atrial rate and worsen the AV nodal block. (B) and (C) are incorrect because they are not part of the treatment of second-degree, Mobitz type II, AV heart block. *(Brady, Paramedic Care 2e, Principles and Practice, Volume 3—Cardiology. Mosby, Paramedic Textbook 3e, Cardiology.)*

372. **The answer is D.** (D) is the correct answer, since this patient is in cardiac arrest, in the PEA algorithm. (A), (B), and (C) are incorrect. *(Brady, Paramedic Care 2e, Principles and Practice, Volume 3—Cardiology. Mosby, Paramedic Textbook 3e, Cardiology.)*

373. **The answer is C.** (C) is correct because IV calcium is an antidote for any calcium-channel blocker overdose. It could potentially return a pulse and blood pressure. (A), (B), and (D) are incorrect. *(Brady, Paramedic Care 2e, Principles and Practice, Volume 3—Cardiology. Mosby, Paramedic Textbook 3e, Cardiology.)*

374. **The answer is C.** (C) is correct because sinus bradycardia is very common in regular long-distance runners. This rhythm should only be treated in patients demonstrating decreased cardiac output, hypotension, angina, or central nervous system symptoms. (A), (B), and (D) are all incorrect in this patient. *(Brady, Paramedic Care 2e, Principles and Practice, Volume 3—Cardiology. Mosby, Paramedic Textbook 3e, Cardiology.)*

375. **The answer is A.** (B), (C), and (D) may be indications for transcutaneous pacing. (A) is not. *(Brady, Paramedic Care 2e, Principles and Practice, Volume 3—Cardiology. Mosby, Paramedic Textbook 3e, Cardiology.)*

376. **The answer is B.** (B) is the correct answer, and, after confirming asystole in more than one lead, the next step is the administration of IV epinephrine 1.0 mg, which can be repeated every 3–5 minutes. (A), (C), and (D) are incorrect and have no place in the treatment of asystole in the cardiac arrest patient. *(Brady, Paramedic Care 2e, Principles and Practice, Volume 3—Cardiology. Mosby, Paramedic Textbook 3e, Cardiology.)*

377. **The answer is A.** (B), (C), (D), and checking the pulse and blood pressure of the patient are all a part of the process of treating a patient with a transcutaneous pacemaker. (A) is incorrect because you should place the patient in the supine position. Explaining the procedure to the patient, administering oxygen, starting an IV line, and ECG monitoring, however are all part of the appropriate care as well. *(Brady, Paramedic Care 2e, Principles and Practice, Volume 3—Cardiology. Mosby, Paramedic Textbook 3e, Cardiology.)*

378. **The answer is D.** (A), (B), and (C) are correct and are examples of ECG manifestations of pacemaker failure. This is true for all types of pacemakers: permanent, temporary, transvenous, and transcutaneous. (D) is incorrect because, whenever the patient's own heart rate is faster than the rate of the pacemaker, there should be no evidence of pacemaker activity. This pacemaker function is known as sensing. *(Brady, Paramedic Care 2e, Principles and Practice, Volume 3— Cardiology. Mosby, Paramedic Textbook 3e, Cardiology.)*

379. **The answer is D.** (A), (B), (C), and failure to sense are all examples of pacemaker failure. (D) is incorrect. *(Brady, Paramedic Care 2e, Principles and Practice, Volume 3—Cardiology. Mosby, Paramedic Textbook 3e, Cardiology.)*

380. **The answer is C.** (A), (B), (D), male sex, diabetes, family history of premature heart disease or stroke, obesity, and lack of exercise are all risk factors. (C) is incorrect because a family history of peptic ulcer disease is unrelated to coronary artery disease. *(Brady, Paramedic Care 2e, Principles and Practice, Volume 3—Cardiology. Mosby, Paramedic Textbook 3e, Cardiology.)*

381. **The answer is A.** (A) is the correct description of the pathophysiology of angina pectoris. (B), (C), and (D) are incorrect. *(Brady, Paramedic Care*

2e, Principles and Practice, Volume 3—Cardiology. Mosby, Paramedic Textbook 3e, Cardiology.)

382. **The answer is D.** (D) is correct and may be accompanied by T-wave inversions. (A), (B), and (C) are incorrect. *(Brady, Paramedic Care 2e, Principles and Practice, Volume 3—Cardiology. Mosby, Paramedic Textbook 3e, Cardiology.)*

383. **The answer is C.** (C) is the correct answer. Most treatment protocols are directed toward the patient with ischemic chest pain, whether due to angina pectoris or an acute MI. (A), (B), and (D) are incorrect. *(Brady, Paramedic Care 2e, Principles and Practice, Volume 3—Cardiology. Mosby, Paramedic Textbook 3e, Cardiology.)*

384. **The answer is A.** (B), (C), (D), putting the patient at ease, putting the patient on a stretcher to rest, beginning an IV, and recording vital signs are the first priorities. (A) is incorrect because, after the first treatment priorities are completed, then a 12-lead ECG can be performed. *(Brady, Paramedic Care 2e, Principles and Practice, Volume 3—Cardiology. Mosby, Paramedic Textbook 3e, Cardiology.)*

385. **The answer is D.** (A), (B), (C), heart failure, cardiogenic shock, syncope, and nonlethal dysrhythmias are some of the complications of an acute MI. (B) is incorrect because skin rashes are unrelated to an acute MI. *(Brady, Paramedic Care 2e, Principles and Practice, Volume 3—Cardiology. Mosby, Paramedic Textbook 3e, Cardiology.)*

386. **The answer is A.** (A) is incorrect because 10–30% of acute MI patients do not have chest pain and are referred to as silent MIs. They may or may not complain of other associated symptoms, such as sweating, shortness of breath, and feeling of impending doom. *(Brady, Paramedic Care 2e, Principles and Practice, Volume 3—Cardiology. Mosby, Paramedic Textbook 3e, Cardiology.)*

387. **The answer is C.** (A); (B); (D); slow, normal, or fast heart rate; regular or irregular pulse rate; and weak or bounding pulse are all hemodynamic states in an acute MI. (C) is incorrect because, even though a normal or increased respiratory rate may be associated with an acute MI, it is not a hemodynamic parameter. *(Brady,*

Paramedic Care 2e, Principles and Practice, Volume 3—Cardiology. Mosby, Paramedic Textbook 3e, Cardiology.)

388. **The answer is A.** (B) is important for detecting hemodynamic changes, and (D) for any evidence of left-sided heart failure. (C) for detecting dysrhythmias, (D) for any evidence of left-sided heart failure. (A) is a useful sign for detecting dehydration but is not a significant parameter to be followed in a patient suffering an acute MI. *(Brady, Paramedic Care 2e, Principles and Practice, Volume 3—Cardiology. Mosby, Paramedic Textbook 3e, Cardiology.)*

389. **The answer is D.** (D) is correct because inverted P waves are not related to an acute MI. ST-segment depression and T-wave inversion may be early signs of an acute MI or just myocardial ischemia. ST-segment elevation is almost always due to acute myocardial injury from an acute MI, but, rarely, coronary artery vasospasm may produce this change as well. (A), (B), (C), tall peaked T waves, and Q waves may all be evolutionary ECG changes seen in an acute MI. *(Brady, Paramedic Care 2e, Principles and Practice, Volume 3—Cardiology. Mosby, Paramedic Textbook 3e, Cardiology.)*

390. **The answer is C.** (A), (B), (D), ventricular aneurysm and coronary artery vasospasm (Prinzmetal's angina) produce ST-segment elevation not due to an acute MI. (C) is incorrect because digoxin toxicity may produce various dysrhythmias but not ST-segment elevation. *(Brady, Paramedic Care 2e, Principles and Practice, Volume 3—Cardiology. Mosby, Paramedic Textbook 3e, Cardiology.)*

391. **The answer is A.** (B), (C), (D), and the patient's being alert and able to give informed consent are all inclusion criteria for thrombolytic therapy. (A) is incorrect because age under 75 years is the correct inclusion criterion. *(Mosby, Paramedic Textbook 3e, Cardiology.)*

392. **The answer is D.** (D) is correct because, with trauma within 2–4 weeks, he is excluded from being treated with thrombolytic therapy. Other exclusion criteria are oral anticoagulants or bleeding disorder, major surgery within 3 weeks,

CPR in progress, uncontrolled high blood pressure, terminal illness, internal bleeding, stroke or intracranial bleeding, intracranial tumor, suspected aortic dissection, thoracic aortic aneurysm, and pregnancy or postpartum state. (A), (B), and (C) are incorrect because this patient shows no evidence of having these exclusion criteria. *(Mosby, Paramedic Textbook 3e, Cardiology.)*

393. **The answer is B.** (B) is correct and is often accompanied by implanting a coronary artery stent in order to keep the previously obstructed coronary artery open. (A), (C), and (D) are incorrect. *(Brady, Paramedic Care 2e, Principles and Practice, Volume 3—Cardiology. Mosby, Paramedic Textbook 3e, Cardiology.)*

394. **The answers are: (A)** 3, **(B)** 6, **(C)** 4, **(D)** 7, **(E)** 5, **(F)** 2, **(G)** 8, **(H)** 1. *(Brady, Paramedic Care 2e, Principles and Practice, Volume 3—Cardiology. Mosby, Paramedic Textbook 3e, Cardiology.)*

395. **The answers are: (A)** 5, **(B)** 3, **(C)** 1, **(D)** 4, **(E)** 2. *(Brady, Paramedic Care 2e, Principles and Practice, Volume 3—Cardiology. Mosby, Paramedic Textbook 3e, Cardiology.)*

396. **The answer is B.** (A), (B), (D), dysrhythmias, and valvular heart disease are all causes of left ventricular congestive heart failure. (B) is incorrect because advanced COPD eventually may result in pulmonary artery hypertension, which may result in right, not left, ventricular heart failure. *(Brady, Paramedic Care 2e, Principles and Practice, Volume 3—Cardiology. Mosby, Paramedic Textbook 3e, Cardiology.)*

397. **The answer is B.** (A), (C), (D), confusion, agitation, and diaphoresis are all symptoms of left ventricular heart failure. (B) is incorrect because headache is not related to left ventricular heart failure. *(Brady, Paramedic Care 2e, Principles and Practice, Volume 3—Cardiology. Mosby, Paramedic Textbook 3e, Cardiology.)*

398. **The answer is C.** (A), (B), and (D) are all signs of acute pulmonary edema due to acute left ventricular heart failure. (C) is incorrect because absent pulses are not considered a sign of acute pulmonary edema. *(Brady, Paramedic Care 2e,*

Principles and Practice, Volume 3—Cardiology. Mosby, Paramedic Textbook 3e, Cardiology.)

399. **The answer is A.** (B), (C), and (D) are possible causes of precipitating pulmonary edema. (A) is incorrect because strep throat will not precipitate acute pulmonary edema. *(Brady, Paramedic Care 2e, Principles and Practice, Volume 3—Cardiology. Mosby, Paramedic Textbook 3e, Cardiology.)*

400. **The answer is D.** (A), (B), and (C) are all a part of the emergent treatment of a patient with acute pulmonary edema. (D) is a correct drug for the treatment of acute pulmonary edema as well; however, the dosage is usually 20–40 mg, not 5 mg, IV bolus. *(Brady, Paramedic Care 2e, Principles and Practice, Volume 3—Cardiology. Mosby, Paramedic Textbook 3e, Cardiology.)*

401. **The answer is D.** (D) is correct because morphine results in less blood returning to the fluid-overloaded failing heart. (A), (B), and (C) are also actions of morphine but are not of prime importance. *(Brady, Paramedic Care 2e, Principles and Practice, Volume 3—Cardiology. Mosby, Paramedic Textbook 3e, Cardiology.)*

402. **The answer is B.** (B) is the correct definition of cardiac tamponade. (A) and (D) are incorrect because, with cardiac tamponade, as blood fills the pericardium, the coronary arteries and aortic and mitral valves are usually not directly affected. (C) is incorrect because, with cardiac tamponade, the blood pressure usually decreases dramatically. *(Brady, Paramedic Care 2e, Principles and Practice, Volume 3—Cardiology. Mosby, Paramedic Textbook 3e, Cardiology.)*

403. **The answer is B.** (A), (C), (D), narrowed pulse pressure, pulsus paradoxicus, and pale, cool, clammy skin are all clinical signs of cardiac tamponade. (B) is incorrect because one of the classic signs of cardiac tamponade is the presence of "muffled" heart sounds, not clear crisp heart sounds. *(Brady, Paramedic Care 2e, Principles and Practice, Volume 3—Cardiology. Mosby, Paramedic Textbook 3e, Cardiology.)*

404. **The answer is D.** (D) is the correct answer because diabetes is unrelated to hypertension.

(A), (B), (C), renal failure, aortic dissection, toxemia of pregnancy, strokes, and intracranial hemorrhage are all examples of end-organ damage, which may be part of the presentation of a hypertensive emergency. *(Brady, Paramedic Care 2e, Principles and Practice, Volume 3—Cardiology. Mosby, Paramedic Textbook 3e, Cardiology.)*

405. **The answer is B.** (A), (C), (D) and sodium nitroprusside are all treatment options available for the prehospital treatment of a hypertensive emergency; however, they usually require prior medical control approval. (B) is incorrect because dilantin is not a part of the treatment of hypertensive emergencies, but is frequently used for treatment of status epilepticus. *(Brady, Paramedic Care 2e, Principles and Practice, Volume 3—Cardiology. Mosby, Paramedic Textbook 3e, Cardiology.)*

406. **The answer is C.** (A), (B), (D), pulmonary congestion, hypoxemia, acidosis, and altered mental status are all signs of cardiogenic shock. (C) is incorrect because marked hypotension, not hypertension, is a sign of cardiogenic shock. *(Brady, Paramedic Care 2e, Principles and Practice, Volume 3—Cardiology. Mosby, Paramedic Textbook 3e, Cardiology.)*

407. **The answer is C.** (C) is correct and then titrate the dose up as needed. Most prehospital protocols recommend dopamine over norepinephrine and other vasopressors because its initial doses maintain renal perfusion, unlike most other agents. (A) is incorrect because, even though it is an agent frequently used for cardiogenic shock patients, it is not felt to be the best initial option. (B) is a medication frequently used for treating patients with hypertensive emergencies and does not have a role in the treatment of cardiogenic shock. (D) is incorrect because the use of pneumatic military antishock trousers (MAST) in cardiogenic shock is truly controversial and is contraindicated if the patient also has acute pulmonary edema. *(Brady, Paramedic Care 2e, Principles and Practice, Volume 3—Cardiology. Mosby, Paramedic Textbook 3e, Cardiology.)*

408. **The answer is A.** (B), (C), and (D) are correct. (A) is incorrect because acute pericarditis causes acute chest pain, sometimes tachydysrhythmias, but not cardiogenic shock. Only if acute pericarditis was accompanied by a large pericardial effusion which could deteriorate into pericardial tamponade, it could result in cardiogenic shock. The cardiogenic shock would be caused by the pericardial tamponade not by acute pericarditis. *(Brady, Paramedic Care 2e, Principles and Practice, Volume 3—Cardiology. Mosby, Paramedic Textbook 3e, Cardiology.)*

409. **The answer is B.** (A), (C), (D), drowning, major trauma, angina, dysrhythmias, and electrocution are some of the emergent conditions that may progress to cardiac arrest. (B) is incorrect because the viral flu syndrome does not usually progress to cardiac arrest. *(Brady, Paramedic Care 2e, Principles and Practice, Volume 3—Cardiology. Mosby, Paramedic Textbook 3e, Cardiology.)*

410. **The answer is C.** (A), (B), (D), and ventricular tachycardia without a pulse are the most common conditions associated with the cardiac arrest patient. (C) is associated with taking digoxin and sometimes with an acute MI. *(Brady, Paramedic Care 2e, Principles and Practice, Volume 3—Cardiology. Mosby, Paramedic Textbook 3e, Cardiology.)*

411. **The answer is D.** (D) is correct because, in the cardiac arrest patient, you immediately need to know the type of cardiac rhythm, so that you can institute the correct cardiac arrest treatment protocol. (A) is incorrect because the patient is apneic and would not benefit at all from an oxygen mask, nor from (B) because assessing the need for defibrillation is the first priority. (C) is incorrect, because IV dextrose is indicated in the treatment of the unconscious patient, but not in the initial treatment of the cardiac arrest patient. *(Brady, Paramedic Care 2e, Principles and Practice, Volume 3—Cardiology. Mosby, Paramedic Textbook 3e, Cardiology.)*

412. **The answer is C.** (A), (B), (D), hypoxia, hypothermia, massive pulmonary embolism, drug overdose, hyperkalemia, acidosis, and massive MI are all potentially correctable causes of PEA. (A) is incorrect because bronchitis is an acute infection of the pulmonary bronchial tissue and unrelated to cardiac arrest and PEA. *(Brady, Paramedic Care 2e, Principles and Practice, Volume 3—Cardiology. Mosby, Paramedic Textbook 3e, Cardiology.)*

413. **The answers are:** (A) 3 or 5, (B) 2, (C) 3 or 5, (D) 4, (E) 1, (F) 6. *(Brady, Paramedic Care 2e, Principles and Practice, Volume 3—Cardiology. Mosby, Paramedic Textbook 3e, Cardiology.)*

414. **The answer is C.** (A), (B), (D), and starting CPR are all critical actions in caring for the cardiac arrest patient. (C) is incorrect because IV calcium is no longer considered useful in the management of the cardiac arrest patient in most cardiac arrest prehospital protocols. However, the use of IV calcium is still believed to be indicated in the cardiac arrest patient with hypocalcemia or with a calcium-blocker medication overdose. *(Brady, Paramedic Care 2e, Principles and Practice, Volume 3—Cardiology. Mosby, Paramedic Textbook 3e, Cardiology.)*

415. **The answer is A.** (B), (C), and (D) are accepted criteria for terminating resuscitative efforts. However, it is very important for you to be aware of your state and local laws, as well as medical direction guidelines, pertaining to this topic. *(Brady, Paramedic Care 2e, Principles and Practice, Volume 3—Cardiology. Mosby, Paramedic Textbook 3e, Cardiology.)*

416. **The answer is A.** (A) is correct. (B) is incorrect because acute phlebitis, also known as deep-vein thrombosis, usually presents as a hot, red, swollen leg with good motion and normal arterial pulses. (C) is incorrect because acute cellulitis usually presents similarly to acute phlebitis. (D) is incorrect because acute arthritis presents with a hot, swollen, tender joint. *(Brady, Paramedic Care 2e, Principles and Practice, Volume 3—Cardiology. Mosby, Paramedic Textbook 3e, Cardiology.)*

417. **The answer is B.** (B) is correct. While this patient may have presented with any of the four rhythms, atrial fibrillation is the only rhythm that is known, over time, to produce thrombus in the atria, which could embolize to an extremity or the brain, resulting in an acute arterial occlusion. (A), (C), and (D) are incorrect because they are not causes of arterial occlusion. *(Brady, Paramedic Care 2e, Principles and Practice, Volume 3—Cardiology. Mosby, Paramedic Textbook 3e, Cardiology.)*

418. **The answer is B.** (B) is correct and usually occurs in an artery. (A) is incorrect because the aneurysm may or may not result in a blocking of a vessel. (C) is incorrect because, even though it may be congenital, it affects the wall of any vessel, not just a vein. (D) is incorrect because an aneurysm is not defined by any curvature of a vessel. *(Brady, Paramedic Care 2e, Principles and Practice, Volume 3—Cardiology. Mosby, Paramedic Textbook 3e, Cardiology.)*

419. **The answer is A.** (A) is correct and is usually intermittent, associated with walking a certain distance and relieved with rest. It is caused by atherosclerosis and results in arterial narrowing to a leg. (B), (C) and (D) are incorrect. *(Brady, Paramedic Care 2e, Principles and Practice, Volume 3—Cardiology. Mosby, Paramedic Textbook 3e, Cardiology.)*

420. **The answer is A.** (B), (C), (D), infectious, and dissecting are types of aneurysms. (A) is incorrect because sometimes aneurysms may produce thrombus, which may on occasion embolize downstream to an artery, but this is not a type of aneurysm. *(Brady, Paramedic Care 2e, Principles and Practice, Volume 3—Cardiology. Mosby, Paramedic Textbook 3e, Cardiology.)*

421. **The answer is D.** (D) is correct because of the ripping quality and the migratory location of the chest pain, but also because of the inequality of the arterial pulses and/or blood pressures in the upper extremities. As the thoracic aorta dissects, the opening to the aortic branches may be sheared off or significantly narrowed, resulting in a significant reduction in arterial blood flow to that affected artery. (A) is incorrect because although an acute gallbladder attack may produce substernal and epigastric pain, it is not associated with varying blood pressures in bilateral arms and does not have a ripping quality. (B) is incorrect because, although the patient had substernal chest pain, it is usually not ripping in quality and usually does not migrate to another area, and usually any effect on the circulation is symmetrical. (C) is incorrect because an arterial occlusion is usually not associated with chest pain. *(Brady, Paramedic Care 2e, Principles and Practice, Volume 3—Cardiology. Mosby, Paramedic Textbook 3e, Cardiology.)*

422. **The answer is D.** (D) is correct. (A) and (B) are incorrect because, while the patient may have severe acute abdominal pain with each, it is usually not with severe hypotension and never with a pulsatile mass. (C) is incorrect because, while the patient may have abdominal pain and a large abdominal mass, which is a distended urinary bladder, it is not pulsatile and is not associated with hypotension. *(Brady, Paramedic Care 2e, Principles and Practice, Volume 3—Cardiology. Mosby, Paramedic Textbook 3e, Cardiology.)*

423. **The answer is C.** (A), (B), (D), and rapid transport are parts of the emergent care of a patient with an abdominal aortic aneurysm. (C) is incorrect because the hypotensive patient may actually have a leaking or a contained rupture of the abdominal aortic aneurysm, and rapid transport is the first priority. The aneurysm needs to be immediately surgically repaired before it fully ruptures, which may result in hemorrhagic shock and/or cardiac arrest. *(Brady, Paramedic Care 2e, Principles and Practice, Volume 3—Cardiology. Mosby, Paramedic Textbook 3e, Cardiology.)*

424. **The answer is A.** (B), (C), (D), obesity, and lack of exercise are all modifiable risk factors for cardiovascular disease. (A), sex, advanced age, and diabetes are nonmodifiable risk factors. However, there is an opinion that good control of diabetes may reduce the risk as well. *(Brady, Paramedic Care 2e, Principles and Practice, Volume 3—Cardiology. Mosby, Paramedic Textbook 3e, Cardiology.)*

425. **The answers are:** (A) 1, (B) 2, (C) 1, (D) 3, (E) 2. *(Brady, Paramedic Care 2e, Principles and Practice, Volume 3—Cardiology. Mosby, Paramedic Textbook 3e, Cardiology.)*

426. **The answer is C.** (C) is correct. (A), (B), and (D) are incorrect. *(Brady, Paramedic Care 2e, Principles and Practice, Volume 3—Cardiology. Mosby, Paramedic Textbook 3e, Cardiology.)*

427. **The answer is B.** (B) is correct with ST-segment elevations in leads V_1-V_6, I, and AVL. (A), (C), and (D) are incorrect. *(Brady, Paramedic Care 2e, Principles and Practice, Volume 3—Cardiology. Mosby, Paramedic Textbook 3e, Cardiology.)*

428. The answer is D. (D) is correct because the 12-lead ECG demonstrates an acute inferior wall MI. Since the right coronary artery supplies the blood to both the inferior wall of the left ventricle and the right ventricle, when there is an acute occlusion (thrombosis) in the right coronary artery, the result is usually an acute inferior wall MI and it occasionally is accompanied by a right ventricular MI as well. (A), (B), and (C) are incorrect. *(Brady, Paramedic Care 2e, Principles and Practice, Volume 3—Cardiology. Mosby, Paramedic Textbook 3e, Cardiology.)*

429. The answers are: (A) 4, **(B)** 2, **(C)** 1, **(D)** 3. *(Brady, Paramedic Care 2e, Principles and Practice, Volume 3—Cardiology.)*

430. The answers are: (A) 2, **(B)** 3, **(C)** 4, **(D)** 1. *(Brady, Paramedic Care 2e, Principles and Practice, Volume 3—Cardiology.)*

MEDICAL NEUROLOGY

431. The answer is A. (A) is correct because changes in the intravascular protein concentration can affect the overall health of all patients but are not often causes of neurologic emergencies. (B) from any traumatic injury to the brain or from a growing brain tumor may increase intracranial pressure and produce a neurologic emergency. (C) Circulatory changes, such as acute cerebrovascular accident or shock of multiple etiologies, are examples of neurologic emergencies. (D), in the form of a penetrating or nonpenetrating trauma, is an example of a neurologic emergency. *(Brady, Paramedic Care 2e, Principles and Practice, Volume 3—Neurology. Mosby, Paramedic Textbook 3e, Neurology.)*

432. The answer is A. (A) is the reason that any increase in intracranial volume results in a significant increase in intracranial pressure. (B), (C), and (D) are incorrect. *(Brady, Paramedic Care 2e, Principles and Practice, Volume 3—Neurology. Mosby, Paramedic Textbook 3e, Neurology.)*

433. The answer is A. (B), (C), and (D) are parts of the primary survey and are the first priority for the treatment of nontraumatic neurologic emergencies. (A) is incorrect because baseline blood work will be helpful but is of little use in the prehospital setting and certainly is not as important as the ABCs. *(Brady, Paramedic Care 2e, Principles and Practice, Volume 3—Neurology. Mosby, Paramedic Textbook 3e, Neurology.)*

434. The answer is D. (A), (B), (C), disorientation, and strange behavior are some examples of patients presenting with an altered mental status. (D) is not an example of a patient with an altered mental status. *(Brady, Paramedic Care 2e, Principles and Practice, Volume 3—Neurology. Mosby, Paramedic Textbook 3e, Neurology.)*

435. The answer is B. (A), (C), and (D) are all part of the pneumonic AEIOU TIPS, which outlines some of the most common causes of coma: A = alcohol or acidosis; E = epilepsy, electrolyte abnormality, or endocrine problem; I = insulin (hypoglycemia); O = overdose; U = uremia; T = trauma or temperature abnormality; I = infection (meningitis); P = psychogenic; S = stroke or space-occupying cerebral lesion. (B) is incorrect because, while antibiotics might produce certain side effects and toxic effects, they are not associated with causing coma. *(Brady, Paramedic Care 2e, Principles and Practice, Volume 3—Neurology. Mosby, Paramedic Textbook 3e, Neurology.)*

436. The answer is B. (A) is important in determining any focal abnormality. (C) is important, since unilateral dilation of a pupil implies pressure on the third cranial nerve, while bilateral midsized pupils are suggestive of a midbrain lesion, and pinpoint pupils may be caused by a lesion in the pons. (D) is important because dysconjugate gaze (eyes looking in different directions) at rest implies a structural brainstem injury. (B) is incorrect because, other than looking for the presence of blood or cerebrospinal fluid in nasal discharge in the head trauma patient, the evaluation of nasal discharge is not important in the comatose patient. *(Brady, Paramedic Care 2e, Principles and Practice, Volume 3—Neurology. Mosby, Paramedic Textbook 3e, Neurology.)*

437. The answer is C. (A), (B), and (D) are parts of the emergent management of the patient with an altered mental status. (C) is incorrect because, if increased intracranial pressure is suspected, hyperventilation will result in lowering the carbon dioxide level in the blood, which will result in cerebral vasoconstriction and will minimize brain swelling. *(Brady, Paramedic Care 2e, Principles and Practice, Volume 3—Neurology. Mosby, Paramedic Textbook 3e, Neurology.)*

438. **The answer is B.** (B) is the correct definition. (A) is incorrect because a seizure is temporary, not permanent. (C) is incorrect because epileptic seizures are not caused by emotional upset. (D) is incorrect because the definition of seizure is unrelated to a cardiac dysrhythmia. *(Brady, Paramedic Care 2e, Principles and Practice, Volume 3—Neurology. Mosby, Paramedic Textbook 3e, Neurology.)*

439. **The answer is D.** (D) is correct because it is accepted as the most common cause of seizures. (A), (B), (C), hypoxia, hypoglycemia, toxins, drugs, drug withdrawal, eclampsia of pregnancy, and idiopathic (unknown cause) are all causes of seizures, but not the most common cause. *(Brady, Paramedic Care 2e, Principles and Practice, Volume 3—Neurology. Mosby, Paramedic Textbook 3e, Neurology.)*

440. **The answer is D.** (D) is correct because there is no such entity as an allergic seizure. (A), (B), (C), and psychomotor are all types of true seizures. Hysterical seizures are demonstrated by patients with psychologic problems. *(Brady, Paramedic Care 2e, Principles and Practice, Volume 3—Neurology. Mosby, Paramedic Textbook 3e, Neurology.)*

441. **The answer is B.** (A); (C); (D); examine the mouth for any evidence of mouth trauma; examine for neck rigidity; examine the extremities for any signs of trauma, medication bracelets, or needle tracks; and examine the patient's clothes and possessions for any evidence of medication vials. (B) is incorrect because leg swelling is usually unrelated to seizures. *(Brady, Paramedic Care 2e, Principles and Practice, Volume 3—Neurology. Mosby, Paramedic Textbook 3e, Neurology.)*

442. **The answer is A.** (B), loss of consciousness, tonic phase, hypertonic phase, (C), postseizure, and (D) are all phases of a generalized, grand mal seizure. (A) is not a phase. *(Brady, Paramedic Care 2e, Principles and Practice, Volume 3—Neurology. Mosby, Paramedic Textbook 3e, Neurology.)*

443. **The answer is A.** (B), (C), (D), administering high-concentration oxygen, and administering 25 g of 50% dextrose are all parts of the treatment of status epilepticus. (C) is incorrect because the correct dosage of 50% dextrose is 25 g, not 100 g. *(Brady, Paramedic Care 2e, Principles and Practice, Volume 3—Neurology. Mosby, Paramedic Textbook 3e, Neurology.)*

444. **The answer is D.** (A) may be suggestive of a cerebrovascular accident or intracerebral (B) may reveal a dramatically rapid or slow pulse, which may be responsible for syncope. (C) may reveal a 20-mmHg drop in systolic blood pressure, associated with a 20 beats per minute increase in pulse rate, which would be diagnostic of postural hypotension. This is associated with hypovolemia from any possible cause, such as recurrent vomiting or diarrhea, bleeding from any source, or use of diuretics. (D) is incorrect because thickening of her toe nails does not provide evidence for a particular cause of syncope. *(Brady, Paramedic Care 2e, Principles and Practice, Volume 3—Neurology. Mosby, Paramedic Textbook 3e, Neurology.)*

445. **The answers are:** (A) 3, (B) 5, (C) 1, (D) 4, (E) 2. While 3 could also be the answer for (C), 1 could not be the answer for (A). *(Brady, Paramedic Care 2e, Principles and Practice, Volume 3—Neurology. Mosby, Paramedic Textbook 3e, Neurology.)*

446. **The answer is D.** (A), (B), (C), transporting the patient in the position of comfort, and treating any specific causes of syncope as well, for example, IV 50% dextrose for hypoglycemia are appropriate prehospital management. (D) is incorrect because a patient with syncope should be transported to the ED in order to determine whether the cause is benign or of a serious nature. *(Brady, Paramedic Care 2e, Principles and Practice, Volume 3—Neurology. Mosby, Paramedic Textbook 3e, Neurology.)*

447. **The answer is D.** (A) is suggestive of possible meningitis (infection of the spinal fluid) until proven otherwise. (B) is always worrisome because one of the potentially most serious

clinical presentations in such patients is an acute intracerebral hemorrhage, resulting in a critical neurologic injury. (C) is strongly suggestive of a structural lesion in the brain, such as a cerebrovascular accident, intracerebral hemorrhage, subdural or epidural hematoma, and so on. (D) is incorrect because these symptoms are suggestive of acute sinusitis that is usually not serious or life threatening. *(Brady, Paramedic Care 2e, Principles and Practice, Volume 3—Neurology. Mosby, Paramedic Textbook 3e, Neurology.)*

448. **The answers are: (A)** 5, **(B)** 1, **(C)** 6, **(D)** 2, **(E)** 7, **(F)** 4, **(G)** 3. *(Brady, Paramedic Care 2e, Principles and Practice, Volume 3—Neurology. Mosby, Paramedic Textbook 3e, Neurology.)*

449. **The answer is C.** (C) is correct, and these changes may also be associated with a recurrent headache. (A) is often the presentation of an intracerebral or subarachnoid hemorrhage. (B) is suspicious for meningitis. (D) is a presentation of acute sinusitis. *(Brady, Paramedic Care 2e, Principles and Practice, Volume 3—Neurology. Mosby, Paramedic Textbook 3e, Neurology.)*

450. **The answer is D.** (D) is correct, since the malignant tumor lies on the right side of the patient's brain and would be expected to produce left-sided weakness. These findings are the same as for an acute cerebrovascular accident on the right side of the brain. (A), (B), and (C) are incorrect. *(Brady, Paramedic Care 2e, Principles and Practice, Volume 3—Neurology. Mosby, Paramedic Textbook 3e, Neurology.)*

451. **The answer is D.** (A) is suggestive of increased intracranial pressure and possible irreversible brain damage. (B) is usually a sign of intracranial bleeding or swelling. (C) is also a sign of an acute medical emergency that may be life threatening. (D) is incorrect because the most common cause of memory deficit is chronic dementia, often from Alzheimer disease or multiple cerebral infarcts. *(Brady, Paramedic Care 2e, Principles and Practice, Volume 3—Neurology. Mosby, Paramedic Textbook 3e, Neurology.)*

452. **The answer is A.** (B) is known for its abrupt onset. (C) is responsible for 60% of all strokes

and is due to atherosclerosis. (D) actually is representative of intracerebral hemorrhage and subarachnoid hemorrhage.(A) is incorrect because, while many malignancies metastasize (spread) to the brain, this mechanism has nothing to do with strokes. *(Brady, Paramedic Care 2e, Principles and Practice, Volume 3—Neurology. Mosby, Paramedic Textbook 3e, Neurology.)*

453. **The answer is D.** (D) is the correct explanation for the cause of the stroke. (A), (B), and (C) are all possible causes of neurologic injury but are not known to produce a stroke. *(Brady, Paramedic Care 2e, Principles and Practice, Volume 3—Neurology. Mosby, Paramedic Textbook 3e, Neurology.)*

454. **The answer is B.** (A), (C), (D), seizures, coma, inappropriate affect, expressive and/or receptive aphasia, dysarthria, irregular pulse, staggering gait, and stiff neck are all possible findings due to a stroke. (B) is unrelated to a stroke. *(Brady, Paramedic Care 2e, Principles and Practice, Volume 3—Neurology. Mosby, Paramedic Textbook 3e, Neurology.)*

455. **The answer is D.** (A), (B), and (C) are correct. (D) is incorrect because a history of cancer is unrelated to an acute stroke. *(Brady, Paramedic Care 2e, Principles and Practice, Volume 3—Neurology. Mosby, Paramedic Textbook 3e, Neurology.)*

456. **The answer is A.** (A) is correct. This presentation is classic for a subarachnoid hemorrhage, which is due to a ruptured cerebral aneurysm. (B) is incorrect because a brain tumor usually causes a very slow and gradual deterioration of mental and physical functioning over months. (C) is incorrect because a thrombosed cerebral vessel usually presents with focal neurologic abnormalities and also causes a slowly progressive deterioration of functions, not abrupt changes, as in this patient. (D) is incorrect because a syncopal episode actually represents an acute loss of consciousness only. *(Brady, Paramedic Care 2e, Principles and Practice, Volume 3—Neurology. Mosby, Paramedic Textbook 3e, Neurology.)*

457. **The answer is D.** (A), (B), and (C) are correct treatment of the patient with an acute ischemic or hemorrhagic stroke. (D) is incorrect because, in the presence of an acute ischemic stroke, the

abrupt lowering of the blood pressure may be dangerous and may actually increase the amount of brain damage. *(Brady, Paramedic Care 2e, Principles and Practice, Volume 3—Neurology. Mosby, Paramedic Textbook 3e, Neurology.)*

458. **The answer is C.** (A) is correct because hypoglycemia may produce an altered mental status sometimes associated with focal neurologic abnormalities. (B) is correct because hyperventilation will produce vasoconstriction of intracerebral blood vessels, which will result in lowering of intracerebral pressure. (D) is correct because the stroke victim, without a gag reflex, is at increased risk of aspiration. Placing the patient on her side will reduce the chance of aspiration. (C) is incorrect because, in the acute stroke victim who is awake, you would try to avoid endotracheal intubation because the attempt may actually cause an increase in intracerebral pressure. *(Brady, Paramedic Care 2e, Principles and Practice, Volume 3—Neurology. Mosby, Paramedic Textbook 3e, Neurology.)*

459. **The answer is C.** (C) is the correct amount of time within which there is total resolution of symptoms, without any residual neurologic deficits. *(Brady, Paramedic Care 2e, Principles and Practice, Volume 3—Neurology. Mosby, Paramedic Textbook 3e, Neurology.)*

460. **The answer is A.** (A) is correct because, usually within 2 years, a patient with a transient ischemic attack will have an acute stroke. (B), (C), and (D) are all unrelated to the patient experiencing a transient ischemic attack. *(Brady, Paramedic Care 2e, Principles and Practice, Volume 3—Neurology. Mosby, Paramedic Textbook 3e, Neurology.)*

461. **The answer is B.** (A), (C), (D), assuring patient safety, hyperventilation if the patient is unconscious, drawing a blood sample or finger-stick glucose determination, protecting paralyzed limbs, patient reassurance, and transport without excessive movement are part of the treatment of both a transient ischemic attack and an acute cerebrovascular accident. The treatment is primarily supportive. (B) is incorrect because, in a thrombotic transient ischemic attack or cerebrovascular accident, any decrease in the blood

pressure may be dangerous and may actually result in worsening of the deficit. *(Brady, Paramedic Care 2e, Principles and Practice, Volume 3—Neurology. Mosby, Paramedic Textbook 3e, Neurology.)*

462. **The answer is D.** (A), (B), (C), hemiplegia, hemiparesis, difficulty in swallowing, aphasia, and dizziness are some examples of symptoms or signs of transient ischemic attacks. (D) is incorrect. *(Brady, Paramedic Care 2e, Principles and Practice, Volume 3—Neurology. Mosby, Paramedic Textbook 3e, Neurology.)*

463. **The answer is C.** (C) is the correct answer, because Bell's palsy is caused by an inflammation of the seventh (7th) cranial nerve, the facial nerve. (A) and (B) are incorrect because a stroke and a transient ischemic attack are usually associated with some focal weakness of the upper and/or lower extremity and without a loss of the forehead wrinkling. (D) is incorrect because sciatica usually presents as acute low back pain which radiates down to one of the legs. *(Brady, Paramedic Care 2e, Principles and Practice, Volume 3—Neurology. Mosby, Paramedic Textbook 3e, Neurology.)*

ENDOCRINOLOGY

464. **The answer is A.** Diabetes mellitus is characterized by decreased secretion of insulin by the pancreas. As a result, blood glucose is unable to enter the cells of the body and builds up in the blood. *(Brady, Paramedic Care 2e, Principles and Practice, Volume 3—Endocrinology. Mosby, Paramedic Textbook 3e, Endocrinology.)*

465. **The answer is B.** (A), (C), and (D) are all characteristics of type I diabetes mellitus. (B) is incorrect because, in type I diabetes mellitus, the patient often presents with dehydration rather than overhydration. *(Brady, Paramedic Care 2e, Principles and Practice, Volume 3—Endocrinology. Mosby, Paramedic Textbook 3e, Endocrinology.)*

466. **The answer is B.** (B) is the manner in which dehydration develops in the type I diabetic patient. (A) is incorrect because an elevated blood sugar level does not routinely produce coma. (C) is incorrect because diabetes does not produce acute kidney damage. Any kidney damage that may occur is a slow, chronic process. (D) is incorrect because an elevated blood sugar level does not always produce a urinary tract infection. Even if a urinary tract infection develops, urinary frequency does not cause dehydration. *(Brady, Paramedic Care 2e, Principles and Practice, Volume 3—Endocrinology. Mosby, Paramedic Textbook 3e, Endocrinology.)*

467. **The answer is C.** (C) is correct because the patient has not been taking his insulin and is dehydrated and hypotensive. After ensuring the airway and breathing and assessing the circulation, the first priority is to provide IV fluid replacement for the dehydrated patient. (A) is incorrect because routine administration of intravenous insulin is not a part of prehospital protocols. However, if there was some reason for a delay in transport, medical control may give you permission to help administer the patient's own insulin. Nevertheless, the dose would never be as much as 20 units IV. Finally, in the acute treatment of uncontrolled diabetes, regular (short-acting) insulin is used, not NPH (long-acting) insulin. (B) and (D) have no place in the initial treatment of an acute diabetic emergency. *(Brady, Paramedic Care 2e, Principles and Practice, Volume 3—Endocrinology. Mosby, Paramedic Textbook 3e, Endocrinology.)*

468. **The answer is D.** (D) is correct because all diabetic patients with severely altered mental status need to have IV glucose administration because of the possibility of hypoglycemia causing an altered mental status. (A) is incorrect because IV glucose is the first priority; then IV 0.9% normal saline solution may be administered. (B) and (C) are not appropriate. *(Brady, Paramedic Care 2e, Principles and Practice, Volume 3—Endocrinology. Mosby, Paramedic Textbook 3e, Endocrinology.)*

469. **The answer is B.** (A), (C), and (D) are all correct. (B) is incorrect because the increased blood sugar levels in type II diabetes mellitus usually occur when obesity causes a decrease in the number of insulin receptors, which become defective and less responsive to insulin. *(Brady, Paramedic Care 2e, Principles and Practice,*

Volume 3—Endocrinology. Mosby, Paramedic Textbook 3e, Endocrinology.)

470. **The answer is A.** (B), (C), and (D) are correct. (A) is incorrect because these are classic symptoms for hyperglycemia (elevated blood sugar) due to diabetes and are unrelated to hypoglycemia. *(Brady, Paramedic Care 2e, Principles and Practice, Volume 3—Endocrinology. Mosby, Paramedic Textbook 3e, Endocrinology.)*

471. **The answer is C.** (A), (B), (D), peripheral neuropathy, and autonomic neuropathy are some of the potential long-term complications of diabetes mellitus. (C) is incorrect because it is unrelated to diabetes and is frequently related to chronic heavy cigarette smoking. *(Brady, Paramedic Care 2e, Principles and Practice, Volume 3—Endocrinology. Mosby, Paramedic Textbook 3e, Endocrinology.)*

472. **The answer is C.** (A), (B), and (D) are correct. (C) is incorrect because an increased intake of carbohydrates usually results in an increase in blood sugar (hyperglycemia) rather than a decrease (hypoglycemia). *(Brady, Paramedic Care 2e, Principles and Practice, Volume 3—Endocrinology. Mosby, Paramedic Textbook 3e, Endocrinology.)*

473. **The answer is A.** (B), (C), (D), and sometimes fever are common signs of diabetic ketoacidosis. (A) is incorrect because classically, in diabetic ketoacidosis, a lack of insulin produces a very high level of blood sugar, which cannot be used by the cells of the body for energy. As a result, the body attempts to compensate by breaking down fats, which generates a large amount of acids and ketones. This results in a severe metabolic acidosis, which the body attempts to compensate for by increasing the respiratory rate and the depth of respirations. This physical finding is known as Kussmaul's respirations and is the body's attempt to blow off carbon dioxide in order to correct the severe metabolic acidosis. *(Brady, Paramedic Care 2e, Principles and Practice, Volume 3—Endocrinology. Mosby, Paramedic Textbook 3e, Endocrinology.)*

474. **The answer is B.** (A), (C), and (D) are common symptoms of patients in diabetic ketoacidosis. Sometimes the severity of the abdominal pain

is mistaken for an acute abdomen, and the patient is considered for an acute laparotomy. As the diabetic ketoacidosis is corrected, the nausea, vomiting, and abdominal pain gradually subside. (B) is incorrect because skin moles are not associated with diabetic ketoacidosis. *(Brady, Paramedic Care 2e, Principles and Practice, Volume 3—Endocrinology. Mosby, Paramedic Textbook 3e, Endocrinology.)*

475. **The answer is B.** (A), (C), (D), increased dietary intake, and decreased metabolic rate are some of the most common reasons for diabetics to develop diabetic ketoacidosis. Less common causes are pregnancy, increased alcohol intake, and severe emotional stress. (B) is incorrect because increased insulin dose usually results in hypoglycemia, not an elevation of blood sugar with ketoacidosis. *(Brady, Paramedic Care 2e, Principles and Practice, Volume 3—Endocrinology. Mosby, Paramedic Textbook 3e, Endocrinology.)*

476. **The answer is C.** (A), (B), and (D) are common causes of hypoglycemia in insulin-dependent diabetics. (C) is incorrect because it is usually not related to hypoglycemia. *(Brady, Paramedic Care 2e, Principles and Practice, Volume 3—Endocrinology. Mosby, Paramedic Textbook 3e, Endocrinology.)*

477. **The answer is B.** (B) is correct, primarily because the brain depends on glucose for most of its energy. (A), (C), and (D) are incorrect; they are potential long-term complications of diabetes mellitus and are unrelated to hypoglycemia. *(Brady, Paramedic Care 2e, Principles and Practice, Volume 3—Endocrinology. Mosby, Paramedic Textbook 3e, Endocrinology.)*

478. **The answer is B.** (A), (C), (D), liver disease, kidney disease, and certain poisonings may also cause hypoglycemic reactions. You must be very careful to note that a lack of a history of diabetes in an unresponsive patient does not eliminate the possibility of hypoglycemia as the possible cause. In this patient, his chronic alcoholism and possible alcoholic liver disease are both potential causes of hypoglycemia. (D) Prostatism is unrelated to hypoglycemia. It often causes increased frequency in urination due to incomplete emptying of the urinary bladder due

to a partial blockage of the urinary tract from an enlarged prostate gland. Because of increased urinary frequency, patients may initially fear that they have diabetes but are reassured by normal results on a finger-stick test or blood sugar evaluation. *(Brady, Paramedic Care 2e, Principles and Practice, Volume 3—Endocrinology. Mosby, Paramedic Textbook 3e, Endocrinology.)*

479. **The answer is A.** (A) is correct, and the elevation in serum potassium level is due to the severity of the acidosis. This hyperkalemia may produce dangerous cardiac arrhythmias. As a result, some medical control physicians would recommend the administration of IV sodium bicarbonate in order to begin to correct the severe acidosis. *(Brady, Paramedic Care 2e, Principles and Practice, Volume 3—Endocrinology. Mosby, Paramedic Textbook 3e, Endocrinology.)*

480. **The answer is B.** (B) is correct. Since the patient is conscious and you suspect that this diabetic's bizarre behavior may be due to hypoglycemia, the treatment of choice is the oral administration of a glucose-containing substance. (A) is incorrect because, as long as the patient is able to take glucose by mouth, the correct route of administration is oral, not IV. (C) is incorrect because the heart rate of 150 beats per minute is probably a sinus tachycardia due to an acute hypoglycemic episode. The treatment of choice is to resolve the hypoglycemia, which will resolve the sinus tachycardia. (D) is not the first step in treatment. *(Brady, Paramedic Care 2e, Principles and Practice, Volume 3—Endocrinology. Mosby, Paramedic Textbook 3e, Endocrinology.)*

481. **The answer is A.** (B), (C), and (D) are correct. (A) is incorrect because, in hyperosmolar hyperglycemic nonketotic coma, there is no production of ketones and acids and thus no acidosis; therefore, there is no need to hyperventilate. Hyperventilation would be used to attempt to compensate for a metabolic acidosis. *(Brady, Paramedic Care 2e, Principles and Practice, Volume 3—Endocrinology. Mosby, Paramedic Textbook 3e, Endocrinology.)*

482. **The answer is D.** (A), (B), (C), insomnia, agitation, paranoia, and fatigue are all signs or symptoms of hyperthyroidism. (D) is incorrect because with hyperthyroidism the patient has heat intolerance. A patient who is hypothyroid (underactive thyroid) has cold intolerance. *(Brady, Paramedic Care 2e, Principles and Practice, Volume 3—Endocrinology. Mosby, Paramedic Textbook 3e, Endocrinology.)*

483. **The answer is B.** (A), (C), (D), weakness, weight gain, and facial bloating are all signs or symptoms of hypothyroidism. (B) is incorrect because the hypothyroid patient has oily skin and hair. *(Brady, Paramedic Care 2e, Principles and Practice, Volume 3—Endocrinology. Mosby, Paramedic Textbook 3e, Endocrinology.)*

484. **The answer is D.** (A), (B), (C), and rapid transport are the basic foundation of the prehospital emergent treatment of hyper- or hypothyroidism. At the ED, the severity of the thyroid disease will dictate the specific treatment of the over- or underactive thyroid gland. (D) is incorrect because usually the treatment of the over- or underactive thyroid gland will resolve most tachy- or bradyarrhythmias. Some hyperthyroid patients will present with atrial fibrillation with a rapid ventricular response. The treatment of choice is usually intravenous calcium blockers, intravenous beta-blockers, such as IV propranolol (Inderal) or metoprolol (Lopressor), not lidocaine. *(Brady, Paramedic Care 2e, Principles and Practice, Volume 3—Endocrinology. Mosby, Paramedic Textbook 3e, Endocrinology.)*

485. **The answer is C.** (A), (B), and (D) are correct. (C) is incorrect because an overactive adrenal gland produces hypokalemia (low potassium level) and weight gain. An underactive adrenal gland (adrenal gland insufficiency, hypoadrenalism) produces hyperkalemia. *(Brady, Paramedic Care 2e, Principles and Practice, Volume 3—Endocrinology. Mosby, Paramedic Textbook 3e, Endocrinology.)*

486. **The answer is C.** (A), (B), (D), weight loss, and hypotension are frequent presenting signs and symptoms of adrenal gland hypofunction. (C) is incorrect because the adrenal gland normally produces and secretes epinephrine and norepinephrine. Adrenal gland hypofunction would produce less of these two essential hormones,

resulting in hypotension. On the other hand, an overactive adrenal gland, known as Cushing syndrome, frequently produces an excess of these two hormones, resulting in hypertension. *(Brady, Paramedic Care 2e, Principles and Practice, Volume 3—Endocrinology. Mosby, Paramedic Textbook 3e, Endocrinology.)*

ALLERGIES AND ANAPHYLAXIS

487. **The answer is A.** (A) is correct. (B) is incorrect because asthma is a chronic inflammatory disorder of the airways that is often aggravated by infections, stress, and certain allergens. (C) and (D) are unrelated to the definition. *(Brady, Paramedic Care 2e, Principles and Practice, Volume 3—Allergy and Anaphylaxis. Mosby, Paramedic Textbook 3e, Allergy and Anaphylaxis.)*

488. **The answer is C.** (C) is correct. (A) is incorrect because immune deficiency is unrelated to allergic reactions. (B) is a mild allergic reaction known as hives. (D) is due to epileptic seizure activity and is not an allergic reaction. *(Brady, Paramedic Care 2e, Principles and Practice, Volume 3—Allergy and Anaphylaxis. Mosby, Paramedic Textbook 3e, Allergy and Anaphylaxis.)*

489. **The answer is A.** (A) is correct. The antigen is usually some form of protein that causes the allergic patient's body to produce antibodies, usually IgE antibodies. These IgE antibodies become attached to the membranes of basophils and mast cells. (B) is one of many substances that act as an antigen and can produce an allergic and/or anaphylactic reaction. (C) is incorrect. (D) is incorrect because the antigen causes the allergic patient's body to produce an antibody, not vice versa. *(Brady, Paramedic Care 2e, Principles and Practice, Volume 3—Allergy and Anaphylaxis. Mosby, Paramedic Textbook 3e, Allergy and Anaphylaxis.)*

490. **The answer is B.** (B) is correct. (A), (C), and (D) are incorrect because they are hormones, not chemical mediators. *(Brady, Paramedic Care 2e, Principles and Practice, Volume 3—Allergy and Anaphylaxis. Mosby, Paramedic Textbook 3e, Allergy and Anaphylaxis.)*

491. The answer is C. (A), (B), and (D) are correct. (C) is incorrect, since there is no direct effect on the coronary arteries. *(Brady, Paramedic Care 2e, Principles and Practice, Volume 3—Allergy and Anaphylaxis. Mosby, Paramedic Textbook 3e, Allergy and Anaphylaxis.)*

492. The answer is A. (B), (C), (D), other medications, foreign proteins, wasps and other Hymenoptera stings, hormones (e.g., insulin), blood products, preservatives, and dextran are some of the agents that may cause anaphylaxis. (A) is incorrect because these substances usually do not produce anaphylaxis. *(Brady, Paramedic Care 2e, Principles and Practice, Volume 3—Allergy and Anaphylaxis. Mosby, Paramedic Textbook 3e, Allergy and Anaphylaxis.)*

493. The answer is D. (A), (B), and (C) are possibly present during an allergic or anaphylactic reaction. (D) is incorrect because most patients are tachycardic with an allergic reaction or anaphylaxis. *(Brady, Paramedic Care 2e, Principles and Practice, Volume 3—Allergy and Anaphylaxis. Mosby, Paramedic Textbook 3e, Allergy and Anaphylaxis.)*

494. The answer is C. (A), (B), and (D) are correct. (C) is incorrect because nosebleeds are not part of an allergic or anaphylactic reaction. *(Brady, Paramedic Care 2e, Principles and Practice, Volume 3—Allergy and Anaphylaxis. Mosby, Paramedic Textbook 3e, Allergy and Anaphylaxis.)*

495. The answer is C. (C) is correct. (A), (B), and (D) are incorrect because they are common methods of access for an allergen to the body, resulting in an anaphylactic reaction. *(Brady, Paramedic Care 2e, Principles and Practice, Volume 3—Allergy and Anaphylaxis. Mosby, Paramedic Textbook 3e, Allergy and Anaphylaxis.)*

496. The answer is D. (A), (B), and (C) are correct. (D) may be seen with both an allergic reaction and an anaphylactic reaction. *(Brady, Paramedic Care 2e, Principles and Practice, Volume 3—Allergy and Anaphylaxis. Mosby, Paramedic Textbook 3e, Allergy and Anaphylaxis.)*

497. The answer is A. (A) is truly the first priority in a patient having an anaphylactic reaction, which is manifested with stridor and threatening the upper airway. (B) and (D) are incorrect, even though of secondary importance in this patient. (C) is incorrect because this would be used for the anaphylactic patient who is demonstrating hypotension. *(Brady, Paramedic Care 2e, Principles and Practice, Volume 3—Allergy and Anaphylaxis. Mosby, Paramedic Textbook 3e, Allergy and Anaphylaxis.)*

498. The answer is D. (D) is correct because this patient, with difficulty breathing, stridor, tachypnea, and a swollen tongue, has a jeopardized airway, and oral endotracheal intubation is the best method not only to establish but also to maintain the airway. (A) is incorrect because a needle cricothyrotomy is usually indicated for complete upper airway obstruction. If this patient's airway is unable to be maintained, he may soon become totally obstructed and require a needle cricothyrotomy. (B) and (C) are incorrect because, with stridor and a swollen tongue, insertion of an oropharyngeal airway may change this obstruction from a partial to a complete one. *(Brady, Paramedic Care 2e, Principles and Practice, Volume 3—Allergy and Anaphylaxis. Mosby, Paramedic Textbook 3e, Allergy and Anaphylaxis.)*

499. The answer is A. (B), (C), and (D) are correct. (A) is incorrect because 0.3–0.5 mg of 1:1000 is the correct dose of SC, not IV, epinephrine. This is the first line of epinephrine treatment in this patient. However, in a severe anaphylactic reaction, medical control may give permission for the administration of 5–10 mL (0.1 mL/kg) of 1:10,000 epinephrine by slow IV push. *(Brady, Paramedic Care 2e, Principles and Practice, Volume 3—Allergy and Anaphylaxis. Mosby, Paramedic Textbook 3e, Allergy and Anaphylaxis.)*

500. The answer is D. (D) is incorrect because IV beta-blockers are not a part of the treatment of anaphylaxis and would be harmful in this situation. (A), (B), and (C) are other correct treatment options for anaphylaxis. *(Brady, Paramedic Care 2e, Principles and Practice, Volume 3—Allergy and Anaphylaxis. Mosby, Paramedic Textbook 3e, Allergy and Anaphylaxis.)*

501. The answers are: (A) 6, (B) 2, (C) 1, (D) 3, (E) 5, (F) 4. *(Brady, Paramedic Care 2e, Principles and Practice, Volume 3—Allergy and Anaphylaxis. Mosby, Paramedic Textbook 3e, Allergy and Anaphylaxis.)*

502. The answer is C. (C) is correct because epinephrine is the treatment of choice for anaphylaxis. (A) is incorrect because this is a corticosteroid that may be an important part of the treatment of anaphylaxis, but not in the initial stage. (B) is used in the initial stage, but not before epinephrine. (D) is incorrect because it is appropriate for every patient with allergic wheezing, but in the patient with anaphylaxis, not before the administration of epinephrine. *(Brady, Paramedic Care 2e, Principles and Practice, Volume 3—Allergy and Anaphylaxis. Mosby, Paramedic Textbook 3e, Allergy and Anaphylaxis.)*

GASTROENTEROLOGY

503. The answer is D. (D) is incorrect because the kidneys are located in the retroperitoneum, behind the abdomen. (A), (B), and (C) are correct because the lower ribs of the thoracic ribcage cover them all. *(Brady, Paramedic Care 2e, Principles and Practice, Volume 3—Gastroenterology. Mosby, Paramedic Textbook 3e, Gastroenterology.)*

504. The answer is C. (C) is a solid abdominal organ, along with the liver, kidneys, pancreas, and the ovaries. (A), (B), (D), the small and large bowel, and the uterus are all hollow abdominal organs. *(Brady, Paramedic Care 2e, Principles and Practice, Volume 3—Gastroenterology. Mosby, Paramedic Textbook 3e, Gastroenterology.)*

505. The answer is A. (A) is correct. It is noted as being diffuse and poorly localized pain, often accompanied by nausea, vomiting, sweating, and tachycardia. (B), (C), and (D) are all incorrect. *(Brady, Paramedic Care 2e, Principles and Practice, Volume 3—Gastroenterology. Mosby, Paramedic Textbook 3e, Gastroenterology.)*

506. The answer is A. (A) is correct and is more localized than visceral pain, sharp, constant, and often worsened by coughing or jarring movements. (B), (C), and (D) are incorrect. *(Brady, Paramedic Care 2e, Principles and Practice, Volume 3—Gastroenterology. Mosby, Paramedic Textbook 3e, Gastroenterology.)*

507. The answer is B. (B) is correct, and an example is when a kidney stone, which is lodged in the ureter, causes pain that usually radiates down the inner thigh and into the genitalia. (A), (C), and (D) are all incorrect. *(Brady, Paramedic Care 2e, Principles and Practice, Volume 3—Gastroenterology. Mosby, Paramedic Textbook 3e, Gastroenterology.)*

508. The answer is B. (A), (C), and (D) are correct. S stands for severity, and Q stands for quality. Some texts precede PQRST with the letter O, which stands for onset. Others add the suffix letter A, which stands for associated symptoms. (B) is incorrect because Q stands for quality, not quantity. *(Brady, Paramedic Care 2e, Principles and Practice, Volume 3—Gastroenterology. Mosby, Paramedic Textbook 3e, Gastroenterology.)*

509. The answer is B. (A), (C), and (D) are the key parts of the abdominal examination. (B) is incorrect because most texts note that it is extremely difficult to perform auscultation of the abdomen in the prehospital setting because of the outside noise interference. *(Brady, Paramedic Care 2e, Principles and Practice, Volume 3—Gastroenterology. Mosby, Paramedic Textbook 3e, Gastroenterology.)*

510. The answer is D. (D) is correct. (A) is incorrect because it is often associated with severe initial periumbilical pain which then localizes in the right lower quadrant. (B) is incorrect because the patient is not vomiting blood and does not have melena (black bowel movements). (C) is incorrect because a patient usually complains of pain on one side, with colicky spasms. *(Brady, Paramedic Care 2e, Principles and Practice, Volume 3—Gastroenterology. Mosby, Paramedic Textbook 3e, Gastroenterology.)*

511. The answer is C. (C) is correct. (A) is incorrect because usually acute duodenal ulcer pain presents as upper abdominal pain, sometimes with vomiting with or without blood, associated with epigastric or right upper abdominal focal tenderness. (B) is incorrect because it usually presents with recurrent bouts of diarrhea. (D) is incorrect because cholecystitis represents an acutely inflamed gallbladder, which usually includes belching, flatus, and right upper abdominal pain sometimes radiating to the back and shoulder, and right upper abdominal tenderness, sometimes with guarding and rebound. (*Brady, Paramedic Care 2e, Principles and Practice, Volume 3—Gastroenterology. Mosby, Paramedic Textbook 3e, Gastroenterology.*)

512. **The answer is B.** (A), (C), (D), keeping the patient supine, and monitoring vital signs and cardiac rhythm are all part of the prehospital emergency management. (B) is incorrect because, since the treatment of the acute abdomen is often a surgical emergency, there should not be any delay in transport to the ED. (*Brady, Paramedic Care 2e, Principles and Practice, Volume 3—Gastroenterology. Mosby, Paramedic Textbook 3e, Gastroenterology.*)

513. **The answer is A.** (A) is correct and may be caused by various conditions, such as a diverticulum of the colon, a ruptured appendix, or a perforated duodenal or gastric ulcer. (B) is incorrect because of an absence of periumbilical pain or right lower quadrant pain, nausea, lack of appetite, and right lower quadrant tenderness. (C) is incorrect because there is usually a history of fatigue, yellow jaundice, dark urine, and light stools, and the physical examination usually only shows right upper quadrant tenderness. (D) is incorrect because of a lack of vomiting blood or melena (black tarry stools). (*Brady, Paramedic Care 2e, Principles and Practice, Volume 3—Gastroenterology. Mosby, Paramedic Textbook 3e, Gastroenterology.*)

514. **The answer is D.** (A), (B), and (C) are correct. (D) is incorrect because it is usually a sign of lower gastrointestinal or rectal bleeding from hemorrhoids, tumor, and so on. (*Brady, Paramedic Care 2e, Principles and Practice, Volume 3—Gastroenterology. Mosby, Paramedic Textbook 3e, Gastroenterology.*)

515. **The answers are: (A)** 2, **(B)** 5, **(C)** 4, **(D)** 6, **(E)** 1, **(F)** 3. (*Brady, Paramedic Care 2e, Principles and Practice, Volume 3—Gastroenterology. Mosby, Paramedic Textbook 3e, Gastroenterology.*)

516. **The answer is C.** (A), (B), (D), ECG monitoring, and rapid transport are all parts of the emergency care. (C) is incorrect because initiating

blood transfusions is part of the care in the ED, not in the prehospital setting. The only exception is for a patient requiring extrication who receives blood transfusions while awaiting extrication. (*Brady, Paramedic Care 2e, Principles and Practice, Volume 3—Gastroenterology. Mosby, Paramedic Textbook 3e, Gastroenterology.*)

517. **The answer is D.** (D) is the correct definition. (A) is incorrect because left lower abdominal pain is usually not accompanied by any gastrointestinal bleeding. (B) is incorrect because urinating blood is known as hematuria. (C) is incorrect because upper gastrointestinal bleeding is defined by vomiting blood. (*Brady, Paramedic Care 2e, Principles and Practice, Volume 3—Gastroenterology. Mosby, Paramedic Textbook 3e, Gastroenterology.*)

518. **The answers are: (A)** 5, **(B)** 2, **(C)** 1, **(D)** 4, **(E)** 6, **(F)** 3. (*Brady, Paramedic Care 2e, Principles and Practice, Volume 3—Gastroenterology. Mosby, Paramedic Textbook 3e, Gastroenterology.*)

519. **The answer is C.** (A), (B), and (D) are correct. (C) is incorrect because, with a lower (or upper) gastrointestinal hemorrhage, the correct IV fluid of choice is two IV lines of Ringer's lactate or normal saline solution. An IV KVO is incorrect, particularly in this patient, who has postural hypotension from lower gastrointestinal hemorrhage. This patient requires aggressive IV fluid administration. (*Brady, Paramedic Care 2e, Principles and Practice, Volume 3—Gastroenterology. Mosby, Paramedic Textbook 3e, Gastroenterology.*)

520. **The answer is B.** (B) is correct. (A) is incorrect because there is no history or evidence of any hematemesis or melena. (C) is incorrect because there is no evidence of periumbilical or right lower quadrant pain or right lower quadrant tenderness. (D) is incorrect because there is no evidence of bloody, mucousy diarrhea. (*Brady, Paramedic Care 2e, Principles and Practice, Volume 3—Gastroenterology. Mosby, Paramedic Textbook 3e, Gastroenterology.*)

521. **The answers are: (A)** 2, **(B)** 4, **(C)** 5, **(D)** 6, **(E)** 1, **(F)** 3. (*Brady, Paramedic Care 2e, Principles and*

Practice, Volume 3—Gastroenterology. Mosby, Paramedic Textbook 3e, Gastroenterology.)

522. **The answer is A.** (A) is correct because it will help to prevent further spread of this outbreak of viral hepatitis. It would also help to have your supervisors discuss notifying the Department of Health who would investigate possible sources of hepatitis at the home. (B) is incorrect because blood work may further define the precise cause of such an outbreak but will not immediately prevent further spread of the hepatitis outbreak. (C) is incorrect because body-substance isolation precautions are the most important steps in preventing the spread of an outbreak of viral hepatitis. Vaccinations may play a role in further limiting the spread of an outbreak. (D) is incorrect because, without body-substance isolation precautions, incorrectly collecting all of the vomitus and stool-stained sheets and clothing may actually cause further spread of the hepatitis to you and/or your partner and the personnel in the laundry. *(Brady, Paramedic Care 2e, Principles and Practice, Volume 3—Gastroenterology. Mosby, Paramedic Textbook 3e, Gastroenterology.)*

523. **The answer is C.** (A), (B), and (D) are correct. (C) is incorrect because all patients with acute abdominal pain, from any number of causes, should never be treated with narcotics, which may relieve the pain but hide the seriousness of the disease and prevent the rapid identification of the cause. This may also delay the emergent treatment of the problem. After thorough examination in the hospital ED, the physician may choose to provide some narcotic pain relief. *(Brady, Paramedic Care 2e, Principles and Practice, Volume 3—Gastroenterology. Mosby, Paramedic Textbook 3e, Gastroenterology.)*

524. **The answer is D.** (A), (B), and (C) are correct. (D) is incorrect, because acute hepatitis is a contagious disease which is transmitted by contact with any of the patient's secretions. It is very important for the Paramedics and EMTs caring for this patient to use body substance isolation procedures. *(Brady, Paramedic Care 2e, Principles and Practice, Volume 3—Gastroenterology. Mosby, Paramedic Textbook 3e, Gastroenterology.)*

RENAL AND UROLOGY

525. **The answer is A.** (A) is correct. (B) is incorrect because difficulty breathing is not a specific sign of acute renal failure, especially in a patient with a known diagnosis of chronic renal failure. (C) is incorrect because urinating blood is the definition of hematuria. (D) is incorrect because it is not the definition. *(Brady, Paramedic Care 2e, Principles and Practice, Volume 3—Urology and Nephrology. Mosby, Paramedic Textbook 3e, Urology.)*

526. **The answer is C.** (C) is the correct sequence for urinary flow. (A), (B), and (D) are incorrect. *(Brady, Paramedic Care 2e, Principles and Practice, Volume 3—Urology and Nephrology. Mosby, Paramedic Textbook 3e, Urology.)*

527. **The answer is B.** (A), (C), and (D) are all common acute urinary disorders. (B) is incorrect because there is no such condition as urinary alkalosis. *(Brady, Paramedic Care 2e, Principles and Practice, Volume 3—Urology and Nephrology. Mosby, Paramedic Textbook 3e, Urology.)*

528. **The answer is A.** (B), (C), and (D) are the three mechanisms for the development of acute renal failure. (A) is incorrect because a urinary tract infection by itself does not cause acute renal failure. *(Brady, Paramedic Care 2e, Principles and Practice, Volume 3—Urology and Nephrology. Mosby, Paramedic Textbook 3e, Urology.)*

529. **The answer is B.** (B) is correct, with total urinary tract obstruction due to an enlarged prostate, which has produced a distended urinary bladder, which appears as a lower abdominal midline mass. The development of fever may have represented an infection, which, if located in the kidneys may actually worsen the acute renal failure. (A) is incorrect because the ingestion of renal toxic medications should not produce urinary tract obstruction with a distended urinary bladder. (C) is incorrect because usually the patient begins by complaining of intense pain on one side of the back or flank. It also would only rarely

produce a distended bladder, if a kidney stone became lodged in the urethra and totally blocked the outflow of urine. (D) is incorrect because a kidney cancer should not lead to acute renal failure because it occurs in only one kidney and would produce acute renal failure only if the patient had only one kidney. (Brady, Paramedic Care 2e, Principles and Practice, Volume 3—Urology and Nephrology. Mosby, Paramedic Textbook 3e, Urology.)

530. **The answer is D.** (D) is correct because the patient is demonstrating the following signs of chronic renal failure: high blood pressure, pasty yellow skin with uremic white frost, decreased urinary output, marked pitting edema, pulmonary edema, and distended neck veins. Other consistent findings are anorexia, nausea, vomiting, and fatigue. (A) is incorrect because, although some of the findings may be present with acute or chronic failure, pulmonary edema and 4+ pitting edema of the legs and abdomen take time to develop. (B) is incorrect because it is anatomically impossible for a woman to get prostate cancer. (C) is incorrect because an acute urinary tract infection simply produces frequent urination, dysuria, nocturia, and sometimes a low-grade fever. (Brady, Paramedic Care 2e, Principles and Practice, Volume 3—Urology and Nephrology. Mosby, Paramedic Textbook 3e, Urology.)

531. **The answer is A.** (A) is correct. Hyperkalemia is an increased serum potassium level, and metabolic acidosis is due to an accumulation of body acids. (B) is incorrect because hypokalemia means a low serum potassium level and metabolic alkalosis, which are usually not signs of chronic renal failure. (C) is incorrect because hypernatremia is an elevated serum sodium level, which is not usually present in the face of fluid overload from chronic renal failure and because patients with chronic renal insufficiency have marked elevations of both serum creatinine and blood urea nitrogen levels. (D) is incorrect because of the reasons given in the previous discussion of hypernatremia and because hypokalemia is not usually a sign of chronic renal failure. (Brady, Paramedic Care 2e, Principles and Practice, Volume 3—Urology and Nephrology. Mosby, Paramedic Textbook 3e, Urology.)

532. **The answer is C.** (A), (B), (D), anxiety, obtundation, and hallucinations are some of the nervous system manifestations of chronic renal failure. (C) is not a sign of chronic renal failure. (Brady, Paramedic Care 2e, Principles and Practice, Volume 3—Urology and Nephrology. Mosby, Paramedic Textbook 3e, Urology.)

533. **The answer is A.** (A) is correct. The two basic types are hemodialysis and peritoneal dialysis. (B) is incorrect because this process is known as gastric lavage. (C) is incorrect because renal dialysis is unrelated to the delivery of antibiotics by any mechanism. (D) is incorrect because renal dialysis is unrelated to the process of urination. (Brady, Paramedic Care 2e, Principles and Practice, Volume 3—Urology and Nephrology. Mosby, Paramedic Textbook 3e, Urology.)

534. **The answer is A.** (B), (C), (D), and air embolism are known complications of renal dialysis. (A) is incorrect because, even though sometimes chronic renal failure patients on dialysis may develop stomach upset with nausea and/or vomiting, this is not due to the development of stomach ulcers. (Brady, Paramedic Care 2e, Principles and Practice, Volume 3—Urology and Nephrology. Mosby, Paramedic Textbook 3e, Urology.)

535. **The answer is A.** (A) is correct. (B) is incorrect because there is no such computer. (C) is incorrect because there is no such formula. (D) is incorrect because other stones, such as gallstones, are unrelated to the functioning of the kidney. (Brady, Paramedic Care 2e, Principles and Practice, Volume 3—Urology and Nephrology. Mosby, Paramedic Textbook 3e, Urology.)

536. **The answer is B.** (B) is correct because this patient's presentation is classic for having renal colic due to a kidney stone lodged in his right renal collecting system (usually in the ureter). Administering IV fluids is a key part of treating this patient because it will increase the amount of urine produced by the kidney, which will help push the stone down the ureter and into the urinary bladder, which will immediately cause the pain to resolve. In the urinary bladder, the stone may dissolve, be passed out of the urethra with urinating, or, rarely, become lodged in

the urethra, where it can be extracted. (A) is incorrect because, although many prehospital protocols will permit Paramedics to administer narcotic analgesics in the field, it is not as important as providing IV fluids. (C) is incorrect because these are not a key part of the treatment of renal colic, even though they would be instituted in the overall care of this patient. (D) is incorrect because this presentation is not related to a drug or toxic ingestion, and syrup of ipecac has no role in the treatment of renal colic. *(Brady, Paramedic Care 2e, Principles and Practice, Volume 3—Urology and Nephrology. Mosby, Paramedic Textbook 3e, Urology.)*

TOXICOLOGY

537. **The answer is C.** (A), (B), (D), and injection are the four routes of exposure for toxicologic emergencies. (C) is incorrect because aspiration occurs when a patient vomits or regurgitates the stomach contents and it passes into the respiratory tract. This often results in pneumonia. However, this is not a toxicologic route of exposure. *(Brady, Paramedic Care 2e, Principles and Practice, Volume 3—Toxicology and Substance Abuse Mosby, Paramedic Textbook 3e, Toxicology.)*

538. **The answer is A.** (B), (C), and (D) are correct. (A) is incorrect because the regional poison centers act in a consultative manner to everyone involved in toxicologic emergencies but routinely do not provide on-site care to the patient. *(Brady, Paramedic Care 2e, Principles and Practice, Volume 3—Toxicology and Substance Abuse. Mosby, Paramedic Textbook 3e, Toxicology.)*

539. **The answer is D.** (D) is correct. *(Brady, Paramedic Care 2e, Principles and Practice, Volume 3—Toxicology and Substance Abuse. Mosby, Paramedic Textbook 3e, Toxicology.)*

540. **The answer is D.** (D) is correct. This tells us that a high percentage of poisonings are preventable. *(Brady, Paramedic Care 2e, Principles and Practice, Volume 3—Toxicology and Substance Abuse. Mosby, Paramedic Textbook 3e, Toxicology.)*

541. **The answer is A.** (B), (C), (D), a patient with a MI, and a patient with certain categories of poisonings, such as corrosives, hydrocarbons, iodides, silver nitrate, and strychnine, are all contraindications to inducing vomiting. If unsure, it is important to call your regional poison control center and/or medical control to discuss the issue. (A) is incorrect because acetaminophen (Tylenol) poisoning is not a contraindication to inducing vomiting. *(Brady, Paramedic Care 2e, Principles and Practice, Volume 3—Toxicology and Substance Abuse. Mosby, Paramedic Textbook 3e, Toxicology.)*

542. **The answer is C.** (A), (B), and (D) are all correct options. (C) is incorrect because colon lavage is not part of a treatment regimen for any toxicologic emergency. *(Brady, Paramedic Care 2e, Principles and Practice, Volume 3—Toxicology and Substance Abuse. Mosby, Paramedic Textbook 3e, Toxicology.)*

543. **The answer is D.** (D) is correct because caustic ingestions can produce soft-tissue damage to the larynx, epiglottis, and/or vocal cords, which may result in upper airway obstruction. (A) and (B) are incorrect in caustic ingestions because, in the process of vomiting, the actual ingested material may produce additional airway and esophageal injury and aspiration. (C) is incorrect because trying to neutralize an alkali ingestion, such as Drano lye, by giving a mild acid generates heat and may produce a thermal injury as well. *(Brady, Paramedic Care 2e, Principles and Practice, Volume 3—Toxicology and Substance Abuse. Mosby, Paramedic Textbook 3e, Toxicology.)*

544. **The answer is D.** (D) is correct because insecticide poisoning (organophosphate) and nerve agent poisoning are similar in how they work producing a cholinergic crisis. The antidotes for treatment are parenteral atropine and pralidoxime. (A), (B), and (C) are incorrect. *(Brady, Paramedic Care 2e, Principles and Practice, Volume 3—Urology and Nephrology. Mosby, Paramedic Textbook 3e, Urology.)*

545. **The answer is C.** (C) is correct because this child with a hydrocarbon ingestion is demonstrating respiratory distress or failure and requires

aggressive airway and breathing management. With hydrocarbon ingestions, the child often aspirates the substance into the lungs. This can result in respiratory distress due to noncardiogenic pulmonary edema. (A) is incorrect because the child needs more aggressive airway and breathing management. (B) is incorrect because routinely you do not want to risk the chance that the vomiting may increase aspiration into the lungs. However, sometimes the poison control consultant may recommend syrup of ipecac if the ingested substance contains a large amount of another toxin. If stomach emptying is recommended, then inducing vomiting is felt to have less risk of aspiration than performing gastric lavage. (D) is incorrect because this is noncardiogenic pulmonary edema, and morphine would not be beneficial and even may be harmful by causing respiratory depression. *(Brady, Paramedic Care 2e, Principles and Practice, Volume 3—Toxicology and Substance Abuse. Mosby, Paramedic Textbook 3e, Toxicology.)*

546. The answer is D. (A), (B), and (C) are correct. (D) is incorrect because, while carbon monoxide causes the most accidental and suicidal deaths from poisoning in the United States each year, it is not a part of each inhalation poisoning. *(Brady, Paramedic Care 2e, Principles and Practice, Volume 3—Toxicology and Substance Abuse. Mosby, Paramedic Textbook 3e, Toxicology.)*

547. The answer is D. (A), (B), (C), methane, ammonia, inert gases, propane, and various hydrocarbons are all causes of inhalation poisoning. (D) is incorrect because alcohol is a common form of poisoning by ingestion. *(Brady, Paramedic Care 2e, Principles and Practice, Volume 3—Toxicology and Substance Abuse. Mosby, Paramedic Textbook 3e, Toxicology.)*

548. The answer is D. (A), (B), (C), and performing primary and secondary assessments are all parts of the emergency care of the carbon monoxide–poisoned patient. (D) is incorrect because you should never enter the toxic environment without respiratory protective breathing apparatus. *(Brady, Paramedic Care 2e, Principles and Practice, Volume 3—Toxicology and Substance Abuse. Mosby, Paramedic Textbook 3e, Toxicology.)*

549. The answer is C. (A), (B), (D), and drunken behavior that resolves rapidly are all possible signs of inhalant abuse. (C) is incorrect and unrelated to an inhaled poison. *(Brady, Paramedic Care 2e, Principles and Practice, Volume 3—Toxicology and Substance Abuse. Mosby, Paramedic Textbook 3e, Toxicology.)*

550. The answer is D. (A), (B), (C), hornet, yellow jacket, ant, scorpion, and snakebites are all examples of injected poisoning. (D) is incorrect because a dog bite may result in an infection or possibly rabies but not usually in poisoning. *(Brady, Paramedic Care 2e, Principles and Practice, Volume 3—Toxicology and Substance Abuse. Mosby, Paramedic Textbook 3e, Toxicology.)*

551. The answer is D. (D) is the correct method for removal of the stinger. (A) and (B) are both incorrect because squeezing of the stinger will only pump more of the venom into the wound. (C) is simply incorrect. *(Brady, Paramedic Care 2e, Principles and Practice, Volume 3—Toxicology and Substance Abuse. Mosby, Paramedic Textbook 3e, Toxicology.)*

552. The answer is B. (A), (C), (D), nausea, vomiting, sweating, seizures, paralysis, hypertension, diminished level of consciousness, and severe back, chest, or shoulder pain with an upper-extremity bite are all possible physical findings. (B) is incorrect because it is unrelated to a black widow spider bite. *(Brady, Paramedic Care 2e, Principles and Practice, Volume 3—Toxicology and Substance Abuse. Mosby, Paramedic Textbook 3e, Toxicology.)*

553. The answer is B. (B) is correct because it encompasses poisoning from all possible drugs. (A) is incorrect because taking prescription drugs too rapidly may or may not cause side effects, but usually not toxic effects. (C) is incorrect because, while many overdoses are combinations of alcohol and other drugs, it usually does not occur with normal doses of prescribed medications. (D) is incorrect because drug overdose pertains to poisoning from legal or illegal drugs. *(Brady, Paramedic Care 2e, Principles and Practice, Volume 3—Toxicology and Substance Abuse. Mosby, Paramedic Textbook 3e, Toxicology.)*

554. **The answer is B.** (A), (C), and (D) are all part of the care of this unresponsive, respiratorily depressed, alcohol (and possible other substances) overdosed patient. (B) is incorrect because you never want to induce vomiting in a patient with a decreased level of consciousness, particularly in a patient without a gag reflex, for fear of aspiration. *(Brady, Paramedic Care 2e, Principles and Practice, Volume 3—Toxicology and Substance Abuse. Mosby, Paramedic Textbook 3e, Toxicology.)*

555. **The answer is D.** Since barbiturate overdoses are basically treated with supportive treatment, (A), (B), (C), ventilatory support if needed, and dopamine if needed are possible parts of the emergency care. (D) is incorrect because, even though the patient has a positive gag reflex, she still has a decreased level of consciousness, with the potential to become much worse, if she truly took 90 phenobarbital (30 mg) tablets. This puts her at risk of aspiration with inducing vomiting. *(Brady, Paramedic Care 2e, Principles and Practice, Volume 3—Toxicology and Substance Abuse. Mosby, Paramedic Textbook 3e, Toxicology.)*

556. **The answer is C.** (A), (B), and (D) are correct for these common complications of a cocaine overdose. (C) is incorrect because, even though flumazenil (Mazecon) is truly the antidote for benzodiazepine overdoses, such as with diazepam (Valium), it should not be given to a patient with a cocaine overdose. The flumazenil antidote would eliminate the benefits of the benzodiazepines in controlling seizures and in calming the patient. *(Brady, Paramedic Care 2e, Principles and Practice, Volume 3—Toxicology and Substance Abuse. Mosby, Paramedic Textbook 3e, Toxicology.)*

557. **The answer is B.** (A), (C), and (D) are all correct. (B) is incorrect because, while a cocaine overdose patient may be euphoric and have dilated pupils, he or she usually has tachycardic heart rhythms, such as sinus tachycardia, supraventricular tachycardia, or even ventricular tachycardia, but usually not bradyarrhythmias. *(Brady, Paramedic Care 2e, Principles and Practice, Volume 3—Toxicology and Substance Abuse. Mosby, Paramedic Textbook 3e, Toxicology.)*

558. **The answers are:** (A) 7, (B) 2, (C) 8, (D) 6, (E) 5, (F) 3, (G) 1, (H) 4. *(Brady, Paramedic Care 2e, Principles and Practice, Volume 3—Toxicology and Substance Abuse. Mosby, Paramedic Textbook 3e, Toxicology.)*

559. **The answer is A.** (A) Since this patient's presentation is most consistent with alcohol withdrawal, the medical control physician may request that you administer IV diazepam (Valium), which may be repeated initially on a 1- to 2-hour basis. The Valium would be administered in order to prevent seizures from delirium tremens (the DTs), which has a significant mortality rate. (B), (C), and (D) are incorrect because they are not the first-line medication administered for alcohol withdrawal. *(Brady, Paramedic Care 2e, Principles and Practice, Volume 3—Toxicology and Substance Abuse. Mosby, Paramedic Textbook 3e, Toxicology.)*

560. **The answer is D.** (A), (B), and (C) are all possible appropriate recommendations from the telemetry physician for a patient presenting with organophosphate poisoning from insecticide spray. (D) is incorrect because, although atropine is actually an antidote for organophosphate poisoning, the dosage in adults is 2–5 mg IV every 10–15 minutes until the secretions are drying up. *(Brady, Paramedic Care 2e, Principles and Practice, Volume 3—Toxicology and Substance Abuse. Mosby, Paramedic Textbook 3e, Toxicology.)*

561. **The answer is B.** (A), (C), and (D) are correct parts of the emergency care rendered by the Paramedic to the patient suffering food poisoning. (B) is incorrect because, while some types of food poisoning, such as paralytic shellfish poisoning, may result in respiratory distress or arrest, this is clearly not the case in this patient. *(Brady, Paramedic Care 2e, Principles and Practice, Volume 3—Toxicology and Substance Abuse. Mosby, Paramedic Textbook 3e, Toxicology.)*

562. **The answer is B.** (B) is correct because flunitrazepam (Rohypnol), commonly known as the "date rape drug," is often slipped into a woman's drink resulting in not only sedation but also amnesia. The treatment is the same as for any benzodiazepine overdose but you must also be careful to report the events to the ED as a possible sexual assault and bring any soiled clothes and sheets with the patient. *(Brady, Paramedic Care 2e, Principles and Practice, Volume 3— Toxicology and Substance Abuse. Mosby, Paramedic Textbook 3e, Toxicology.)*

HEMATOLOGY

563. **The answer is B.** (A), (C), and (D) are correct. (B) is incorrect because, in the fetus, blood cell production occurs in the liver (A) and the spleen (D). After birth, the red bone marrow (C) takes over the production. As the body matures, some of the red bone marrow becomes replaced by fat. This is known as the yellow bone marrow, which is inactive. *(Brady, Paramedic Care 2e, Principles and Practice, Volume 3—Hematology. Mosby, Paramedic Textbook 3e, Hematology.)*

564. **The answer is A.** (B), (C), and (D) are correct. (A) is incorrect because hemoglobin, not myoglobin, is the key molecule in RBCs and is responsible for the blood's efficient transport of oxygen. *(Brady, Paramedic Care 2e, Principles and Practice, Volume 3—Hematology. Mosby, Paramedic Textbook 3e, Hematology.)*

565. **The answer is D.** (A), (B), and (C) are correct. (D) is incorrect because, in the adult, chronic blood loss is the most common cause of anemia. *(Brady, Paramedic Care 2e, Principles and Practice, Volume 3—Hematology. Mosby, Paramedic Textbook 3e, Hematology.)*

566. **The answer is B.** (A), (C), and (D) are correct. (B) is incorrect because a patient with suspected anemia, particularly one with orthostatic signs, should be treated with high-concentration oxygen by nonrebreather mask. *(Brady, Paramedic Care 2e, Principles and Practice, Volume 3—Hematology. Mosby, Paramedic Textbook 3e, Hematology.)*

567. **The answer is A.** (B), (C), and (D) are correct. (A) is incorrect because WBCs act in the tissues and are transported by the blood. *(Brady, Paramedic Care 2e, Principles and Practice, Volume 3—Hematology. Mosby, Paramedic Textbook 3e, Hematology.)*

568. **The answer is C.** (A), (B), and (D) are correct. (C) is incorrect because anemia is a RBC disorder. *(Brady, Paramedic Care 2e, Principles and Practice, Volume 3—Hematology. Mosby, Paramedic Textbook 3e, Hematology.)*

569. **The answer is B.** (A), (C), and (D) are correct. (B) is incorrect even though, at the hospital, a patient having a sickle cell crisis will be treated with narcotics. However, it is essential that the patient's chest, abdominal, and extremity pain be evaluated in the ED prior to the administration of narcotics in order to rapidly diagnose and properly treat emergent conditions, such as acute appendicitis and pneumothorax. *(Brady, Paramedic Care 2e, Principles and Practice, Volume 3—Hematology. Mosby, Paramedic Textbook 3e, Hematology.)*

570. **The answer is A.** (B), (C), and (D) are all correct possibilities. (B) Acute leukemia is a disease characterized by abnormal increases in the number and immaturity of WBCs, which interfere with the production of platelets and can cause bleeding. (C) Warfarin (Coumadin) is an anticoagulant, which can result in severe bleeding if too much is taken. (D) Hemophilia is a hereditary disease caused by a lack of one or more factors necessary for coagulation of the blood. This case presentation is most typical of a patient suffering from hemophilia. (A) is incorrect because bleeding causes anemia, not vice versa. *(Brady, Paramedic Care 2e, Principles and Practice, Volume 3—Hematology. Mosby, Paramedic Textbook 3e, Hematology.)*

571. **The answer is C.** (A), (B), and (D) are correct. (C) is incorrect because platelets are disk-shaped fragments and are not cells. *(Brady, Paramedic Care 2e, Principles and Practice, Volume 3—Hematology. Mosby, Paramedic Textbook 3e, Hematology.)*

572. **The answer is A.** (A) With the onset of acute leukemia the patient's bone marrow continues to overproduce (causing bone pain) a certain type of WBC which proceeds to wipe out the precursor cells for making RBCs and platelets. As a result, the patient becomes very anemic and weak, as well as having very low platelet counts which result in frequent bruising and petechiae (small punctate purplish spots in various places

over the skin). With acute leukemia there are also several large swollen lymph nodes all over the body and a very enlarged liver and spleen. Even though there is usually a tremendous number of a certain type of WBC, they are ineffective WBCs and therefore do not help to fight infections as well. While parts of the patient's presentation sound suspicious for (B), (C), and (D), they are incorrect. *(Brady, Paramedic Care 2e, Principles and Practice, Volume 3—Hematology. Mosby, Paramedic Textbook 3e, Hematology.)*

ENVIRONMENTAL EMERGENCIES

573. **The answer is D.** (D) is correct. Being able to recognize them promptly and understanding their causes can lead to your rapid treatment of these various conditions. (A), (B), and (C) are incorrect. *(Brady, Paramedic Care 2e, Principles and Practice, Volume 3—Environmental Emergencies. Mosby, Paramedic Textbook 3e, Environmental Conditions.)*

574. **The answer is C.** (A), (B), (D), and pressure disorders are some environmental factors that may affect care. (C) is incorrect because it is not an environmental factor, even though it certainly could have an affect on the care. *(Brady, Paramedic Care 2e, Principles and Practice, Volume 3—Environmental Emergencies. Mosby, Paramedic Textbook 3e, Environmental Conditions.)*

575. **The answer is D.** (D) is correct. (B) is incorrect because heat cramps present as painful cramps in the fingers, arms, legs, or abdominal muscles following strenuous activity in a hot environment. (C) is incorrect because heat exhaustion is usually seen in a patient who is working or exercising in a hot environment with a low fluid intake and has signs of dehydration: orthostatic hypotension, dizziness, syncope, headache, nausea, vomiting, diarrhea, muscle cramps, and moist cool skin. (A) is also incorrect. *(Brady, Paramedic Care 2e, Principles and Practice, Volume 3—Environmental Emergencies. Mosby, Paramedic Textbook 3e, Environmental Conditions.)*

576. **The answer is D.** (A), (B), (C), 100% oxygen, and monitoring core temperature are correct.

(D) is incorrect because the patient requires 100% oxygen by nonrebreather mask or assisted by a bag-valve-mask if the patient's respirations are shallow. *(Brady, Paramedic Care 2e, Principles and Practice, Volume 3—Environmental Emergencies. Mosby, Paramedic Textbook 3e, Environ-mental Conditions.)*

577. **The answer is B.** (A), (C), and (D) are correct. Also, modest hypothermia is associated with a temperature between 86 and 94°F. (B) is incorrect because there is no such category as lethal hypothermia. *(Brady, Paramedic Care 2e, Principles and Practice, Volume 3—Environmental Emergencies. Mosby, Paramedic Textbook 3e, Environmental Conditions.)*

578. **The answer is C.** (A), (B), (D), prolonged and/or intense exposure, and weather conditions are all predisposing factors for heat and cold disorders. (C) is incorrect because one's religious affiliation is not. *(Brady, Paramedic Care 2e, Principles and Practice, Volume 3—Environmental Emergencies. Mosby, Paramedic Textbook 3e, Environmental Conditions.)*

579. **The answer is A.** (A) is correct. (B), (C), and (D) may be associated with the cold weather, but they are all incorrect. *(Brady, Paramedic Care 2e, Principles and Practice, Volume 3—Environmental Emergencies. Mosby, Paramedic Textbook 3e, Environmental Conditions.)*

580. **The answer is C.** (C) is correct. (A) is incorrect because it represents localized injury. (B) is incorrect because patients suffering from severe hypothermia stop shivering and proceed from confusion to stupor and coma. (D) is incorrect because, without signs of alcohol on the patient's breath and any signs of recent alcohol intake, this alone is unlikely. *(Brady, Paramedic Care 2e, Principles and Practice, Volume 3—Environmental Emergencies. Mosby, Paramedic Textbook 3e, Environmental Conditions.)*

581. **The answer is A.** (A) is the best definition. (B) is incorrect because frostbite is a localized injury that may or may not be accompanied by hypothermia. (C) and (D) are incorrect because frostbite is unrelated to any kind of a bite and may occur in any freezing climate, not

only frosty. *(Brady, Paramedic Care 2e, Principles and Practice, Volume 3—Environmental Emergencies. Mosby, Paramedic Textbook 3e, Environmental Conditions.)*

582. **The answer is B.** (B) is correct. (A) is incorrect because superficial frostbite produces blisters, which turn into black eschar, while deep frostbite produces mottled blue or gray skin, which later forms a black eschar. (C) is incorrect because superficial frostbite rewarming is extremely painful, and, in deep frostbite, deep purple blisters may appear in 1–3 weeks. (D) is incorrect because in superficial frostbite the patient feels coldness and numbness, and in deep frostbite the foot remains cold, mottled, and blue or gray after rewarming. *(Brady, Paramedic Care 2e, Principles and Practice, Volume 3—Environmental Emergencies. Mosby, Paramedic Textbook 3e, Environmental Conditions.)*

583. **The answer is D.** (A), (B), (C), and changing all of the patient's restrictive and wet clothing in order to prevent hypothermia are all parts of the emergency care. (D) is incorrect because vigorous rubbing is ineffective and potentially harmful. Also, partial slow rewarming with blankets is injurious. *(Brady, Paramedic Care 2e, Principles and Practice, Volume 3—Environmental Emergencies. Mosby, Paramedic Textbook 3e, Environ-mental Conditions.)*

584. **The answer is A.** (A) is correct. (B) and (C) are incorrect because near-drowning is unrelated to being near another drowning victim. (D) is incorrect because usually death does not occur or occurs after 24 hours in near-drowning. *(Brady, Paramedic Care 2e, Principles and Practice, Volume 3—Environmental Emergencies. Mosby, Paramedic Textbook 3e, Environmental Conditions.)*

585. **The answer is A.** (A) is correct because, in 10–15% of drownings, a patient dies during laryngospasm, which is a part of the body's response to a very small amount of water being aspirated into the larynx. (B), (C), and (D) are all incorrect. *(Brady, Paramedic Care 2e, Principles and Practice, Volume 3—Environmental Emergencies. Mosby, Paramedic Textbook 3e, Environmental Conditions.)*

586. **The answer is C.** (A), (B), and (D) are correct. (C) is incorrect because performing the Heimlich maneuver in the drowning patient will not remove water from the lungs but may displace water from the stomach into the lungs. *(Brady, Paramedic Care 2e, Principles and Practice, Volume 3—Environmental Emergencies. Mosby, Paramedic Textbook 3e, Environmental Conditions.)*

587. **The answer is B.** (B) is correct. (A), (C), and (D) are incorrect. *(Brady, Paramedic Care 2e, Principles and Practice, Volume 3—Environmental Emergencies. Mosby, Paramedic Textbook 3e, Environmental Conditions.)*

588. **The answer is D.** (D) is the classic presentation of decompression sickness, initially with joint aches, known as *the bends*, with multiple sensory and motor abnormalities due to cerebral dysfunction, staggering gait due to cerebellar dysfunction, and finally paraplegia due to spinal cord dysfunction. (A) is incorrect because a patient suffering from an air embolism usually presents as a diver having a sudden loss of consciousness immediately on surfacing. (B) is incorrect because, with a cerebrovascular accident, a patient would present with an acute focal neurologic weakness or paralysis. (C) is incorrect because there was no historical evidence suggesting any seizure activity. *(Brady, Paramedic Care 2e, Principles and Practice, Volume 3—Environmental Emergencies. Mosby, Paramedic Textbook 3e, Environmental Conditions.)*

589. **The answer is C.** (C) is correct, even though (A) and (B) are a part of the emergency care of the patient with decompression sickness. (A) and (B) are incorrect because they are not the most important part of the emergency care. (D) is incorrect because IV naloxone (Narcan) is not related to the care of the patient with decompression sickness. *(Brady, Paramedic Care 2e, Principles and Practice, Volume 3—Environmental Emergencies. Mosby, Paramedic Textbook 3e, Environmental Conditions.)*

590. **The answer is A.** (B), (C), (D), assessing the ABCs, and considering the administration of IV corticosteroids are correct parts of the emergency care of a patient suffering an air embolism. Also, if the patient requires air transport, it is very important to use pressurized airplanes or to fly at a low altitude. (A) is incorrect because, even though the patient is tachypneic,

it is important to place the patient in the left lateral Trendelenburg position. This position keeps air bubbles away from the brain and coronary arteries. *(Brady, Paramedic Care 2e, Principles and Practice, Volume 3—Environmental Emergencies. Mosby, Paramedic Textbook 3e, Environmental Conditions.)*

591. **The answer is D.** (D) is the correct definition. (B), (C), and (D) all may occur in the setting described but do not represent high-altitude sickness. *(Brady, Paramedic Care 2e, Principles and Practice, Volume 3—Environmental Emergencies. Mosby, Paramedic Textbook 3e, Environmental Conditions.)*

592. **The answer is B.** (A), (C), and (D) are correct. (B) is incorrect because it usually occurs after rapid ascent to elevations above 8000 feet. *(Brady, Paramedic Care 2e, Principles and Practice, Volume 3—Environmental Emergencies. Mosby, Paramedic Textbook 3e, Environmental Conditions.)*

593. **The answer is D.** (A), (B), (C), and use of a portable hyperbaric chamber are all correct. (D) is incorrect because, in high-altitude pulmonary edema, the mainstay of treatment is immediate descent to a lower altitude. *(Brady, Paramedic Care 2e, Principles and Practice, Volume 3—Environmental Emergencies. Mosby, Paramedic Textbook 3e, Environmental Conditions.)*

594. **The answer is D.** (A), (B), and (C) are correct. (D) is incorrect because, even though 100% oxygen is a very important part of the treatment of high-altitude cerebral edema, descent to a lower altitude is the most important part of the emergency care. *(Brady, Paramedic Care 2e, Principles and Practice, Volume 3—Environmental Emergencies. Mosby, Paramedic Textbook 3e, Environmental Conditions.)*

INFECTIOUS AND COMMUNICABLE DISEASES

595. **The answer is C.** (A), (B), (D), fungi, protozoans, and helminths (worms) are all possible causes. (C) is incorrect because carcinoma is the medical word for cancer, which is not infectious or communicable. *(Brady, Paramedic Care 2e,*

Principles and Practice, Volume 3—Infectious Disease. Mosby, Paramedic Textbook 3e, Infectious and Communicable Diseases.)

596. **The answer is B.** (A), (C), and (D) are parts of the human body's defense. T and B lymphocytes are a part of the body's immune system. The lymphatic system is a network of lymph ducts and nodes, which help to fight infections as well. (B) is incorrect because the circulatory system is a key part of the body but does not play a direct role in fighting infections. *(Brady, Paramedic Care 2e, Principles and Practice, Volume 3—Infectious Disease. Mosby, Paramedic Textbook 3e, Infectious and Communicable Diseases.)*

597. **The answer is D.** (A), (B), (C), and foodborne are some of the potential routes. (D) is incorrect because exposure is to patients who have a communicable disease, not to someone who was only exposed to a communicable disease. *(Brady, Paramedic Care 2e, Principles and Practice, Volume 3—Infectious Disease. Mosby, Paramedic Textbook 3e, Infectious and Communicable Diseases.)*

598. **The answer is C.** (A), (B), and (D) are included. (C) is incorrect because, even though vaccinations may prevent the acquisition of certain communicable diseases, they are not considered a part of universal precautions. *(Brady, Paramedic Care 2e, Principles and Practice, Volume 3—Infectious Disease. Mosby, Paramedic Textbook 3e, Infectious and Communicable Diseases.)*

599. **The answer is C.** (A), (B), (D), and cerebrospinal fluid may transmit HIV infection. HIV may be also transmitted by tears, saliva, breast milk, amniotic fluid, and urine, but such transmissions are uncommon. (C) is incorrect. *(Brady, Paramedic Care 2e, Principles and Practice, Volume 3—Infectious Disease. Mosby, Paramedic Textbook 3e, Infectious and Communicable Diseases.)*

600. **The answer is A.** (B), (C), and (D) are correct. (A) is incorrect because used needles should never be recapped, because of the high incidence of needle-stick injuries. *(Brady, Paramedic Care 2e, Principles and Practice, Volume 3—Infectious Disease. Mosby, Paramedic Textbook 3e, Infectious and Communicable Diseases.)*

601. **The answer is C.** (C) is correct because all EMS professional exposures should be immediately reported to the infectious disease control officer (IDCO) so that immediate medical follow-up care and counseling for the Paramedic can be undertaken. This will also facilitate immediate attempts to acquire follow-up testing for the identified source patient as well. *(Brady, Paramedic Care 2e, Principles and Practice, Volume 3—Infectious Disease. Mosby, Paramedic Textbook 3e, Infectious and Communicable Diseases.)*

602. **The answer is D.** (A), (B), and (C) are correct. (D) is incorrect because it is essential for the Paramedics caring for this patient to wear disposable masks in order to decrease the chance of acquiring and spreading this infection. In this case, pulmonary tuberculosis and other causes of pneumonia are possible diagnoses. *(Brady, Paramedic Care 2e, Principles and Practice, Volume 3—Infectious Disease. Mosby, Paramedic Textbook 3e, Infectious and Communicable Diseases.)*

603. **The answer is D.** (A), (B), and (C) are very important in order to prevent the spread of a possible case of acute meningitis. Meningitis is primarily spread through airborne droplets released by coughing or sneezing. (D) is incorrect because, even though this is very important, it is performed after the patient has been taken to the hospital. *(Brady, Paramedic Care 2e, Principles and Practice, Volume 3—Infectious Disease. Mosby, Paramedic Textbook 3e, Infectious and Communicable Diseases.)*

604. **The answer is B.** (A), (C), (D), wearing disposable gloves, and using universal precautions are important parts of the emergency care of this child with an animal bite and possible rabies exposure. (B) is incorrect because it is essential to wear disposable gloves in order to prevent possibly acquiring and spreading the rabies virus. *(Brady, Paramedic Care 2e, Principles and Practice, Volume 3—Infectious Disease. Mosby, Paramedic Textbook 3e, Infectious and Communicable Diseases.)*

605. **The answers are:** (A) 1, (B) 3, (C) 4, (D) 2, (E) 5. *(Brady, Paramedic Care 2e, Principles and Practice, Volume 3—Infectious Disease. Mosby, Paramedic Textbook 3e, Infectious and Communicable Diseases.)*

606. **The answers are:** (A) 4, (B) 8, (C) 7, (D) 5, (E) 2, (F) 10, (G) 6, (H) 3, (I) 1, (J) 9. *(Brady, Paramedic Care 2e, Principles and Practice, Volume 3—Infectious Disease. Mosby, Paramedic Textbook 3e, Infectious and Communicable Diseases.)*

607. **The answer is A.** (B), (C), (D), and hand washing are all appropriate parts of the emergency care of this child with chickenpox (varicella). (A) is incorrect because it is very important to notify the ED of the diagnosis and arrival of this patient so that an isolation room can be designated for her. This will decrease the exposure of other patients, families, visitors, staff, and, particularly, any pregnant women to this patient. *(Brady, Paramedic Care 2e, Principles and Practice, Volume 3—Infectious Disease. Mosby, Paramedic Textbook 3e, Infectious and Communicable Diseases.)*

608. **The answer is B.** (B) is the correct definition of the MMR vaccine. (A) is incorrect because MMR does not prevent meningitis or rabies. (C) is incorrect because measles is the same as rubeola, and the *R* stands for rubella. (D) is incorrect for the reasons previously stated. *(Brady, Paramedic Care 2e, Principles and Practice, Volume 3—Infectious Disease. Mosby, Paramedic Textbook 3e, Infectious and Communicable Diseases.)*

609. **The answer is A.** (A) is correct. (B) and (D) are incorrect because active genital herpes does not require isolation, since it is only transmitted by direct contact with the lesions. (C) is incorrect because the use of forceps is unrelated to the pregnant mother with active herpes genitalis. It is also very important, in this case, to carefully bag all of the linens and sterilize the stretcher and mattress, since the patient's water broke and the herpes simplex II virus has contaminated the amniotic fluids. *(Brady, Paramedic Care 2e, Principles and Practice, Volume 3—Infectious Disease. Mosby, Paramedic Textbook 3e, Infectious and Communicable Diseases.)*

610. **The answer is C.** (A), (B), and (D) are correct. (C) is incorrect because patients with lice do not require isolation. The staff members treating the patient only need protective gloves, gowns, and headgear. *(Brady, Paramedic Care 2e, Principles and Practice, Volume 3—Infectious Disease. Mosby,*

Paramedic Textbook 3e, Infectious and Communicable Diseases.)

611. **The answer is A.** (A) is correct because acute viral gastroenteritis usually presents as a viral infection that causes inflammation of the stomach (nausea and/or vomiting) and the intestines (diarrhea) associated with fairly normal physical examination findings. Gastroenteritis less commonly may be caused by bacteria, parasites, or other toxins. (B) is incorrect because peptic ulcer disease usually presents with severe upper abdominal pain, and sometimes with vomiting of blood, associated with significant upper abdominal tenderness (epigastric area). (C) is incorrect because acute appendicitis usually presents with severe abdominal pain that is initially periumbilical and then moves down to the right lower quadrant, and abdominal examination findings of a very tender right lower quadrant. (D) is incorrect because acute diverticulitis usually presents with acute focal (usually lower) abdominal pain and focal tenderness. *(Brady, Paramedic Care 2e, Principles and Practice, Volume 3—Infectious Disease. Mosby, Paramedic Textbook 3e, Infectious and Communicable Diseases.)*

612. **The answer is D.** (A), (B), and (C) are correct. (D) is incorrect because it is not associated with Lyme disease. *(Brady, Paramedic Care 2e, Principles and Practice, Volume 3—Infectious Disease. Mosby, Paramedic Textbook 3e, Infectious and Communicable Diseases.)*

613. **The answer is D.** (A), (B), (C), and eye protection are all parts of the PPE for Paramedics and EMTs in caring for a severe acute respiratory syndrome (SARS) patient. The patient should be encouraged to use a nonrebreather face mask or a surgical mask. Procedures which encourage patients to cough, such as nebulizer treatments, should be avoided. (D) is incorrect because despite being mandatory equipment in caring for patients in certain toxicology, bioterrorism, or decontamination situations, it is not part of the PPE required for treating SARS patients. *(Brady, Paramedic Care 2e, Principles and Practice, Volume 3—Infectious Disease. Mosby, Paramedic Textbook 3e, Infectious and Communicable Diseases.)*

BEHAVIORAL AND PSYCHIATRIC DISORDERS

614. **The answer is D.** (D) is correct, with the key point being that the patient's behavior appears to be dangerous to him- or herself or to others. (A), (B), and (C) are incorrect because, even though the behavior may be different from that to which we are accustomed, it does not contain the elements of a psychiatric or behavioral emergency. *(Brady, Paramedic Care 2e, Principles and Practice, Volume 3—Psychiatric and Behavioral Disorders. Mosby, Paramedic Textbook 3e, Behavioral and Psychiatric Disorders.)*

615. **The answers are:** (A) 4, (B) 6, (C) 2, (D) 3, (E) 5, (F) 1. *(Brady, Paramedic Care 2e, Principles and Practice, Volume 3—Psychiatric and Behavioral Disorders. Mosby, Paramedic Textbook 3e, Behavioral and Psychiatric Disorders.)*

616. **The answer is A.** (A) is correct. (B), (C), and (D) are all incorrect reasons for asking to have anyone removed from the scene of an emotionally disturbed patient. *(Brady, Paramedic Care 2e, Principles and Practice, Volume 3—Psychiatric and Behavioral Disorders. Mosby, Paramedic Textbook 3e, Behavioral and Psychiatric Disorders.)*

617. **The answer is B.** (A), (C), (D), asking effective questions, and correcting cognitive misconceptions or distortions are some of the useful interviewing techniques. (B) is incorrect because the patient should be encouraged to express his or her feelings. *(Brady, Paramedic Care 2e, Principles and Practice, Volume 3—Psychiatric and Behavioral Disorders. Mosby, Paramedic Textbook 3e, Behavioral and Psychiatric Disorders.)*

618. **The answer is D.** (D) is correct. At the hospital, if the psychiatrist has the same impression, he or she may hospitalize the patient against his or her will for a limited period of time. (A), (B), and (C) are incorrect because, even though you may be called on to evaluate similar patients, you would be expected to transport the patient against his or her will only if the patient appeared to be a danger to him- or herself or others. *(Brady, Paramedic Care 2e, Principles and*

Practice, Volume 3—Psychiatric and Behavioral Disorders. Mosby, Paramedic Textbook 3e, Behavioral and Psychiatric Disorders.)

619. **The answer is B.** (A), (C), and (D) are some of the more common techniques used to restrain the emotionally disturbed patient. (B) is incorrect because mouth gagging is not a restraint technique and is potentially very dangerous to the patient. *(Brady, Paramedic Care 2e, Principles and Practice, Volume 3—Psychiatric and Behavioral Disorders. Mosby, Paramedic Textbook 3e, Behavioral and Psychiatric Disorders.)*

620. **The answer is D.** (A), (B), (C), expressing suicidal thoughts and concrete suicide plans; being single, widowed, or divorced; social isolation; alcohol or drug abuse; recent loss of spouse or significant relationship; chronic debilitating illness; and family history of suicide and schizophrenia are all risk factors for suicide. (D) is incorrect because being a male over 55 years of age is a risk factor for suicide. *(Brady, Paramedic Care 2e, Principles and Practice, Volume 3—Psychiatric and Behavioral Disorders. Mosby, Paramedic Textbook 3e, Behavioral and Psychiatric Disorders.)*

621. **The answer is A.** (A) is correct. (B) is incorrect because the patient does not appear to be agitated or need to be forcibly restrained. (C) is incorrect because you should never leave a possibly suicidal patient at home. (D) is incorrect because you should never leave this possibly suicidal patient alone, for fear that he may harm himself. *(Brady, Paramedic Care 2e, Principles and Practice, Volume 3—Psychiatric and Behavioral Disorders. Mosby, Paramedic Textbook 3e, Behavioral and Psychiatric Disorders.)*

622. **The answer is C.** (A), (B), (D), and the loudness, intensity, and content of vocal activity are all factors which help to determine the potential for a violent episode. (C) is incorrect because the location of the call does not provide any additional insight into the potential for a violent episode. *(Brady, Paramedic Care 2e, Principles and Practice, Volume 3—Psychiatric and Behavioral Disorders. Mosby, Paramedic Textbook 3e, Behavioral and Psychiatric Disorders.)*

GYNECOLOGY

623. **The answers are:** (A) 7, (B) 5, (C) 2, (D) 8, (E) 3, (F) 4, (G) 6, (H) 1. *(Brady, Paramedic Care 2e, Principles and Practices, Volume 3—Gynecology. Mosby, Paramedic Textbook 3e, Gynecology.)*

624. **The answer is D.** (A), (B), and (C) are common symptoms of gynecologic emergencies. (D) is incorrect because dysuria and increased urinary frequency are symptoms of a urinary tract infection. *(Brady, Paramedic Care 2e, Principles and Practices, Volume 3—Gynecology. Mosby, Paramedic Textbook 3e, Gynecology.)*

625. **The answer is B.** (A), (C), and (D) are parts of the emergency care rendered to patients with gynecologic emergencies. (B) is incorrect because gynecologic emergencies associated with excessive bleeding should be treated as "load and go" in order to arrive at the hospital before the development of shock. This is also done in order to be able to surgically treat the cause of the bleeding, which cannot occur in the prehospital setting. *(Brady, Paramedic Care 2e, Principles and Practices, Volume 3—Gynecology. Mosby, Paramedic Textbook 3e, Gynecology.)*

626. **The answer is A.** (B), (C), and (D) are all gynecologic emergencies that could present in a similar manner to this patient. The triad of abdominal pain, vaginal bleeding, and amenorrhea are most suggestive of an ectopic pregnancy. (A) is incorrect because this is a gastrointestinal disease and usually presents with epigastric or right upper quadrant pain associated with nausea, vomiting, and occasionally hematemesis. *(Brady, Paramedic Care 2e, Principles and Practices, Volume 3—Gynecology. Mosby, Paramedic Textbook 3e, Gynecology.)*

627. **The answer is A.** (B), (C), (D), handling clothing as little as possible, not examining the victim's perineal area, using brown paper bags to collect bloodstained articles separately, and not allowing the victim to comb her hair or clean her fingernails are all part of the care rendered to a sexual assault victim. (A) is incorrect because this will be performed at the hospital and later by the police officers. *(Brady, Paramedic Care 2e, Principles and Practices, Volume 3—Gynecology. Mosby, Paramedic Textbook 3e, Gynecology.)*

628. **The answer is D.** (A), (B), and (C) are correct. (D) is incorrect because all bloodstained articles are to be collected in brown paper bags. *(Brady, Paramedic Care 2e, Principles and Practices, Volume 3—Gynecology. Mosby, Paramedic Textbook 3e, Gynecology.)*

OBSTETRICS

629. **The answer is A.** (B), (C), and (D) are correct. (A) is incorrect because a prematurely born fetus has a good chance of surviving at 28 weeks. *(Brady, Paramedic Care 2e, Principles and Practices, Volume 3—Obstetrics. Mosby, Paramedic Textbook 3e, Obstetrics.)*

630. **The answer is D.** (A), (B), and (C) are correct. (D) is incorrect because orthostatic vital signs are very important in evaluating the obstetric patient. They are very helpful in diagnosing early bleeding or fluid loss. *(Brady, Paramedic Care 2e, Principles and Practices, Volume 3—Obstetrics. Mosby, Paramedic Textbook 3e, Obstetrics.)*

631. **The answer is A.** (B), (C), and (D) are correct. (A) is incorrect because breech delivery is an obstetrical emergency that occurs during delivery, not in the predelivery period. *(Brady, Paramedic Care 2e, Principles and Practices, Volume 3—Obstetrics. Mosby, Paramedic Textbook 3e, Obstetrics.)*

632. **The answer is D.** (D) is correct because third-trimester vaginal bleeding associated with abdominal pain is more likely due to abruptio placenta. (A) is incorrect because eclampsia presents as seizures associated with hypertension, edema, and protein in the urine without vaginal bleeding. (B) is incorrect because placenta previa is usually painless. It is defined as the placentas being located partially or completely in front of the cervix. (C) is incorrect because postpartum hemorrhage is vaginal bleeding that occurs after delivery, not during pregnancy. *(Brady, Paramedic Care 2e, Principles and*

Practices, Volume 3—Obstetrics. Mosby, Paramedic Textbook 3e, Obstetrics.)

633. **The answer is D.** (A), (B), and (C) are correct. (D) is incorrect because the third stage of labor is from the delivery of the baby until the delivery of the placenta. *(Brady, Paramedic Care 2e, Principles and Practices, Volume 3—Obstetrics. Mosby, Paramedic Textbook 3e, Obstetrics.)*

634. **The answer is B.** (A), (C), and (D) are correct. (B) is incorrect because you should position the mother in the supine position (on her back) with her legs apart. *(Brady, Paramedic Care 2e, Principles and Practices, Volume 3—Obstetrics. Mosby, Paramedic Textbook 3e, Obstetrics.)*

635. **The answer is D.** (A), (B), and (C) are correct. (D) is incorrect because, after the head has been delivered and before the next contraction, you should try to suction the baby's mouth and nose. After the completed delivery, you should clean the baby's airway with sterile gauze and repeat suctioning of the mouth and nose. *(Brady, Paramedic Care 2e, Principles and Practices, Volume 3—Obstetrics. Mosby, Paramedic Textbook 3e, Obstetrics.)*

636. **The answer is D.** (A), (B), and (C) are correct. (D) is incorrect because, with a baby presenting with probable meconium aspiration, you need to proceed with endotracheal intubation and suctioning immediately, without contacting medical control. *(Brady, Paramedic Care 2e, Principles and Practices, Volume 3—Obstetrics. Mosby, Paramedic Textbook 3e, Obstetrics.)*

637. **The answer is C.** (A) is correct. The Brady text recommends that the first clamp be 10 cm from the baby and the second clamp 15 cm. (B), (C), and (D) are incorrect. *(Brady, Paramedic Care 2e, Principles and Practices, Volume 3—Obstetrics. Mosby, Paramedic Textbook 3e, Obstetrics.)*

638. **The answer is B.** (A), (C), and (D) are correct. (B) is incorrect because, in neonates, the correct dose for fluid administration is 10 mL/kg. In the pediatric population, the correct dose is 20 mL/kg. *(Brady, Paramedic Care 2e, Principles and Practices, Volume 3—Obstetrics. Mosby, Paramedic Textbook 3e, Obstetrics.)*

639. **The answer is B.** (B) is correct because, if necessary, the Paramedic may assist the mother in safely delivering a buttocks breech delivery. (A), (C), and (D) are incorrect because all must be delivered at the hospital by cesarean section. *(Brady, Paramedic Care 2e, Principles and Practices, Volume 3—Obstetrics. Mosby, Paramedic Textbook 3e, Obstetrics.)*

640. **The answer is B.** (A), (C), (D), and rapid transport are correct. (B) is incorrect because you should never insert packs into the vagina. If the patient is hemorrhaging from perineal tears, provide firm external pressure on the site of bleeding. *(Brady, Paramedic Care 2e, Principles and Practices, Volume 3—Obstetrics. Mosby, Paramedic Textbook 3e, Obstetrics.)*

641. **The answer is D.** (A), (B), and (C) are correct. (D) is incorrect because rapid assessment, stabilization, and rapid transport to the hospital are also essential in the care of this patient. *(Brady, Paramedic Care 2e, Principles and Practices, Volume 3—Obstetrics. Mosby, Paramedic Textbook 3e, Obstetrics.)*

Special Considerations

The following topics are covered in Section VI:

- Neonatology
- Pediatrics
- Geriatrics
- Abuse and Assault
- Acute Interventions for Chronic Care Patients

Questions

NEONATOLOGY

DIRECTIONS: Each item below contains four suggested responses. Select the one best response to each item.

642. Neonates are defined as

    (A) an infant up to 1 month old
    (B) a term newborn from time of birth to 1 week old
    (C) an infant up to 3 months old
    (D) a preterm newborn child

643. You arrive on the scene of a full-term woman in labor, the woman states that she is actually 2 weeks overdue and that when her bag of waters broke, there was a green fluid that leaked out. During your examination, you notice that she has begun crowning. The greenish tint of the fluid is most likely

    (A) meconium
    (B) postpartum infection
    (C) placental remnant
    (D) normal

644. Based on your assessment, you decide that you should begin suctioning. When should you begin this process?

    (A) as soon as the head is delivered and before the first breath
    (B) after the child is delivered but before the first breath
    (C) after the child is delivered and after administering the first breath
    (D) after drying, warming, and providing tactile stimulation to initiate spontaneous respiration

645. You are in the process of delivering a newborn. While you are suctioning with a bulb syringe, you notice thick meconium in the airway. What is the next immediate step you would take?

    (A) Administer 100% oxygen via "blow by."
    (B) Immediately perform endotracheal intubation and attach to suction to clear the airway of meconium.
    (C) Ventilate with 100% oxygen via bag-valve-mask.
    (D) Perform tactile stimulation to increase respiratory effort.

646. One minute after delivering a newborn, the child has a pink body and cyanotic extremities, a pulse rate of 160 beats per minute, a grimace, some flexion of the extremities, and a strong cry. What is the initial APGAR (**A**ctivity, **P**ulse, **G**rimace, **A**ppearance, and **R**espiration) score for this newborn?

    (A) 7
    (B) 8
    (C) 9
    (D) 10

647. A neonate is defined as premature when it meets which of the following criteria?

    (A) born at less than 38 weeks' gestation *or* weighing less than 2500 g
    (B) born at less than 28 weeks' gestation *or* weighing less than 2500 g
    (C) born at less than 38 weeks' gestation *and* weighing less than 2500 g
    (D) born at less than 28 weeks' gestation *and* weighing less than 2500 g

648. Based on the inverted resuscitation pyramid, the next appropriate step after drying, warming, and tactile stimulation would be

    (A) chest compressions
    (B) ventilation via bag-valve-mask
    (C) administration of oxygen
    (D) administration of medications

649. Which of the following is *not* considered a complication of pregnancy (delivery)?

    (A) breech presentation
    (B) pre-eclampsia
    (C) multiple pregnancy (twins)
    (D) antepartum hemorrhage

650. The umbilical cord contains vessels that the Paramedic may cannulate in order to administer medications to the neonate. How many of each vessel is in the umbilical cord, and which one would the Paramedic use to cannulate for administration of medication?

    (A) two veins, one artery; vein is cannulated
    (B) one artery, one vein; artery is cannulated
    (C) two arteries, one vein; artery is cannulated
    (D) two arteries, one vein; vein is cannulated

651. You are called to the scene of an ill neonate, the history of present illness suggests that the child has been vomiting, has high fever, and has had diarrhea for several days. The diaper, which has been on all day, is still dry. The child has sunken eyes and fontanelle. Which of the following is the most likely diagnosis?

    (A) meningitis
    (B) influenza
    (C) dehydration
    (D) chicken pox

652. Based on the child's condition, which of the following fluid replacement regimens is indicated?

    (A) 10 mL/kg
    (B) 12 mL/kg
    (C) 15 mL/kg
    (D) 20 mL/kg

653. The neonatal dose of naloxone is

    (A) 1 mg
    (B) 1 mg/kg
    (C) 0.01 mg/kg
    (D) 0.1 mg/kg

PEDIATRICS

DIRECTIONS: Each item below contains four suggested responses. Select the one best response to each item.

654. The pediatric age group most likely to suffer from fear of mutilation is

    (A) school-aged children (6–11 years)
    (B) infants and toddlers (birth to 3 years)
    (C) preschoolers (4–5 years)
    (D) adolescents (12–18 years)

655. The age group most likely to suffer from separation anxiety is

    (A) school-aged children (6–11 years)
    (B) adolescents (12–18 years)
    (C) infants and toddlers (birth to 3 years)
    (D) preschoolers (4–5 years)

656. A Paramedic must deal with the child's caregiver as well as with the patient. Which of the following actions would be beneficial in managing the child's caregiver?

    (A) Explain to the caregiver that you must do your job and he or she must leave.
    (B) Give the caregiver a role in assisting in the care of the child.
    (C) Tell the caregiver to relax and you will take care of everything.
    (D) Have a spouse or family member remove the caregiver from the room.

657. The Paramedic who is treating an adolescent should

    (A) Discuss all interventions with the patient and allow his or her input into the treatment.
    (B) Discuss all interventions with the parent, and inform the patient of the parent's decision.
    (C) Inform the adolescent that your interventions are necessary and he or she must agree to the treatment protocol.
    (D) Transport the patient without intervention if he or she becomes disagreeable with your treatments due to lack of information.

658. Of the following, which set of vital signs would the Paramedic expect to find while assessing a 6-month-old child?

    (A) pulse 100–160 beats per minute, systolic blood pressure 50–75, respiration 30–60 breaths per minute
    (B) pulse 90–120 beats per minute, systolic blood pressure 80–100, respiration 25–40 breaths per minute
    (C) pulse 60–90 beats per minute, systolic blood pressure 90–120, respiration 15–20 breaths per minute
    (D) pulse 70–110 beats per minute, systolic blood pressure 80–110, respiration 18–25 breaths per minute

659. You are treating an injured 3-year-old child, the normal range of vital signs for that age group are most likely

    (A) pulse 80–120 beats per minute, systolic blood pressure 80–110, respiration 20–30 breaths per minute
    (B) pulse 90–120 beats per minute, systolic blood pressure 80–100, respiration 25–40 breaths per minute
    (C) pulse 60–90 beats per minute, systolic blood pressure 90–120, respiration 15–20 breaths per minute
    (D) pulse 100–160 beats per minute, systolic blood pressure 50–70, respiration 30–60 breaths per minute

660. In contrast to an adult, the assessment of infants and small children should be complete in what order?

    (A) head to toe, as in the adult
    (B) only if absolutely necessary
    (C) toe to head
    (D) only in the areas affected by illness or injury

661. You are on the scene of a pediatric patient with difficulty breathing. Your partner forgot the pediatric blood pressure cuff in the vehicle and is taking the patient's blood pressure with an adult cuff. What would be an appropriate response to this intervention?

    (A) Estimate the patient's blood pressure using pulse points.
    (B) Accept your partner's blood pressure reading as accurate.
    (C) Reduce the systolic blood pressure by 10 mmHg due to cuff size.
    (D) Inform your partner that it is inappropriate to obtain pediatric blood pressure with an adult cuff.

662. Pulse assessment in an infant should be done for _____ seconds.

    (A) 15
    (B) 30
    (C) 45
    (D) 60

663. Which of the following is *not* a common fracture found in children?

    (A) comminuted fractures
    (B) bend fractures
    (C) buckle fractures
    (D) greenstick fractures

664. Which of the following is *not* a complicating factor in pediatric intubation?

    (A) The tongue is larger in relation to the remainder of the upper airway.
    (B) The cricoid ring has the smallest diameter of all the airway structures.
    (C) The tracheal cartilage is hard and bony, allowing for easier intubation.
    (D) The smaller structures of the larynx and trachea make visualization more difficult.

665. Bronchiolitis is most commonly seen in which pediatric age group?

    (A) 1–3 years old
    (B) 6–12 months old
    (C) 3–5 years old
    (D) 6–12 years old

666. You respond to a call for a 5-year-old child with difficulty breathing. She is sitting in a tripod position; in the sniffing position with her chin thrust upward. Her mother explains that she was fine this morning and then developed a high fever and cannot speak. The child looks extremely scared, and you notice she will not swallow and is drooling. The most appropriate diagnosis is

    (A) epiglottitis
    (B) foreign-body obstruction
    (C) caustic ingestion
    (D) croup

667. You are dispatched to a scene of a respiratory arrest. On your arrival, the mother is hysterical and tells you that she placed the child in for a nap about an hour ago. When she went to wake him, he was not responsive and she called 911. She states that the child is 2 months old and has been perfectly healthy. You begin cardiopulmonary resuscitation (CPR) and transport the child to the hospital. The most appropriate cause of the child's condition is

    (A) child abuse
    (B) sudden infant death syndrome (SIDS)
    (C) choking
    (D) an undiagnosed respiratory infection

668. In the case of SIDS where the child has obviously been dead for several hours and is cold and lifeless, the main responsibility of the Paramedic is

(A) Begin CPR and transport the child.
(B) Tell the parents what they should have done to help prior to your arrival.
(C) Assist the parents in their grief and offer to contact relatives, priest or rabbi, or family and friends.
(D) Notify the police department and leave the premises after you have done the appropriate paperwork.

669. All of the following factors have been identified to cause seizures in the pediatric patient *except*:

(A) dysrhythmia
(B) fever
(C) trauma
(D) Reye syndrome

670. The Paramedic's initial action in the treatment of the seizing child is

(A) administer diazepam 0.3 mg/kg IV
(B) administer 25% dextrose 1 mL/kg IV
(C) establish airway
(D) administer 100% oxygen

671. You are treating a 6-month-old child with high fever. On your arrival, the mother explains that the child has had a recent upper respiratory and ear infection. Your examination of the child reveals that the child is irritable, with high fever, lethargy, and a bulging anterior fontanelle. The father states that the child has not been eating well at all. You suspect

(A) epiglottitis
(B) croup
(C) meningitis
(D) bronchiolitis

672. Which of the following children is having the most severe asthma attack?

(A) A 7-year-old child with mild end-expiratory wheezes who is awake and alert.
(B) A 6-year-old child who has loud wheezes in all fields and is lethargic.
(C) A 9-year-old child who is in the tripod position, is lethargic, has wheezes in all lung fields, and has accessory muscle use.
(D) A 6-year-old child who is sleepy, has a silent chest, and has accessory muscle use.

673. Which of the following is not a beta$_2$-adrenergic agonist used in the treatment of pediatric asthma?

(A) methylprednisolone
(B) epinephrine
(C) albuterol
(D) terbutaline

674. The most common dysrhythmia found in the pediatric patient is

(A) supraventricular tachycardia
(B) ventricular tachycardia
(C) asystole
(D) bradycardia

675. All of the following children should receive a rapid cardiopulmonary assessment to recognize and prevent decompensation and cardiac arrest *except*:

(A) a 6-year-old child with a closed fracture of the radius and/or ulna
(B) a 6-year-old child with respiratory distress and cyanosis
(C) a 6-year-old child with a heart rate of 58 beats per minute
(D) a 6-year-old child with an open femur fracture

676. Which of the following people would most likely fit the description of a person capable of child abuse?

   (A) an unemployed factory worker
   (B) a decorated police captain
   (C) a caring mother of four children
   (D) all of the above

677. All of the following are common injuries that suggest an abused child *except*:

   (A) a wrist fracture in a 6-year-old child in which the mother states "he fell off his bicycle"
   (B) injuries in various stages of healing
   (C) obvious fractures in children less than 2 years old
   (D) bruises or burns with particular patterns

678. You respond to an unconscious child. On your arrival, you find a 7-year-old male unconscious with an open head injury in the occipital region. Further investigation reveals greenish-yellow facial bruising in the orbital area as well as various bruises on his arms and legs. On questioning, the father states that the child was playing near the top of the stairs and fell down on his head. Your number one priority should be to

   (A) further question the father about the abusive injury pattern
   (B) stabilize the child's cervical spine and assess the airway, breathing, and circulation (ABCs)
   (C) have your partner care for the child while you hold the father until police arrive
   (D) contact medical control for instructions

679. Intraosseous (IO) needle insertion is an appropriate intervention until _____.

   (A) 3 years of age
   (B) 4 years of age
   (C) 5 years of age
   (D) 6 years of age

680. Hypotensive pediatric patients should receive volume replacement at which of the following rates?

   (A) 5 mL/kg
   (B) 10 mL/kg
   (C) 20 mL/kg
   (D) 30 mL/kg

681. In asystole, the Paramedic should administer epinephrine to the pediatric patient at which of the following doses?

   (A) 1.0 mg of a 1:10,000 solution
   (B) 0.1 mg/kg of a 1:10,000 solution
   (C) 0.01 mg/kg of a 1:10,000 solution
   (D) 0.1 mg/kg of a 1:1,000 solution

682. In pediatric bradycardia, the *initial* dose of atropine is

   (A) 2.0 mg/kg
   (B) 0.2 mg/kg
   (C) 0.02 mg/kg
   (D) 0.02 μg/kg

683. Bradycardia in an infant is defined as a

   (A) heart rate less than 60 beats per minute
   (B) heart rate less than 70 beats per minute
   (C) heart rate less than 80 beats per minute
   (D) heart rate less than 90 beats per minute

GERIATRICS

DIRECTIONS: Each item below contains four suggested responses. Select the one best response to each item.

684. All of the following statements are true about the difficulties in assessing the geriatric patient *except*:

(A) The geriatric patient may fail to report initial symptoms.

(B) Emotional factors may make geriatric assessment difficult.

(C) The geriatric patient has a lack of temperature-regulatory mechanisms.

(D) Many geriatric patients suffer from several chronic problems, making diagnosis more difficult.

685. You respond to an 86-year-old male who has been disoriented for a few days. On your arrival, you find that the patient has been complaining of seeing a yellow haze and is just "not feeling right." At the hospital, the patient is diagnosed with digitalis toxicity. All of the following are common accidental causes of medication reactions in the elderly patient *except*:

(A) Geriatric patients have changes in drug absorption and metabolism.

(B) Geriatric patients use medications in an attempt to end their lives.

(C) Due to memory deterioration, the geriatric patients may accidentally overdose on medication.

(D) Geriatric patients may see more than one physician and have duplicate medications.

686. Which of the following is the number one cause of decreased cardiac output in the otherwise healthy geriatric patient?

(A) deterioration of the electrical conduction system of the heart

(B) cardiac hypertrophy

(C) hypertension

(D) arteriosclerosis

687. Which of the following is *not* a typical age-related physiologic change?

(A) degeneration of the joints

(B) decreased respiratory vital capacity

(C) decreased renal function

(D) increase in brain mass

688. All of the following are common complaints in the elderly *except*:

(A) chest pain

(B) dizziness

(C) fatigue

(D) falls

689. You are dispatched to an 84-year-old female who has fallen on the sidewalk. On your arrival, you find the woman lying on the ground, alert, and oriented. You notice a large hematoma in the occipital region with little external bleeding. Which of the following would lead you to a high index of suspicion for brain injury in this patient?

(A) Due to decreased brain mass, elderly patients are prone to head injuries.

(B) Based on mental status, there is no evidence of brain injury.

(C) Little external bleeding with a hematoma usually means it is bleeding internally.

(D) The occipital region is prone to internal injuries.

690. You respond to a 78-year-old male with a syncopal episode. On your arrival, you find the male awake and lying on a couch. The patient has a heart rate of 40 beats per minute, a blood pressure of 86/62, and a respiratory rate of 20 breaths per minute. The patient states that he is okay when lying down but feels faint when he stands. In fact, he passed out before. You acquire an ECG, which shows a third-degree heart block. The type of syncope associated with heart blocks is known as

    (A) cardiogenic syncope
    (B) orthostatic syncope
    (C) psychogenic syncope
    (D) Stokes-Adams syncope

691. Your patient is a 72-year-old female who has just suffered a seizure. On arrival, you find that the patient is postictal. Family members on the scene tell you that she has no history of medical problems and is quite physically fit. As a matter of fact, she fell and hit her head recently while rollerblading and got right back up and continued skating. Based on this information, what would be the most likely cause of this seizure activity?

    (A) alcohol withdrawal
    (B) hypoglycemia
    (C) subdural hematoma
    (D) epilepsy

692. You arrive at a well-kept residence to find an 87-year-old woman who has multiple bruises about her face and arms. The family members who are present state that she has been a burden and has been falling constantly. The patient, who is alert and answers your questions, states that they are trying to kill her and hit her all the time. The family states that she is senile and has no idea what she is talking about. After medically treating the patient, the Paramedic may suspect

    (A) The patient is embarrassed about her falls and is confabulating a story.
    (B) The patient is a victim of elder abuse.
    (C) The patient suffers from senile dementia.
    (D) The patient may be suffering from head injuries due to the fall.

ABUSE AND ASSAULT

DIRECTIONS: Each item below contains four suggested responses. Select the one best response to each item.

693. All of the following are categories of abuse *except*:

    (A) drug abuse
    (B) sexual abuse
    (C) elderly abuse
    (D) child abuse

694. All of the following are characteristics associated with the profile of a typical adult abuser *except*:

    (A) usually outgoing and very sociable
    (B) frequently jealous, irritable, and explosive
    (C) poorly educated
    (D) likely alcohol and drug user

695. You are waved down by a young child who requests that you please come and help his mother, who is bleeding. On your entering the patient's apartment, you find a 40-year-old female holding her right arm, with multiple facial bruises and active bleeding from the mouth. The patient's husband has alcohol on his breath and claims that his wife slipped on the floor and hit herself on the kitchen table. As you begin to assess the patient and treat her wounds, you are very suspicious that this may represent an example of

(A) adult abuse
(B) child abuse
(C) geriatric abuse
(D) drug abuse

696. Which of the following is the correct number of women beaten by a spouse or partner each year in the United States?

(A) 250,000
(B) 750,000
(C) 1.5 million
(D) 4 million

697. You are sent to the home of a 79-year-old male who has been injured. As you walk into the house, a younger man who claims to be the patient's son greets you. He has alcohol on his breath and proceeds to tell you that the patient has fallen and hit his chin on the desk. He also tells you that his father is losing his memory, is often combative, and is incontinent of urine day and night. He tells you that he has lost his job recently and is unable to look for another one because of his father's condition. He then begins to become angry and rants about being sick and tired of babysitting his father. When you finally are led to the patient, you find him lying in bed, disheveled, confused, with a swollen and ecchymotic left chin, as well as red finger marks on his right cheek. As you approach the patient, he withdraws from you and proceeds to cover his head with his arms. He also is grossly incontinent of urine. Which of the following best describes this presentation?

(A) child abuse
(B) drug abuse
(C) adult abuse
(D) elder abuse

698. All of the following are characteristics of a typical abuser of the elder *except*:

(A) usually does not have any financial responsibility for the elder
(B) frequently abuses alcohol and drugs
(C) angry and under any stress
(D) usually does not allow the elder to visit alone with a health care provider

699. You are dispatched to an injured 3-year-old boy. As you arrive at the child's home, his 7-year-old sister leads you to the child. She states that her mother is busy washing clothes and her father is at work. As you enter the room, you notice that the child is sitting on the floor, with several bruises on his arms and legs. All of the following are consistent with this representing a case of child abuse *except*:

(A) The child's sister states that he has always been a little slow and that he gets hurt a lot.

(B) The child seems apathetic and does not cry, even with examination of the bruises.

(C) The child's mother approaches you and demonstrates little interest in her child.

(D) The child only has fresh bruises, without any old scars or burns.

700. All of the following are typical characteristics of an abusive parent *except*:

(A) acts abusively often in response to stresses or losses, such as loss of a job or a divorce

(B) often does not demonstrate any cuddling or closeness to the child

(C) usually offers a clear, detailed description of each injury to the child

(D) frequently involved with alcohol or drugs

701. You are dispatched to a 26-year-old female who has been sexually assaulted. As you arrive at the patient's apartment, you find the patient crying and very upset. She states that a man must have followed her home and quickly put his foot in her apartment door just after she opened it. Then, using the threat of a knife, he raped her. All of the following are parts of the approach to treating this patient *except*:

(A) Always allow and encourage the patient to shower and use the bathroom to clean up before going to the hospital.

(B) Only examine the patient's vaginal area if she is heavily bleeding.

(C) Attempt to gather any evidence of the patient's sexual assault, such as bloodstained clothing.

(D) Examine the patient for any signs of serious trauma.

702. All of the following are parts of the correct method of documenting the ambulance call report in a suspected rape case *except*:

(A) State, in the patient's own words, exactly what occurred.

(B) Carefully describe the patient's appearance and emotional state.

(C) Complete the report by offering your opinion as to whether the patient has or has not been raped.

(D) Carefully document the patient's injuries.

ACUTE INTERVENTIONS FOR CHRONIC CARE PATIENTS

Directions: Each item below contains four suggested responses. Select the one best response to each item.

703. All of the following are categories of vascular access devices used in home health care *except*:

    (A) implanted ports
    (B) central venous catheters
    (C) arterial lines
    (D) peripheral inserted central catheters

704. All of the following are characteristics of a central venous catheter *except*:

    (A) manufactured by Broviac, Hickman, Groshong, or Corcath
    (B) a small cap covering each lumen
    (C) are tunneled under the subcutaneous tissue to the venous entrance site
    (D) only come with a single lumen

705. You are dispatched to a 54-year-old female who is complaining of substernal chest pain. As you approach the patient, she tells you that she has had 2 hours of substernal chest pain radiating down her left arm. She has a history of angina and has not had chest pain as severe as she has experienced today. She also tells you that she had a mastectomy 4 months ago, is in the process of receiving outpatient chemotherapy, and has a Broviac central venous catheter in place. According to your protocol, you have begun ECG monitoring and high-concentration oxygen by nonrebreather face mask, and have administered sublingual nitroglycerin, without relief. You attempt to begin an IV line, but the patient tells you that she has awful veins. Despite additional nitroglycerin, the patient continues to have chest pain and is also short of breath. You have received medical control permission to administer IV 3 mg morphine sulfate. All of the following are parts of the approach to accessing the central venous catheter *except*:

    (A) Clamp the catheter with a smooth hemostat.
    (B) Use aseptic technique, with sterile gloves.
    (C) If an infusion is going in one of the multiple lumens, a free lumen may be used.
    (D) Never accept advice from a patient, family member, or caregiver concerning the use of the catheter.

706. All of the following are possible complications of accessing vascular access devices *except*:

    (A) toe gangrene
    (B) infection at the catheter's access site
    (C) thrombosis in the catheter
    (D) air embolism

707. All of the following are possible complications and emergencies associated with patients who have tracheostomies *except*:

    (A) respiratory distress
    (B) tracheal stenosis
    (C) sepsis
    (D) skin rash on both arms

708. You are dispatched to the home of a 76-year-old male who is having difficulty breathing. However, as you enter the patient's bedroom, you become aware that the patient has a tracheostomy and is connected to a ventilator. The patient's nurse states that the patient has been having an increase in secretions for the past few days. Then, this morning, the patient began to have difficulty breathing. The nurse also stated that she was having difficulty suctioning the patient today. Your assessment reveals that the patient's respiratory rate is 28 breaths per minute, his pulse rate is 120 beats per minute, and his blood pressure is 162/78. In addition, the patient has circumoral and peripheral cyanosis. Which of the following is the best way to proceed in providing emergency care for this patient?

    (A) Contact medical control to discuss various treatment options.
    (B) Place the patient and the portable ventilator on the stretcher and transport both to the hospital.
    (C) Disconnect the patient from the ventilator and begin to ventilate the patient with a bag-valve-mask attached to the tracheostomy tube.
    (D) Administer 100% oxygen by nonrebreather face mask.

709. All of the following are possible complications occurring with the use of gastrostomy feeding tubes *except*:

    (A) pulmonary aspiration
    (B) dehydration
    (C) headache
    (D) diarrhea

710. You are sent to the home of an 86-year-old female with bleeding from a gastrostomy tube site. The patient's home health aide tells you that she was in the process of turning the patient when the patient's gastrostomy tube became caught on the bed. The patient then was noted to begin bleeding from the gastrostomy tube sight. Which of the following is the correct way to care for this patient?

    (A) Package the patient, and transport her to the hospital.
    (B) Apply direct pressure with a sterile dressing to the bleeding site.
    (C) Try to flush the gastrostomy tube with 500 mL saline solution.
    (D) Try to maneuver the catheter by pushing it further into the abdomen.

Answers and Explanations

NEONATOLOGY

642. The answer is A. The neonate is best described as an infant less than 1 month of age. *(Brady, Paramedic Care 2e, Principles and Practice, Volume 5—Neonatology. Mosby, Paramedic Textbook 3e, Neonatology.)*

643. The answer is A. Meconium, a greenish substance, is a waste product from the newborn. It usually occurs in term and "late" pregnancies as the newborn is more developed. Meconium is usually dispelled during labor and becomes an aspirated hazard during birth. Meconium can be aspirated into the newborn's lungs and create respiratory infections. *(Brady, Paramedic Care 2e, Principles and Practice, Volume 5—Neonatology. Mosby, Paramedic Textbook 3e, Neonatology.)*

644. The answer is A. Meconium staining is a serious complication and the Paramedic should focus on immediate suctioning of the newborn's airway. Suctioning should begin as soon as the head delivers and should continue until all meconium is aspirated. *(Brady, Paramedic Care 2e, Principles and Practice, Volume 5—Neonatology. Mosby, Paramedic Textbook 3e, Neonatology.)*

645. The answer is B. During meconium suctioning, the Paramedic should avoid administering any ventilation. Attempts at ventilation will force meconium deeper into the airways and could result in a life-threatening illness. All efforts should be aimed at a rapid suctioning of the airway and replacement of the endotracheal tube with a fresh tube after every attempt. This is a rarely performed skill that should be practiced regularly in order to retain proficiency. *(Brady, Paramedic Care 2e, Principles and Practice, Volume 5—Neonatology. Mosby, Paramedic Textbook 3e, Neonatology.)*

646. The answer is A. The child has a 1-minute APGAR score of 7. Pink body and cyanotic extremities scores 1. The pulse rate over 100 beats per minute scores 2. The grimace scores 1. Some flexion of the extremities scores 1, and a strong cry scores 2. It is suggested that the Paramedic be very familiar with APGAR scoring. APGAR scoring is performed at 1 and 5 minutes after birth. *(Brady, Paramedic Care 2e, Principles and Practice, Volume 5—Neonatology. Mosby, Paramedic Textbook 3e, Neonatology.)*

647. The answer is A. A neonate is defined as premature when birth occurs at less than 38 weeks' gestation and less than 2500 grams. Premature neonates are prone to respiratory disorders, hypothermia, volume depletion, and cardiovascular problems. *(Brady, Paramedic Care 2e, Principles and Practice, Volume 5—Neonatology. Mosby, Paramedic Textbook 3e, Neonatology.)*

648. The answer is C. Administration of oxygen, ventilation via bag-valve-mask, chest compressions, and the administration of medications all follow the primary resuscitation efforts of drying, warming, and tactile stimulation. *(Brady, Paramedic Care 2e, Principles and Practice, Volume 5—Neonatology. Mosby, Paramedic Textbook 3e, Neonatology.)*

649. The answer is A. Breech presentations create special problems during the birth of the neonate, but it is a problem that occurs, not during pregnancy, but during actual childbirth. Antepartum hemorrhage, pre-eclampsia, and multiple pregnancy are all factors that affect birth. *(Brady, Paramedic Care 2e, Principles and Practice, Volume 5—Neonatology. Mosby, Paramedic Textbook 3e, Neonatology.)*

650. **The answer is D.** The umbilical cord contains three vessels: two arteries and one vein. Cannulation of the umbilical vein is an excellent pathway for the delivery of medication to the neonate. (A), (B), and (C) are incorrect. *(Brady, Paramedic Care 2e, Principles and Practice, Volume 5—Neonatology. Mosby, Paramedic Textbook 3e, Neonatology.)*

651. **The answer is C.** This is clearly a case of dehydration. Infants are susceptible to cases of dehydration secondary to viral illness. This child has neither eaten nor has taken in any fluids. The resulting dehydration has affected urine output, which is evidenced by the dry diaper. Meningitis would result in a bulging fontanelle and chicken pox would have an associated rash. Influenza virus may cause dehydration but the primary treatable diagnosis is dehydration. *(Brady, Paramedic Care 2e, Principles and Practice, Volume 5—Neonatology. Mosby, Paramedic Textbook 3e, Neonatology.)*

652. **The answer is A.** The neonate who is hypovolemic for any reason (e.g., dehydration due to vomiting, diarrhea, or hemorrhage) should receive 10 mL/kg of a volume expander to increase intravascular volume. In this example, volume expanders include whole blood, albumin, Ringer's lactate, and normal saline solution; 20 mL/kg is the correct volume for a child over 1 month old. *(Brady, Paramedic Care 2e, Principles and Practice, Volume 5—Neonatology. Mosby, Paramedic Textbook 3e, Neonatology.)*

653. **The answer is C.** The neonatal dose of naloxone (Narcan) is 0.01 mg/kg. Keep in mind that this dosage is only for infants less than 1 month of age. Children over the age of 1 month use a different dosing regimen. *(Brady, Paramedic Care 2e, Principles and Practice, Volume 5—Neonatology. Mosby, Paramedic Textbook 3e, Neonatology.)*

PEDIATRICS

654. **The answer is C.** Preschool age children have fears of mutilation and bleeding to death. These are simplistic fears and they are very prone to suggestive comments by adults. EMS professionals should always consider whether their comments would exacerbate these fears. *(Brady, Paramedic Care 2e, Principles and Practice, Volume 5—Pediatrics. Mosby, Paramedic Textbook 3e, Pediatrics.)*

655. **The answer is C.** Separation anxiety is extremely common in infants and toddlers. The Paramedic would be well served to allow the parent to hold the child during the assessment and transport if this would not interfere with the care of the patient. *(Brady, Paramedic Care 2e, Principles and Practice, Volume 5—Pediatrics. Mosby, Paramedic Textbook 3e, Pediatrics.)*

656. **The answer is B.** In many cases, parents feel a sense of guilt when their child is ill. It assists the Paramedic and the parent greatly when the parent is invited to participate in the care of the child. As previously discussed in this section, allowing the parent to hold the child during assessment and care will also reduce separation anxiety. *(Brady, Paramedic Care 2e, Principles and Practice, Volume 5—Pediatrics. Mosby, Paramedic Textbook 3e, Pediatrics.)*

657. **The answer is A.** Adolescents have fear of loss of control as well as altered body image. If the Paramedic allows the adolescent to have input in his or her care, this will serve to alleviate his or her fears and assist the Paramedic in properly performing the duties. *(Brady, Paramedic Care 2e, Principles and Practice, Volume 5—Pediatrics. Mosby, Paramedic Textbook 3e, Pediatrics.)*

658. **The answer is B.** (B) would be the most appropriate vital signs set for the 6-month-old child. (A) would be the normal range of vital signs for the newborn. (C) is the normal range of vital signs for children over 10 years of age. (D) gives the normal vital signs for a 6-year-old patient. *(Brady, Paramedic Care 2e, Principles and Practice, Volume 5—Pediatrics. Mosby, Paramedic Textbook 3e, Pediatrics.)*

659. **The answer is A.** (A) would be the most appropriate vital signs for the 3-year-old child. (B) would be most appropriate for the 6-month-old child. (C) would be most appropriate for the 10-year-old child, and (D) would be most appropriate for a newborn. *(Brady, Paramedic Care 2e, Principles and Practice, Volume 5—Pediatrics. Mosby, Paramedic Textbook 3e, Pediatrics.)*

660. **The answer is C.** Between infancy and 24 months, a child may easily become apprehensive. Head to toe examination will help to alleviate this anxiety. *(Brady, Paramedic Care 2e, Principles and Practice, Volume 5—Pediatrics. Mosby, Paramedic Textbook 3e, Pediatrics.)*

661. **The answer is D.** It is entirely inappropriate to assess pediatric vital signs with adult equipment. You should advise your partner that adult equipment use could result in an inaccurate assessment and improper care. As a professional, a Paramedic is responsible for obtaining and maintaining the appropriate assessment tools. *(Brady, Paramedic Care 2e, Principles and Practice, Volume 5—Pediatrics. Mosby, Paramedic Textbook 3e, Pediatrics.)*

662. **The answer is B.** Pediatric patients tend to have variations in heart rate; therefore, it is suggested that a pulse be checked for *no less* than 30 seconds. *(Brady, Paramedic Care 2e, Principles and Practice, Volume 5—Pediatrics. Mosby, Paramedic Textbook 3e, Pediatrics.)*

663. **The answer is A.** Comminuted fractures are not commonly seen in pediatric patients. (B) Bend fractures (angulation and deformity with break), (C) buckle fractures (raised or bulging projection at fracture site), and (D) greenstick fractures (incomplete break in the bone) are all common and due to the softness of the bone because of growth plates being open. *(Brady, Paramedic Care 2e, Principles and Practice, Volume 5—Pediatrics. Mosby, Paramedic Textbook 3e, Pediatrics.)*

664. **The answer is C.** In a child, the tracheal cartilage is softer, not harder, and may hinder intubation attempts. *(Brady, Paramedic Care 2e, Principles and Practice, Volume 5—Pediatrics. Mosby, Paramedic Textbook 3e, Pediatrics.)*

665. **The answer is B.** In the 6- to 12-month age group, bronchiolitis is a common viral infection that presents very much like that of asthma. This infection is caused by the respiratory syncytial virus (RSV). Since this virus presents similarly to asthma, many doctors will delay the diagnosis of asthma until after 1 year of age. Field treatment is supportive and may consist of aerosolized medications or humidified oxygen. *(Brady, Paramedic Care 2e, Principles and Practice, Volume 5—Pediatrics. Mosby, Paramedic Textbook 3e, Pediatrics.)*

666. **The answer is A.** Epiglottitis is a bacterial infection that usually presents in children between 2 and 6 years of age. It is characterized by an abrupt onset of high fever, severe sore throat, difficulty swallowing, drooling, tripod positioning, and muffled speech. Epiglottitis is considered a true emergency and is a severe airway threat. *(Brady, Paramedic Care 2e, Principles and Practice, Volume 5—Pediatrics. Mosby, Paramedic Textbook 3e, Pediatrics.)*

667. **The answer is B.** SIDS affects approximately 10,000 infants a year in the United States. This is an unexplained event that occurs in otherwise healthy infants. It is typical that the child is put to sleep and the parent finds the child not breathing and pulseless. The cause of SIDS is generally unknown; however, it may be connected with sleep position. Autopsy reveals no apparent causative agent for the child's death. Historically, this is not the cause of the cardiac arrest. *(Brady, Paramedic Care 2e, Principles and Practice, Volume 5—Pediatrics. Mosby, Paramedic Textbook 3e, Pediatrics.)*

668. **The answer is C.** In cases where a child is obviously dead and no CPR effort has been begun, the Paramedic should turn his or her attention to the parents. The parents have now become the patients, since they are suffering from overwhelming emotional grief as well as feelings of guilt and helplessness. They need assistance in dealing with this type of loss, and it is the Paramedic's job to provide such assistance. *(Brady, Paramedic Care 2e, Principles and Practice, Volume 5—Pediatrics. Mosby, Paramedic Textbook 3e, Pediatrics.)*

669. **The answer is A.** Of all the many causes of seizure in children, such as Reye syndrome, fever, and head trauma, cardiac dysrhythmia does not directly result in seizure activity. (*Brady, Paramedic Care 2e, Principles and Practice, Volume 5—Pediatrics. Mosby, Paramedic Textbook 3e, Pediatrics.*)

670. **The answer is C.** Most pediatric deaths from seizure are secondary to hypoxic events. With that knowledge, the Paramedic should seek to manage airway and breathing of pediatric seizure patients as a high priority. Blow-by oxygen is also indicated, but only after the Paramedic is comfortable with the status of the patient's airway. (*Brady, Paramedic Care 2e, Principles and Practice, Volume 5—Pediatrics. Mosby, Paramedic Textbook 3e, Pediatrics.*)

671. **The answer is C.** Children with meningitis present with high fever, headache, joint pain, photophobia, poor feeding, and, in the case of the infant, bulging fontanelle due to meningeal swelling. Treatment is supportive, with fluid replacement indicated for dehydration. Meningitis may be viral (aseptic), which is usually self-limiting, or bacterial which can be deadly. (*Brady, Paramedic Care 2e, Principles and Practice, Volume 5—Pediatrics. Mosby, Paramedic Textbook 3e, Pediatrics.*)

672. **The answer is D.** In all patients with asthma, a silent chest is an ominous sign. The Paramedic should be aware that a child with a silent chest requires immediate intervention, ventilation, and oxygenation to prevent cardiac arrest. (*Brady, Paramedic Care 2e, Principles and Practice, Volume 5—Pediatrics. Mosby, Paramedic Textbook 3e, Pediatrics.*)

673. **The answer is A.** Methylprednisolone, although used in the treatment of asthmatic patients, is not a beta$_2$-adrenergic agonist. Methylprednisolone (Solu-Medrol) is classified as a corticosteroid. (*Brady, Paramedic Care 2e, Principles and Practice, Volume 5—Pediatrics. Mosby, Paramedic Textbook 3e, Pediatrics.*)

674. **The answer is D.** Bradycardia is by far the most common dysrhythmia found in the pediatric patient. It results from hypoxia, hypotension, and acidosis. Supraventricular tachycardia, although not common, may be seen in the pediatric patient. Ventricular tachycardia is rarely seen in the pediatric patient unless that patient has a congenital abnormality. Asystole is a common cardiac arrest rhythm encountered in pediatric patient. Most commonly, the child in respiratory distress will develop bradycardia and then degenerate into asystole. (*Brady, Paramedic Care 2e, Principles and Practice, Volume 5—Pediatrics. Mosby, Paramedic Textbook 3e, Pediatrics.*)

675. **The answer is A.** Isolated closed radius fractures do not meet the criteria for a cardiopulmonary assessment. Respiratory distress, bradycardia, and open fractures may all result in cardiovascular compromise and collapse and warrant a complete assessment. (*Brady, Paramedic Care 2e, Principles and Practice, Volume 5—Pediatrics. Mosby, Paramedic Textbook 3e, Pediatrics.*)

676. **The answer is D.** There is no racial or economic social typecast of a child abuser. The typical child abuser could possibly be under financial, marital, or occupational stress. In addition, the child abuser may have been abused as a child. (*Brady, Paramedic Care 2e, Principles and Practice, Volume 5—Pediatrics. Mosby, Paramedic Textbook 3e, Pediatrics.*)

677. **The answer is A.** (A) The child with an isolated wrist fracture does not immediately fall into the category of child abuse. Wrist fractures are commonly seen in injuries sustained from falls, and the statement of the mother indicates a very possible scenario. (B), (C), and (D) are all indicative of abuse patterns and should be investigated further. The Paramedic should keep in mind that the main priority is the treatment of the child and not the questioning or accusation of the parents or caregivers. (*Brady, Paramedic Care 2e, Principles and Practice, Volume 5—Pediatrics. Mosby, Paramedic Textbook 3e, Pediatrics.*)

678. **The answer is B.** The Paramedic should always focus first on the treatment of the patient. Cervical spine stabilization and monitoring the ABCs should take precedence over investigative questioning. The Paramedic should avoid confrontation with the parents and document all findings. The primary goal is to get the child to a definitive care facility and report your findings for further evaluation. *(Brady, Paramedic Care 2e, Principles and Practice, Volume 5—Pediatrics. Mosby, Paramedic Textbook 3e, Pediatrics.)*

679. **The answer is D.** IO infusion is only indicated in patients under 6 years of age. It should be attempted only when attempts at peripheral access have failed and the patient is unconscious. Indications for necessary IO attempts are severe shock, cardiac arrest, status asthmaticus, and prolonged seizures. *(Brady, Paramedic Care 2e, Principles and Practice, Volume 5— Pediatrics. Mosby, Paramedic Textbook 3e, Pediatrics.)*

680. **The answer is C.** Fluid loss in the pediatric patient is always treated with an initial fluid bolus of 20 mL/kg. This can usually be repeated twice. In a neonate, the bolus is reduced to 10 mL/kg. *(Brady, Paramedic Care 2e, Principles and Practice, Volume 5—Pediatrics. Mosby, Paramedic Textbook 3e, Pediatrics.)*

681. **The answer is C.** (C) In cases of asystole, the initial pediatric dosage of epinephrine is 0.01 mg/kg of a 1:10,000 solution. (A), (B), and (D) are incorrect, although answer (D) is the initial endotracheal dose of epinephrine in asystole. *(Brady, Paramedic Care 2e, Principles and Practice, Volume 5—Pediatrics. Mosby, Paramedic Textbook 3e, Pediatrics.)*

682. **The answer is C.** In bradycardia, the initial dose of atropine in the pediatric patient is 0.02 mg/kg. The minimum individual dose is 0.1 mg, and the maximum individual dose is 0.5 mg for a child and 1.0 mg for an adolescent. (A), (B), and (D) are incorrect. *(Brady, Paramedic Care 2e, Principles and Practice, Volume 5—Pediatrics. Mosby, Paramedic Textbook 3e, Pediatrics.)*

683. **The answer is C.** In an infant, bradycardia is defined as a heart rate of less than 80 beats per minute. The Paramedic should be alert for respiratory causes of bradycardia. Respiratory arrest and distress is the number one cause of bradycardia in children. *(Brady, Paramedic Care 2e, Principles and Practice, Volume 5—Pediatrics. Mosby, Paramedic Textbook 3e, Pediatrics.)*

GERIATRICS

684. **The answer is C.** (C) Although the temperature-regulatory mechanism in the geriatric patients may be depressed, they do not lack this ability. (A) Geriatric patients are prone to not complain of initial symptoms for fear of hospitalization and other issues. (B) Psychologic and emotional factors may impede the Paramedic from obtaining a good history. (D) Because geriatric patients may suffer from several chronic problems, it makes it more difficult for the Paramedic to accurately diagnose the etiology of the current problem. *(Brady, Paramedic Care 2e, Principles and Practice, Volume 5—Geriatric Emergencies. Mosby, Paramedic Textbook 3e, Geriatrics.)*

685. **The answer is B.** (B) Although the incidence of suicide in geriatric patients amounts to approximately 25% of all suicides, this is not an accidental cause of medication reactions. It is intentional. (A), (C), and (D) are all common causes of accidental medication reactions in the elderly patient. *(Brady, Paramedic Care 2e, Principles and Practice, Volume 5—Geriatric Emergencies. Mosby, Paramedic Textbook 3e, Geriatrics.)*

686. **The answer is B.** (B) Cardiac hypertrophy is enlargement of the cardiac muscle. This is common and naturally occurring in the geriatric patient. Hypertrophy is considered to be caused by stiffening of blood vessels. Hypertrophy causes decreased cardiac output even in normally healthy patients. (A), (C), and (D), while all normal in the physiologic process of aging, are not the primary causes of decreased cardiac output. *(Brady, Paramedic Care 2e, Principles and Practice, Volume 5—Geriatric Emergencies. Mosby, Paramedic Textbook 3e, Geriatrics.)*

687. **The answer is D.** (D) Increase in brain mass is not a normal age-related physiologic change. Some age-related changes are decreased brain mass, decreased cardiac stroke volume and rate, (A) degeneration of the joints, (B) decreased respiratory vital capacity, (C) decreased renal function, and decreased total body water. *(Brady, Paramedic Care 2e, Principles and Practice, Volume 5—Geriatric Emergencies. Mosby, Paramedic Textbook 3e, Geriatrics.)*

688. **The answer is A.** Elderly patients generally have common complaints for which they call for assistance. For example, (B) dizziness and (C) fatigue are some of the most common complaints in the elderly patients. (D) Falls are another common complaint, and the Paramedic must be cautious not to rule out other causes that may have lead to the patient's falling (e.g., syncopal events). (A) Due to decreased nerve conduction velocity and deterioration of the nervous system, many elderly patients may have no complaint of chest pain, even during a cardiac event. Paramedics should be alert to other signs and symptoms of cardiac events in these cases. (*Brady, Paramedic Care 2e, Principles and Practice, Volume 5—Geriatric Emergencies. Mosby, Paramedic Textbook 3e, Geriatrics.*)

689. **The answer is A.** (A) is correct. Elderly patients are prone to severe internal head injuries due to decreased brain mass. This allows free movement of the brain in the cranial cavity, increasing the incidence of injury. In addition, the patient cannot be diagnosed on (B) mental status alone because brain injuries in the elderly, especially bleeding, may not be symptomatic due to increased capacity of the cranial cavity, which may lead to the delay of signs of increasing intercranial pressure. (C) and (D) are incorrect. (*Brady, Paramedic Care 2e, Principles and Practice, Volume 5—Geriatric Emergencies. Mosby, Paramedic Textbook 3e, Geriatrics.*)

690. **The answer is D.** (D) Stokes-Adams syncope is commonly associated with heart blocks, and the patient will generally not produce enough cardiac output to support a stable mental status. This patient, when lying down, will have enough perfusion to remain conscious, but the decreased cardiac output due to the heart block will not produce enough perfusion to the brain while standing. (B) Orthostatic syncope usually occurs due to decreased hypovolemic states, which are commonly caused by dehydration, certain medications, and prolonged bed rest. (A) and (C) are incorrect. (*Brady, Paramedic Care 2e, Principles and Practice, Volume 5—Geriatric Emergencies. Mosby, Paramedic Textbook 3e, Geriatrics.*)

691. **The answer is C.** (C) Based on the patient's history in this scenario, this patient is most likely suffering from a subdural hematoma. Due to increased capacity of the cranial cavity, geriatric patients may be slow to develop symptoms from bleeding in the head. (A) Although alcohol withdrawal, (B) hypoglycemia, and (D) epilepsy are all common causes of seizure in the elderly, there is no significant historical information that can support these diagnoses. Other causes of new-onset seizures can be mass brain lesions and stroke. (*Brady, Paramedic Care 2e, Principles and Practice, Volume 5—Geriatric Emergencies. Mosby, Paramedic Textbook 3e, Geriatrics.*)

692. **The answer is B.** (B) Elder abuse knows no socioeconomic boundaries. This patient has appeared to you in a properly alert fashion and answered your questions correctly. Her story of abuse should not be disregarded due to statements from family members. Paramedics must remember that the geriatric person is the patient and should be questioned about his or her condition. Although (A) confabulation and (C) senile dementia are real scenarios, this patient is awake and alert. (D) Subdural bleeding in this case may be possible, but mental status and injury patterns suggest otherwise. (*Brady, Paramedic Care 2e, Principles and Practice, Volume 5—Geriatric Emergencies. Mosby, Paramedic Textbook 3e, Geriatrics.*)

ABUSE AND ASSAULT

693. **The answer is A.** (B), (C), (D), and adult abuse are some of the categories of abuse. Domestic violence is another frequently used term to describe the use of force by one family member against another with the intent to inflict harm or even death. (A) is incorrect because, even though it may be abusive behavior toward oneself, it is not considered a category of abuse. Abuse is primarily considered as being perpetrated by one individual on another. (*Brady, Paramedic Care 2e, Principles and Practice, Volume 5—Abuse and Assault. Mosby, Paramedic Textbook 3e, Abuse and Neglect.*)

694. The answer is A. (B), (C), and (D) are correct. (A) is incorrect because an adult abuser usually lacks self-confidence and is socially isolated. *(Brady, Paramedic Care 2e, Principles and Practice, Volume 5—Abuse and Assault. Mosby, Paramedic Textbook 3e, Abuse and Neglect.)*

695. The answer is A. (A) is correct. It may also be referred to as spousal abuse. (B), (C), and (D) are incorrect. *(Brady, Paramedic Care 2e, Principles and Practice, Volume 5—Abuse and Assault. Mosby, Paramedic Textbook 3e, Abuse and Neglect.)*

696. The answer is D. (D) is correct; however, estimates of less than 10% of these episodes are reported to the police. *(Brady, Paramedic Care 2e, Principles and Practice, Volume 5—Abuse and Assault. Mosby, Paramedic Textbook 3e, Abuse and Neglect.)*

697. The answer is D. (D) is correct. The four main types of elder abuse are: physical abuse, physical neglect, psychologic abuse, and material abuse. This presentation demonstrates the first three. (A), (B), and (C) are all incorrect. *(Brady, Paramedic Care 2e, Principles and Practice, Volume 5—Abuse and Assault. Mosby, Paramedic Textbook 3e, Abuse and Neglect.)*

698. The answer is A. (B), (C), and (D) are correct. (A) is incorrect because frequently the elder is financially dependent on the abuser. *(Brady, Paramedic Care 2e, Principles and Practice, Volume 5—Abuse and Assault. Mosby, Paramedic Textbook 3e, Abuse and Neglect.)*

699. The answer is D. (A), (B), and (C) are correct. (D) is incorrect because usually an abused child demonstrates evidence of old scars, burns, or deformities in addition to the new injuries. *(Brady, Paramedic Care 2e, Principles and Practice, Volume 5—Abuse and Assault. Mosby, Paramedic Textbook 3e, Abuse and Neglect.)*

700. The answer is C. (A), (B), and (D) are correct. (C) is incorrect because the abusive parent usually is evasive and offers very little information about what happened to the child. *(Brady, Paramedic Care 2e, Principles and Practice, Volume 5—Abuse and Assault. Mosby, Paramedic Textbook 3e, Abuse and Neglect.)*

701. The answer is A. (B), (C), and (D) are correct. (A) is incorrect because, if at all possible, you should gently encourage the patient not to use the bathroom or shower, so that emergency department personnel are better able to gather evidence for the police. *(Brady, Paramedic Care 2e, Principles and Practice, Volume 5—Abuse and Assault. Mosby, Paramedic Textbook 3e, Abuse and Neglect.)*

702. The answer is C. (A), (B), and (D) are correct. (C) is incorrect because, since the ambulance call report is a legal document, you should never offer your opinion as to whether the patient was or was not raped. *(Brady, Paramedic Care 2e, Principles and Practice, Volume 5—Abuse and Assault. Mosby, Paramedic Textbook 3e, Abuse and Neglect.)*

ACUTE INTERVENTIONS FOR CHRONIC CARE PATIENTS

703. The answer is C. (A), (B), and (D) are correct. (C) is incorrect because, while arterial lines are vascular access devices, they are not used in the home health care setting. They are usually accessed only in the hospital setting. *(Brady, Paramedic Care 2e, Volume 5—Acute Interventions for the Chronic Care Patient. Mosby, Paramedic Textbook 3e, Acute Interventions for the Home Health Care Patient.)*

704. The answer is D. (A), (B), and (C) are correct. (D) is incorrect because central venous catheters come in single or multiple lumens. *(Brady, Paramedic Care 2e, Volume 5—Acute Interventions for the Chronic Care Patient. Mosby, Paramedic Textbook 3e, Acute Interventions for the Home Health Care Patient.)*

705. The answer is D. (A), (B), and (C) are correct. (D) is incorrect because you should always be open to accepting advice from the patient, family members, and caregivers who have been routinely accessing the catheter. *(Brady, Paramedic Care 2e, Volume 5—Acute Interventions for the Chronic Care Patient. Mosby, Paramedic Textbook 3e, Acute Interventions for the Home Health Care Patient.)*

706. The answer is A. (B), (C), (D), sepsis, and a torn or leaking catheter are all possible complications of accessing vascular access devices. (A) is not. *(Brady, Paramedic Care 2e, Volume 5—Acute Interventions for the Chronic Care Patient. Mosby, Paramedic Textbook 3e, Acute Interventions for the Home Health Care Patient.)*

707. The answer is D. (A), (B), (C), site infection, necrosis, fistula, and subcutaneous or mediastinal emphysema are sometimes complications and emergencies. (D) is incorrect because it has nothing to do with a patient who has a tracheostomy. *(Brady, Paramedic Care 2e, Volume 5— Acute Interventions for the Chronic Care Patient. Mosby, Paramedic Textbook 3e, Acute Interventions for the Home Health Care Patient.)*

708. The answer is C. (C) is correct. (A) is incorrect because, if permitted by your medical control, you should begin to administer advanced life support to the patient with difficulty breathing. (B) is incorrect because the patient is already cyanotic and having difficulty breathing while being connected to the ventilator. (D) is incorrect because administering 100% oxygen by nonrebreather face mask is useless, since the patient is breathing through the tracheostomy tube opening in his neck. *(Brady, Paramedic Care 2e, Volume 5—Acute Interventions for the Chronic Care Patient. Mosby, Paramedic Textbook 3e, Acute Interventions for the Home Health Care Patient.)*

709. The answer is C. (A), (B), (D), nausea, bacterial contamination, electrolyte imbalance, and tube displacement are all possible complications of gastrostomy tubes. (C) is incorrect. *(Brady, Paramedic Care 2e, Volume 5—Acute Interventions for the Chronic Care Patient. Mosby, Paramedic Textbook 3e, Acute Interventions for the Home Health Care Patient.)*

710. The answer is B. (B) is correct. (A) is incorrect because the bleeding site should be treated immediately. (C) is incorrect because the bleeding is coming from the gastrostomy tube site, not from inside the stomach. Therefore, flushing the gastrostomy tube is of no benefit. (D) is incorrect because a gastrostomy tube should never be pushed further into the abdomen blindly. *(Brady, Paramedic Care 2e, Volume 5—Acute Interventions for the Chronic Care Patient. Mosby, Paramedic Textbook 3e, Acute Interventions for the Home Health Care Patient.)*

Operations

The following topics are covered in Section VII:

- Ambulance Operations
- Medical Incident Command
- Rescue Awareness
- Hazardous Materials Incidents

Questions

AMBULANCE OPERATIONS

DIRECTIONS: Each item below contains four suggested responses. Select the one best response to each item.

711. Of the following examples, which is *not* a scenario in which air medical transport should be considered?

    (A) lengthy extrication times
    (B) lengthy ground transport time
    (C) spinal injury
    (D) lengthy manual transport out of a remote area

712. All of the following patients meet air medical transport criteria *except*:

    (A) A 22-year-old female who has suffered a fall of 42 feet while rock climbing.
    (B) A 30-year-old male who was thrown from his car in a motor vehicle accident on a desolate highway.
    (C) A woman with major trauma who is 30 minutes from the hospital by ground transport.
    (D) A 4-year-old female who has overdosed on her mother's hypertension medication.

713. Which of the following law defines the minimum qualifications of those who may perform various health services, the skills that each type of practitioner is legally permitted to use and the levels of certification for various categories of health care professionals?

    (A) EMS Certification Act
    (B) Good Samaritan Act
    (C) Negligence Act
    (D) Medical Practice Act

714. On your arrival at a motor vehicle collision, you find a female about 28 years old. She appears quite intoxicated and is argumentative. She was involved in a one-car collision with a guardrail. Your partner states the patient has no significant injuries, although the patient is complaining of neck pain. The patient demands to go to the hospital because her neck is sore. You transport but do not immobilize her and seat her in the crew chair of your vehicle. The patient is later diagnosed with a cervical spine fracture and is now suffering from paralysis. You and your partner may face charges of

(A) assault

(B) negligence

(C) battery

(D) slander

715. Based on the 1974 KKK-A-1822 standards, match the following ambulances with the correct description.

(A) type 1

(B) type 2

(C) type 3

1. Conventional cab and chassis with a modular ambulance body. There is no passageway between the driver's compartment and the patient's compartment.

2. Specialty van with forward cab and integral body. There is a passageway between the driver's compartment and the patient's compartment.

3. Van-type vehicle, possibly with a raised roof. There is a passageway between the driver's compartment and the patient's compartment.

MEDICAL INCIDENT COMMAND

DIRECTIONS: Each item below contains four suggested responses. Select the one best response to each item.

716. Which of the following is *not* an objective of the incident command system?

(A) It defines lines of responsibility and authority.

(B) It provides an organized plan designed to effectively manage needs.

(C) It allows all responding agencies to work independently of each other.

(D) It offers performance evaluation criteria.

717. Which type of mass casualty incident would necessitate an emergency operations center and secondary levels of management?

(A) a high-impact incident

(B) a low-impact incident

(C) a disaster or catastrophic incident

(D) a terrorist event

718. Define a *mass casualty incident*.

(A) an incident that can be managed by the initial responding unit

(B) an incident that overwhelms local resources

(C) an incident involving multiple-response agencies

(D) a terrorist event

719. Which of the following is a responsibility of the treatment sector at a major incident?

(A) tagging patients according to their injuries

(B) establishing immediate and delayed areas

(C) coordinating procurement of medical supplies from hospitals

(D) establishing a helicopter landing zone

720. The command structure at a major incident is described as

(A) a structure in which a single person is in command of the entire incident with sector commanders reporting their status to the incident commander

(B) a structure in which all sectors have separate commanders who report directly to the communications center

(C) a structure with independent commanders representing each agency on the scene

(D) a structure in which commanders are assigned based on patient count

721. When responding to a major incident, which area should you respond to initially?

(A) triage
(B) treatment
(C) support
(D) staging

722. At a mass casualty incident, when should responders identify a command post and incident commander?

(A) immediately on identification of a potential large incident
(B) on the arrival of the police department
(C) on the arrival of the fire department
(D) on the arrival of a chief officer

723. On the scene of a major incident, you attempt to open a patient's airway and find that she is not breathing. You take the appropriate corrective actions, and there is still no respiratory effort. Using the START (simple triage and rapid treatment) triage system, what category would you place this patient in?

(A) black
(B) yellow
(C) green
(D) red

724. Which of the following is *not* a component of the START method of triage?

(A) respiratory status
(B) motor status
(C) hemodynamic status
(D) mental status

725. You have begun your assessment of a patient and have found his respiratory system intact, with a respiratory effort under 30 breaths per minute. What should be your next step in the triage of this patient?

(A) transport to the treatment area
(B) assess mental status
(C) assess hemodynamic status
(D) administer oxygen

726. You have completed your hemodynamic status evaluation of a patient, and you are ready to move on to the next step in the START triage method. What would you assess next?

(A) motor function
(B) airway
(C) breathing
(D) mental status

RESCUE AWARENESS

DIRECTIONS: Each item below contains four suggested responses. Select the one best response to each item.

727. All of the following reflect a component of the Paramedic's role in a rescue operation *except*:

(A) evaluation of scene hazards
(B) gaining access to the patient
(C) extrication of the patient and continued treatment
(D) securing hazardous materials leaks

728. While operating on a major interstate, traffic flow is moving dangerously close to your area of operations. What would be your safest choice in the control of the traffic situation to ensure scene safety?

(A) Continue to let the traffic flow as it is so that the road remains open.

(B) Divert the traffic around the scene, allowing cars to pass.

(C) Completely block traffic flow until the operations are complete.

(D) Detour the traffic from the main roadway at the previous exit.

729. All of the following statements regarding a confined space rescue are true *except*:

(A) Confined space rescuers may encounter hazardous atmospheres.

(B) Exposed electrical wiring may be a hidden danger to the rescuer.

(C) Confined space rescuers may encounter a potential for engulfment.

(D) Paramedics may enter a confined space without safety equipment as long as they are accompanied by trained rescuers.

730. Which of the following is *not* an acceptable sacrifice of extrication procedure in order to facilitate positive patient outcome?

(A) a patient trapped in a car which was pinned up against a tree in a flash flood with a rapidly rising water level

(B) a patient pinned in a car under a leaking gasoline tanker

(C) a patient who has fallen from a cliff side and is at the bottom of a steep slope

(D) a chemical worker lying unconscious in a chemical holding tank

731. You are called to the scene of a 22-year-old female who was last seen crawling into a dense area of brush. On your arrival, her friends explain that she wanted to "check out" this thick area for nesting animals. It has been about an hour since she was last seen. What should you request from communications to assist you in this search?

(A) helicopter support with high-intensity lighting

(B) specially trained dogs and experienced search managers

(C) a high-angle rescue team

(D) four-wheel drive vehicles

732. When would you consider it safe to operate within the area of the downed power line?

(A) when the power line stops sparking

(B) when the fire department arrives and moves the power line off the vehicle with a hook

(C) when the patient's condition warrants a rapid extrication

(D) when the local power company arrives on scene and advises that power has been cut to that line

733. All of the following vehicle collisions would not require vehicle stabilization *except*:

(A) an overturned vehicle

(B) a vehicle that has hit a wall

(C) a vehicle that has struck a bridge support

(D) all vehicles are considered unstable until properly supported

734. A vehicle is leaking gasoline after a collision. You notice a build-up of gasoline fumes in the area. Which of the following actions should be avoided in the interest of scene safety?

(A) turning off the ignition

(B) cutting the battery cable

(C) securing the area of all bystanders

(D) minimizing the use of tools that may cause sparks

735. Which of the following should be done first to attempt to gain access to remove your patient from a vehicle when the driver's door is crushed and will not open?

(A) Have the extrication team come in and open the door with a power tool.

(B) Break the glass and enter the vehicle through the window, and then alert the extrication team.

(C) Try the undamaged door on the other side to see if will offer access.

(D) Remove the roof of the vehicle.

736. You arrive on the scene of a patient who is trapped in rapidly rising and fast moving water. Which of the following would be the best way to mitigate this situation?

(A) Attempt to reach the patient only after you are secured to a rope.

(B) Try to climb down to the patient from the bridge.

(C) Don a life vest and attempt to swim to the patient.

(D) Alert a swift-water rescue team and stand by until they arrive.

737. Which of the following situations would a Paramedic be correct in bypassing portions of the assessment and treatment process in the interest of safety?

(A) A patient in a vehicle that was involved in a head-on collision.

(B) A patient who is in a tank and overcome by toxic gases.

(C) A patient who is trapped in a collapsed trench.

(D) A patient who is inside a burning vehicle but complaining of numbness in his or her extremities.

738. The greatest hazard of a deployed supplemental restraint system (SRS), or air bag, is

(A) The inflated SRS will hinder airway management interventions.

(B) The deployed SRS has a residue on it that may cause burns.

(C) The deployed SRS will reduce the area in which the rescuer has to operate.

(D) The deployed SRS will produce no hazard to the rescuer.

739. What is the most appropriate intervention in the prevention of burns from an SRS, or air bag deployment system?

(A) As this is a toxic chemical, all rescuers should be completely decontaminated after coming in contact with an SRS.

(B) The rescuer should seek treatment in the emergency department for possible treatment of irritation.

(C) Rescuers who have come in contact with SRS should contact poison control for further instructions.

(D) The rescuer should thoroughly wash all exposed areas as soon as possible.

740. All of the following are appropriate response procedures for the Paramedic when dealing with an undeployed air bag *except*:

(A) Disconnect the battery cable.

(B) Avoid placing body in the direct path of a possibly deploying SRS.

(C) Avoid placing any heat in the area of the steering wheel hub.

(D) Drill into the SRS module to release the charge.

741. Which of the following is *not* in the National Standard Curriculum as Paramedic standard of care during a prolonged extrication?

(A) on-scene amputation of limbs to initiate rescue on critical patients

(B) fluid therapy

(C) pain management

(D) removal of impaled objects

742. You arrive at the scene of a car which has been driven over the side of a cliff. You call for a specially trained team of rescuers who can gain access to the patient. This type of rescue is identified as

(A) vertical rescue

(B) technical rescue

(C) team rescue

(D) rappelling rescue

743. Which of the following *best* describes disentanglement?

(A) mitigation of all scene hazards to ensure rapid extrication

(B) removal of the entrapping section of the vehicle from the patient

(C) removal of the patient from the entrapping section of the vehicle

(D) the effort of the Paramedic to avoid becoming trapped in the vehicle with the patient

744. On your arrival at a call for an emotionally disturbed person, you are told that the patient has barricaded himself in his house and a police officer has been shot. The officer is located on the front lawn in direct view of the patient. The commander at the scene informs you that he will provide you with a "cover" team to assist you in the extrication of the wounded police officer from the lawn. You should

(A) Prepare your equipment for a rapid patient removal.

(B) Advise the commander that you are not trained in tactical rescue and await his decision.

(C) Attempt to talk with the gunman to "make a deal" in order to remove the policeman.

(D) Protect yourself and your partner by refusing this assignment, since it could lead to additional casualties.

745. Which of the following is the primary means of gaining information for rapidly locating patients trapped in a building collapse?

(A) alerting the proper agencies for specialized equipment to locate trapped building occupants

(B) performing a rapid, blind search of the building

(C) sending in large independent teams to sweep all areas

(D) interviewing witnesses and building employees for building occupancy areas

746. While treating a patient who has been removed after being trapped under heavy debris, the number one concern of the Paramedic is

(A) open fractures

(B) rapid cardiovascular collapse

(C) cavitation injuries

(D) impaled objects

HAZARDOUS MATERIALS INCIDENTS

DIRECTIONS: Each item below contains four suggested responses. Select the one best response to each item.

747. Which of the following is *not* a responsibility of the hazardous materials first responder?

(A) knowledge of hazardous materials and the risks associated with them in case of an accident

(B) entry to the hot zone and mitigation of the incident

(C) an understanding of the potential outcomes of a hazardous materials emergency

(D) the ability to recognize the need for specialty resources

748. You respond to an overturned truck on the freeway. On your arrival, you notice that the truck has a placard that has white and red stripes. This truck is most likely carrying

(A) flammable liquids
(B) flammable solids
(C) explosives
(D) oxidizers

749. The guidebook that the EMS responder would most likely use to identify a hazardous material by its UN number as well as obtain safety information is

(A) the shipper's manifest
(B) a Paramedic hazardous materials textbook
(C) U.S. Department of Transportation (DOT) truck placard chart
(D) DOT emergency response guidebook

750. All EMS operations at a hazardous materials incident should take place in the

(A) hot zone
(B) warm zone
(C) cold zone
(D) wherever the largest number of patients are

751. While on the scene of a hazardous materials incident, in order to get additional information regarding a specific chemical product (agent), the responder may call

(A) Federal Emergency Management Agency (FEMA)
(B) the Centers for Disease Control
(C) Chemical Transportation Emergency Center (CHEMTREC)
(D) poison control

752. The type of personal protective equipment that provides the highest level of protection at a hazardous materials incident is known as

(A) level A
(B) level B
(C) level C
(D) level D

753. The initial approach to a chemically contaminated patient should include

(A) cervical spine management and decontamination
(B) pharmacologic intervention
(C) cardiac monitoring
(D) a complete history and physical examination assessment of the airway, breathing, and circulation (ABCs)

754. The Occupational Safety and Health Administration (OSHA) requirement that all members of a hazardous materials entry team receive a complete assessment prior to and after "suiting up" is known as

(A) medical surveillance
(B) team assessment
(C) provider guidelines
(D) DOT protection clause

Answers and Explanations

AMBULANCE OPERATIONS

711. **The answer is C.** (C) Spinal injury is not considered critical criteria in itself for air medical transport. However, the patient who may have multiple traumas in addition to spinal injury may fall into the category for air medical transport. (A), (B), and (D) are all criteria for patient removal by air. *(Brady, Paramedic Care 2e, Principles and Practice, Volume 5—Ambulance Operations. Mosby, Paramedic Textbook 3e, Ambulance Operations.)*

712. **The answer is D.** (D) A 4-year-old female who has overdosed does not meet air medical transport criteria. This patient should be monitored and taken by ground transport to the closest hospital. Most critical traumas, especially those with long access or extended ground transport times easily meet air medical transport criteria. *(Brady, Paramedic Care 2e, Principles and Practice, Volume 5—Ambulance Operations. Mosby, Paramedic Textbook 3e, Ambulance Operations.)*

713. **The answer is D.** (D) The Medical Practice Act defines the levels of training and certification as well as the minimum qualifications to become certified at any level of care provider. This act is partially responsible for EMS training curricula at all provider levels. The Good Samaritan Act is a protective act for prehospital providers who render aid in good faith to patients in emergent situations. *(Brady, Paramedic Care 2e, Principles and Practice, Volume 5—Ambulance Operations. Mosby, Paramedic Textbook 3e, Ambulance Operations.)*

714. **The answer is B.** (B) best describes your situation. Negligence occurs when the following conditions are met: (1) there was an injury, (2) the Paramedic had a duty to act, (3) the Paramedic breached that duty to act, and (4) an injury occurred due to that breach of duty. Although the patient was injured prior to the arrival of the crew, aggravation of his injury may have been prevented by early intervention and proper immobilization of the patient. This crew may face charges of negligence for failure to treat the patient in a proper fashion. *(Brady, Paramedic Care 2e, Principles and Practice, Volume 5—Ambulance Operations. Mosby, Paramedic Textbook 3e, Ambulance Operations.)*

715. **The answers are:** (A) 1. Type 1 has a conventional cab and chassis with a modular ambulance body. There is no passageway between the driver's compartment and the patient's compartment. (B) 3. Type 2 is a van-type vehicle, possibly with a raised roof. There is a passageway between the driver's compartment and the patient's compartment. (C) 2. Type 3 is a specialty van with forward cab and integral body. There is a passageway between the driver's compartment and the patient's compartment. *(Brady, Paramedic Care 2e, Principles and Practice, Volume 5—Ambulance Operations. Mosby, Paramedic Textbook 3e, Ambulance Operations.)*

MEDICAL INCIDENT COMMAND

716. **The answer is A.** (A) is incorrect, since it states exactly the opposite of what the incident command system is designed to accomplish. It provides (B) a definition of responsibility and authority, (C) an organized plan to effectively manage needs, and (D) performance evaluation criteria. In addition, it provides a framework that groups similar functions, provides an orderly means of communication, and establishes a common terminology to reduce the probability of confusion during a large incident. *(Brady, Paramedic Care 2e, Principles and Practice, Volume 5—Medical Incident Command. Mosby, Paramedic Textbook 3e, Medical Incident Command.)*

717. The answer is C. (C) A disaster or catastrophic incident will tax the resources of a region and necessitate the implementation of an emergency operations center and secondary levels of management. (A) A high-impact incident will necessitate mutual assistance from EMS agencies within the region. (B) A low-impact incident will usually be handled and mitigated by local EMS responder and does not require mutual aid or assistance from outside agencies. (D) Although the probabilities are high that a terrorist incident will probably tax the region in which it occurs, it will not always generate a large patient count; therefore, (D) is incorrect. *(Brady, Paramedic Care 2e, Principles and Practice, Volume 5—Medical Incident Command. Mosby, Paramedic Textbook 3e, Medical Incident Command.)*

718. The answer is B. (B) An incident that overwhelms local resources is a mass casualty incident. These incidents are defined in three categories: low impact, high impact, and disaster or catastrophic incident. (A) does not describe a mass casualty incident, since any incident that can be managed by a single unit does not produce large numbers of patients. (C) Mass casualty incidents will most likely involve multiple agencies; however, not all multiple agency responses produce large numbers of patients. (D) Terrorist events may produce large numbers of patients, but some terrorist events are targeted at structures and not people. *(Brady, Paramedic Care 2e, Principles and Practice, Volume 5—Medical Incident Command. Mosby, Paramedic Textbook 3e, Medical Incident Command.)*

719. The answer is B. (B) Establishing immediate and delayed treatment areas is a responsibility of the treatment sector. This allows for the most serious injuries to be treated first. (A) Tagging patients is the responsibility of the triage sector. (C) Procurement of hospital supplies is a responsibility of the support sector. (D) Establishment of the helicopter landing zone is a role of the transportation sector. *(Brady, Paramedic Care 2e, Principles and Practice, Volume 5—Medical Incident Command. Mosby, Paramedic Textbook 3e, Medical Incident Command.)*

720. The answer is A. (A) The command structure is based on a single individual who is in control of all operations. This individual will have dedicated commanders in each sector who will generate progress reports to the command post for incident evaluation. (B) is incorrect because sector commanders do not communicate with the communications center. (C) Although each responding agency would probably have a commander with it, those commanders would report to the incident commander for assignment. (D) is incorrect; there is no assignment of commanders based on patient count. *(Brady, Paramedic Care 2e, Principles and Practice, Volume 5—Medical Incident Command. Mosby, Paramedic Textbook 3e, Medical Incident Command.)*

721. The answer is D. (D) All responding vehicles and personnel should always report initially to the staging sector for direction. From there they will be assigned to a sector where their resources are needed. *(Brady, Paramedic Care 2e, Principles and Practice, Volume 5—Medical Incident Command. Mosby, Paramedic Textbook 3e, Medical Incident Command.)*

722. The answer is A. (A) The first arriving unit, on identification of a major incident, should set up a command post and direct responding units as well as identify the needs for resources. Command may be passed on the arrival of a ranking officer; however, the officer may decide to maintain an advisory role to maintain continuity of the initial command structure. (B), (C), and (D) are all incorrect, since the incident command system should be implemented immediately following the identification of a mass casualty incident. *(Brady, Paramedic Care 2e, Principles and Practice, Volume 5—Medical Incident Command. Mosby, Paramedic Textbook 3e, Medical Incident Command.)*

723. The answer is A. (A) Patients who have no respiratory effort after corrective actions are tagged black (dead or unsalvageable). These incidents do not allow for long-term resuscitative efforts that may use additional resources, making them unavailable to assist other patients. *(Brady, Paramedic Care 2e, Principles and Practice, Volume 5—Medical Incident Command. Mosby, Paramedic Textbook 3e, Medical Incident Command.)*

724. The answer is B. (B) The START method of triage evaluates (A) respiratory, (C) hemodynamic, and (D) mental status and does not include the patient's motor status. The patient is evaluated for respiration; if there are no respirations, the patient is marked dead or unsalvageable. If the respirations are above 30 breaths per minute and/or the patient needs airway maintenance, the patient is marked critical/immediate. If the patient has a respiratory rate less than 30 breaths per minute, the Paramedic should begin the hemodynamic assessment. *(Brady, Paramedic Care 2e, Principles and Practice, Volume 5—Medical Incident Command. Mosby, Paramedic Textbook 3e, Medical Incident Command.)*

725. The answer is C. (C) If your patient's respiratory status is intact and supporting ventilation, you should move on to the hemodynamic assessment. This assessment will consist of monitoring a radial pulse. If the radial pulse is present, then the Paramedic will move on to the assessment of mental status. If a radial pulse is absent, the Paramedic will attempt to control all bleeding and mark the patient immediate. (A) is incorrect, since the patient is not sent to the treatment area until after initial triage is completed. (B) Assessment of mental status is not begun until the completion of hemodynamic assessment. (D) is incorrect. In the triage area, no adjunctive treatment is completed. *(Brady, Paramedic Care 2e, Principles and Practice, Volume 5—Medical Incident Command. Mosby, Paramedic Textbook 3e, Medical Incident Command.)*

726. The answer is D. (D) Mental status is the third step in the START method of triage. If the patient has an impaired mental status and fails to follow simple commands, he or she is marked immediate. If the patient is responsive and alert, he or she is marked delayed. (A) Motor function is not part of the START method, since mental status is assessed only. The AVPU (alert, voice, pain, unresponsive) scale is used in the START method of triage as a mental status indicator. (B) Airway and (C) breathing are both evaluated during the respiratory step of the START method. *(Brady, Paramedic Care 2e, Principles and Practice, Volume 5—Medical Incident Command. Mosby, Paramedic Textbook 3e, Medical Incident Command.)*

RESCUE AWARENESS

727. The answer is D. Paramedics are a patient care resource and are normally not the primary responder for hazardous materials mitigation. Their primary role includes evaluation of scene safety, searching for the location of all patients, gaining access, initial care of the patient, extrication, continued care, and finally, transportation of the patient to a definitive care facility. Personnel who are untrained in hazardous materials mitigation should never attempt to secure a hazardous materials scene. *(Brady, Paramedic Care 2e, Principles and Practice, Volume 5—Rescue Awareness and Operations. Mosby, Paramedic Textbook 3e, Rescue Awareness and Operations.)*

728. The answer is C. Complete shutdown of the roadway is always the safest option when operating on a fast moving highway. There are other options, such as flare patterns, engaging police to divert traffic at the previous exit, or around the scene. Any situation which continues to permit traffic flow at unsafe speeds through the accident area is not acceptable. *(Brady, Paramedic Care 2e, Principles and Practice, Volume 5—Rescue Awareness and Operations. Mosby, Paramedic Textbook 3e, Rescue Awareness and Operations.)*

729. The answer is D. A Paramedic should *never* enter a confined space without the appropriate training and equipment. The fact that they are with trained team members does nothing for their personal safety. Rescuers in confined spaces may encounter hazardous atmospheres, specifically, low oxygen levels and toxins. Unprotected rescuers also risk engulfment by falling debris, grain, and other materials at the scene. Exposed electrical wiring may also be an inherent danger to the untrained rescuer. *(Brady, Paramedic Care 2e, Principles and Practice, Volume 5—Rescue Awareness and Operations. Mosby, Paramedic Textbook 3e, Rescue Awareness and Operations.)*

730. **The answer is C.** The patient at the bottom of a steep slope does not pose any risk to rescuers should they delay extrication for initial care. Any patient who is in a hazardous situation, such as imminent fire impingement, hazardous chemical exposure, or rapidly running water, needs immediate extrication. *(Brady, Paramedic Care 2e, Principles and Practice, Volume 5—Rescue Awareness and Operations. Mosby, Paramedic Textbook 3e, Rescue Awareness and Operations.)*

731. **The answer is B.** In thick brush, even the most well-trained rescuer could be easily disoriented. The use of search dogs may be required to track the movements of your patient. Although (A) helicopters with high-intensity lighting are usually a great asset, if the patient is lost in thick brush, it is possible that the helicopter will have no visibility of the ground. (C) A high-angle rescue team is not required, since you are in brush and not dealing with angles, hills, and slopes. (D) Four-wheel drive vehicles will not work in thick brush. This is a slow-moving, coordinated search using dogs and/or sensitive equipment for location of the patient. *(Brady, Paramedic Care 2e, Principles and Practice, Volume 5—Rescue Awareness and Operations. Mosby, Paramedic Textbook 3e, Rescue Awareness and Operations.)*

732. **The answer is D.** The only time it is safe to operate in the area of a downed power line is after the power company confirms that the power is off. The fire department and other rescue agencies might be able to secure the area, but only the power company can ensure the Paramedic's safety by shutting the power down to the appropriate pole. *(Brady, Paramedic Care 2e, Principles and Practice, Volume 5—Rescue Awareness and Operations. Mosby, Paramedic Textbook 3e, Rescue Awareness and Operations.)*

733. **The answer is D.** All vehicles can become easily unstable after a collision. Any vehicle which has been hit can have its center of balance altered. Even the most harmless looking situations can become deadly in the presence of an unstable vehicle. *(Brady, Paramedic Care 2e, Principles and Practice, Volume 5—Rescue Awareness and Operations. Mosby, Paramedic Textbook 3e, Rescue Awareness and Operations.)*

734. **The answer is B.** Cutting of the battery cable in an atmosphere of high gasoline fumes could create a spark large enough to ignite a fire in the vehicle, and the surrounding area. The paramedic should remain aware of all potential hazards of the scene, and the potential for any intervention to be a catalyst for a dangerous situation. *(Brady, Paramedic Care 2e, Principles and Practice, Volume 5—Rescue Awareness and Operations. Mosby, Paramedic Textbook 3e, Rescue Awareness and Operations.)*

735. **The answer is C.** Sometimes the simplest solution is the one that is the most logical. The Paramedic should always check the other doors of a vehicle before resorting to hydraulic and/or power tools. This reduces the risk of injury, but more importantly, expedites patient care. *(Brady, Paramedic Care 2e, Principles and Practice, Volume 5—Rescue Awareness and Operations. Mosby, Paramedic Textbook 3e, Rescue Awareness and Operations.)*

736. **The answer is D.** If the Paramedic is not trained in water rescue, then a specially trained swift water rescue team should be requested. Rapidly moving water can overcome even the most experienced rescuers if they do not have the appropriate equipment. As with any situation, rescuer safety is the highest priority. *(Brady, Paramedic Care 2e, Principles and Practice, Volume 5—Rescue Awareness and Operations. Mosby, Paramedic Textbook 3e, Rescue Awareness and Operations.)*

737. **The answer is A.** Although the patient who has been in a head-on collision could be quite critical, this patient would warrant a full assessment as well as proper stabilization. Patients overcome by toxic gases in chemical tanks, trapped in an unstable collapse zones and those

trapped inside a burning vehicle will benefit from immediate extrication from the area. *(Brady, Paramedic Care 2e, Principles and Practice, Volume 5— Rescue Awareness and Operations. Mosby, Paramedic Textbook 3e, Rescue Awareness and Operations.)*

738. The answer is B. Older deployed SRS contain either cornstarch or talcum powder mixed with sodium hydroxide, which will cause nonhazardous irritation to unprotected skin. Rescuers should wear gloves and eye protection while operating near deployed SRS. *(Brady, Paramedic Care 2e, Principles and Practice, Volume 5—Rescue Awareness and Operations. Mosby, Paramedic Textbook 3e, Rescue Awareness and Operations.)*

739. The answer is D. Rescuers and patients who come in contact with SRS lubricant should wash thoroughly with soap and water to alleviate the possibility of irritation and burns. Generally, these lubricants do not cause serious burns, but as with any chemical exposure, should be dealt with appropriately. *(Brady, Paramedic Care 2e, Principles and Practice, Volume 5— Rescue Awareness and Operations. Mosby, Paramedic Textbook 3e, Rescue Awareness and Operations.)*

740. The answer is D. The rescuer should never drill into an SRS module; this action could deploy the SRS system and injure the rescuer as well as the patient. *(Brady, Paramedic Care 2e, Principles and Practice, Volume 5—Rescue Awareness and Operations. Mosby, Paramedic Textbook 3e, Rescue Awareness and Operations.)*

741. The answer is A. The field amputation is the role of a surgeon, and although a lifesaving procedure in the rarest of occasions, it is *not* part of the Paramedic scope of practice. The Paramedic should request a specialty surgical team to the scene of this type of event. Paramedics should however be prepared to assist in the procedure, as long as they remain within their scope of practice. *(Brady, Paramedic Care 2e, Principles and Practice, Volume 5—Rescue Awareness and Operations. Mosby, Paramedic Textbook 3e, Rescue Awareness and Operations.)*

742. The answer is A. (A) Anytime a rescue team must contend with the forces of gravity, the operation is known as a vertical rescue. These specially trained teams require special equipment and constant training to affect a successful rescue. The untrained and unequipped Paramedic should not attempt these types of rescues. (B), (C), and (D) are all aspects of this type of rescue. Rappelling is used to gain access; it is a team effort, and it is certainly a technical rescue, but it is also part of the picture of a vertical rescue and not its definition. *(Brady, Paramedic Care 2e, Principles and Practice, Volume 5— Rescue Awareness and Operations. Mosby, Paramedic Textbook 3e, Rescue Awareness and Operations.)*

743. The answer is B. Disentanglement is defined as removing the vehicle from around the patient. The damaged vehicle could cause serious soft tissue or exacerbate serious injury. Removal of sharp or entrapping vehicle parts ensures that the patient can be removed from the wreckage without further injury. *(Brady, Paramedic Care 2e, Principles and Practice, Volume 5—Rescue Awareness and Operations. Mosby, Paramedic Textbook 3e, Rescue Awareness and Operations.)*

744. The answer is D. Most police departments have tactical Paramedics who are trained in these situations and will remove the patient for you. Police departments also have their own negotiators who will talk to the gunman to remedy the situation. At no time should an untrained Paramedic crew move into the line of fire. The common goal of this, as in any event, is rescuer safety. *(Brady, Paramedic Care 2e, Principles and Practice, Volume 5—Rescue Awareness and Operations. Mosby, Paramedic Textbook 3e, Rescue Awareness and Operations.)*

745. The answer is D. Conducting witness interviews is an essential component in establishing the location of patients trapped in "use areas" of collapsed buildings. These interviews can assist the rescuer in understanding exactly where the highest occupancy areas of the building are located. Specialized equipment will be needed in these situations, but rescue efforts should not be delayed awaiting their arrival. *(Brady, Paramedic Care 2e, Principles and Practice, Volume 5— Rescue Awareness and Operations. Mosby, Paramedic Textbook 3e, Rescue Awareness and Operations.)*

746. The answer is B. Cardiovascular collapse and subsequent cardiac arrest are the primary concerns for a patient with crush syndrome after a building collapse. Acidosis and hyperkalemia should be treated immediately to prevent this occurrence. Although cavitation injuries, open fractures, and impaled objects all require priority management, treatment and maintenance of cardiovascular function are of the highest priority. *(Brady, Paramedic Care 2e, Principles and Practice, Volume 5—Rescue Awareness and Operations. Mosby, Paramedic Textbook 3e, Rescue Awareness and Operations.)*

HAZARDOUS MATERIALS INCIDENTS

747. The answer is B. (B) Hazardous materials first responders are not trained in the mitigation of a hazardous materials incident. Hazardous materials technicians and specialists accomplish mitigation. The first responder is responsible for knowledge of the risks associated with hazardous materials, the ability to recognize the need for special resources, and understanding potential outcomes. Hazardous materials first responders are responsible to protect nearby life, property, and environmental issues. They do not attempt to control the release of the agent. *(Brady, Paramedic Care 2e, Principles and Practice, Volume 5—Hazardous Materials Awareness and Operations. Mosby, Paramedic Textbook 3e, Hazardous Materials Incidents.)*

748. The answer is B. (B) The DOT placard system identifies flammable solids with a white and red striped placard. The EMS responder should be aware that shippers are only required to place a placard on a vehicle if it is carrying more than 1001 pounds of an agent. Responders should take great caution in approaching any shipping container that has no placard. (A), (C), and (D) are incorrect. *(Brady, Paramedic Care 2e, Principles and Practice, Volume 5—Hazardous Materials Awareness and Operations. Mosby, Paramedic Textbook 3e, Hazardous Materials Incidents.)*

749. The answer is D. (D) The DOT emergency response guidebook will allow the first responder to identify the type of hazardous material involved in the incident. It is also a resource to obtain information on safety distances and evacuation. In addition, it will provide basic emergency care information to assist in patient care. Although a Paramedic textbook may have good information on hazardous materials, it will usually not have specific information on all materials. The DOT placard chart explains the types of agents but does not break it down into specifics. The shipper's manifest is an excellent resource for the cargo information, but it may not be readily available during an emergency. If the driver is injured or unconscious, or there is a leak of product, the provider will not have access to the manifest. *(Brady, Paramedic Care 2e, Principles and Practice, Volume 5—Hazardous Materials Awareness and Operations. Mosby, Paramedic Textbook 3e, Hazardous Materials Incidents.)*

750. The answer is C. (C) All EMS operations are to be provided in the cold zone to patients after they are decontaminated. Individuals properly trained in personal protective equipment should do decontamination. Decontamination is usually done in the warm zone with a corridor into the cold zone. EMS providers should remain in the cold zone regardless of the situation at the scene unless they are properly trained and outfitted in personal protective equipment. (A) Hot zone is the actual incident. (B) Warm zone requires personal protective equipment and is usually set up as a decontamination area. (D) The patient locations have no effect on the location of the cold zone. *(Brady, Paramedic Care 2e, Principles and Practice, Volume 5—Hazardous Materials Awareness and Operations. Mosby, Paramedic Textbook 3e, Hazardous Materials Incidents.)*

751. The answer is C. (C) CHEMTREC is a 24-hour hotline designed to provide trained experts to assist in hazardous materials incident mitigation. A call to 1-800-CHEMTREC will allow responders to obtain comprehensive information regarding specific chemicals and their effects on the body. CHEMTREC will also provide fire officials with information on product mitigation and decontamination. (A), (B), and (D) are all incorrect. *(Brady, Paramedic Care 2e, Principles and Practice, Volume 5—Hazardous Materials Awareness and Operations. Mosby, Paramedic Textbook 3e, Hazardous Materials Incidents.)*

752. **The answer is A.** (A) Level A protection provides a fully encapsulating chemical resistant suit with self-contained breathing apparatus. (B) Level B provides the same respiratory protection but not the same mucous membrane protection. (C) Level C provides an air-purifying respirator and chemical-resistant clothing. (D) Level D provides no respiratory protection and minimal mucous membrane protection. *(Brady, Paramedic Care 2e, Principles and Practice, Volume 5—Hazardous Materials Awareness and Operations. Mosby, Paramedic Textbook 3e, Hazardous Materials Incidents.)*

753. **The answer is D.** (D) The treatment of a chemically contaminated patient should be minimized to ABCs and cervical spine maintenance prior to decontamination. It is important to stress that the Paramedic should not be in contact with contaminated patients unless he or she is trained in the use of personal protective equipment. After the patient is decontaminated, the Paramedic can perform a complete history and physical examination, begin pharmacologic intervention, and monitor the ECG for any irregularities. *(Brady, Paramedic Care 2e, Principles and Practice, Volume 5—Hazardous Materials Awareness and Operations. Mosby, Paramedic Textbook 3e, Hazardous Materials Incidents.)*

754. **The answer is A.** (A) Medical surveillance is conducted on all members of an entry team prior to suiting up in personal protective equipment. This physical examination includes assessment of pulse, temperature, respiration, blood pressure, cardiac rhythm, weight, cognitive and motor skills, and hydration. This assessment is done after exit to determine whether the provider is or is not capable of reentry to the scene. (A), (C), and (D) are all incorrect. *(Brady, Paramedic Care 2e, Principles and Practice, Volume 5—Hazardous Materials Awareness and Operations. Mosby, Paramedic Textbook 3e, Hazardous Materials Incidents.)*

CBRNE

The following topics are covered in Section VIII:

- Chemical Agents and Dissemination
- Biological Agents
- Radiological and Nuclear Incidents
- Explosive and Incendiary Devices

Questions

CHEMICAL AGENTS AND DISSEMINATION

DIRECTIONS: Each item below contains four suggested responses. Select the one best response to each item.

755. All of the following are identified as toxic industrial chemicals *except*:

   (A) anhydrous ammonia
   (B) chlorine
   (C) sarin
   (D) hydrogen cyanide

756. Sarin, tabun, soman, and VX agents are all classified as _____.

   (A) choking agents
   (B) nerve agents
   (C) blister agents
   (D) incapacitating agents

757. You would expect the patient with exposure to chemical nerve agent to exhibit all of the following symptoms *except*:

   (A) dry mouth
   (B) runny eyes
   (C) vomiting
   (D) dyspnea

758. Your unit is dispatched to a movie theatre for a "smoke inhalation case." On your arrival, you find a large crowd of people running from the theatre and holding their faces. Many of the people have runny eyes, some are vomiting, and others seem to be having trouble breathing. Your first action should be:

   (A) leave the vehicle and set up a triage area
   (B) radio for police assistance before beginning triage
   (C) retreat from the scene to a safe distance and radio for additional resources
   (D) open your ambulance doors and allow as many people who can fit to enter, then drive them to a safe zone and request additional ambulances for the rest of the patients

759. As you begin your assessment of a patient from question 758 she tells you she was sitting in the theatre and heard a bang, then smelled something foul which made her begin to wheeze and made her eyes tear "like running water." As you assess her, you find her vital signs to be BP 160/90, pulse 120, respirations 22. You hear bilateral end-expiratory wheezes and notice that her pupils are dilated. She has most likely been exposed to:

    (A) chemical nerve agents
    (B) riot control agent
    (C) incapacitating agent
    (D) blister agents

760. You would treat this patient with all of the following *except*:

    (A) oxygen
    (B) supportive care
    (C) decontamination
    (D) several Mark-1 antidote kits

761. Exposure to lewisite would most likely be self-limiting because it produces an immediate effect on the eyes and skin.

    (A) true
    (B) false

762. Your ambulance is dispatched to a basement lab where the police stop you and advise you that there was a chemical release. As the hazardous materials response team (HAZMAT) brings you a patient, you are advised that there are three people dead from the same area as your patient. The patient, who is extremely cyanotic, manages to advise you that he was watching TV while his friends were "playing with some chemical." The last thing he remembers was a bitter smell like almonds and then he passed out. He is complaining of difficulty breathing and his vital signs are BP 100/90, pulse 130, respirations are labored at 26. You suspect

    (A) chlorine poisoning
    (B) illicit drug abuse
    (C) carbon monoxide poisoning
    (D) cyanide poisoning

763. In the absence of a cyanide antidote kit, the Paramedic should

    (A) request an antidote kit be transported to the scene
    (B) manage airway and ventilation in a supportive fashion
    (C) establish an IV and administer epinephrine to prevent cardiac arrest
    (D) await decontamination before attempting any intervention

764. A Paramedic can operate in an Immediately Dangerous to Life and Health (IDLH) unknown environment for extended periods as long as he or she has level C protective equipment and is trained in its use.

    (A) true
    (B) false

BIOLOGICAL AGENTS

DIRECTIONS: Each item below contains four suggested responses. Select the one best response to each item.

765. Smallpox, Marburg, and Lassa fever are all caused by a _____.

    (A) bacterial infection
    (B) viral infection
    (C) enterotoxin
    (D) man-made organisms

766. Anthrax is classified as a

    (A) bacterial infection
    (B) viral infection
    (C) enterotoxin
    (D) man-made organism

767. Two weeks after attending a conference, 15 people begin to experience low-grade fevers and body aches. All of the affected people begin to develop a rash that begins on their chest and spreads all over their bodies. As the disease progresses, new eruptions of the rash occur. Two people are hospitalized for complications, you suspect:

(A) pneumonic plague

(B) smallpox

(C) chicken pox

(D) anthrax

768. You are dispatched to the home of a patient who is complaining of flu-like symptoms and difficulty breathing. He states that several days ago he was at a friend's house and opened a letter which contained "white powder." He thought nothing of it until he began feeling sick. Based on the history, you should immediately decontaminate this patient before treatment.

(A) true

(B) false

769. On a regularly quiet day, the emergency medical service (EMS) providers in your response area begin to receive several calls for patients with double vision, dry mouth, dysphagia, and descending flaccid paralysis. One crew had to ventilate their patient on the way to the hospital as respiratory arrest developed. You should suspect

(A) *Salmonella* poisoning

(B) *Shigella*

(C) botulinum toxin

(D) nerve agent exposure

770. You are assigned to the emergency department triage desk when over the period of an hour, 14 people come in complaining of weakness, fever, and cough. They all report that they were shopping in the mall 2 days earlier when a guy in a clown suit ran through the mall spraying what he called "fairy dust." The patients thought nothing of the incident and went home. Within 18 hours, all began to become symptomatic. Several hours after their arrival, they continue to deteriorate and develop pulmonary edema and severe hypoxemia. Within 12 hours, three patients die and six more are on ventilators, you suspect

(A) ricin agent

(B) anthrax exposure

(C) botulinum toxins

(D) viral hemorrhagic fever

771. What would be your expected course of treatment for the patients in question 770?

(A) supportive care

(B) Cipro or doxycycline

(C) atropine

(D) fluid therapy

772. Which of the following biological agents has the capability of being transmitted person to person?

(A) anthrax

(B) tularemia

(C) brucellosis

(D) smallpox

773. Biological events are relatively rare, and in fact, prior to 1936 there were no documented cases of intentional dissemination of biological agents.

(A) true

(B) false

774. A widened mediastinum on a chest x-ray is a hallmark finding of _____.

(A) anthrax
(B) plague
(C) tularemia
(D) brucellosis

RADIOLOGICAL AND NUCLEAR INCIDENTS

DIRECTIONS: Each item below contains four suggested responses. Select the one best response to each item.

775. All of the following are forms of ionizing radiation *except*:

(A) neutron
(B) beta
(C) gamma
(D) rem

776. You respond to a large explosion in a busy rail station. The fire department's HAZMAT team states that they are picking up high levels of radiation in the blast area. You suspect

(A) nuclear detonation
(B) improvised explosive device (IED) with C4 (C4 can emit radiation)
(C) IED with radiation source
(D) faulty equipment

777. During response to the detonation of a "dirty bomb" inside a building, which of the following is not a concern for rescuers?

(A) falling debris and broken glass
(B) secondary devices
(C) fallout
(D) inhalation hazards

778. Which of the following is not the way responders can protect themselves from the hazards of ionizing radiation exposure?

(A) reducing time in the contaminated area
(B) showering after irradiation
(C) staying a good distance from the radiation source
(D) using structures and protective clothing as shielding

779. You respond to a call for a patient who was in the vicinity of a package that later was identified as emitting high levels of radiation. Your patient is exhibiting early signs of radiation exposure, such as nausea and vomiting. This patient is the victim of what type of radiation exposure?

(A) irradiation
(B) internal contamination
(C) external contamination
(D) area contamination

780. You respond to an explosion in a coffee shop, on your arrival, you find several patients who are walking in the parking lot and are slightly disoriented from the blast. One patient, a 42-year-old female approaches you and is bleeding from the head. She tells you that a man walked in and threw a package into the shop while shouting "you'll be glowing for years" and ran out. She tells you that she is dizzy, she is also extremely nauseous and begins to vomit. Based on her presentation, you should suspect all of the following *except*:

(A) acute radiation sickness
(B) blast injuries
(C) head trauma
(D) hypotension

781. Immediate treatment of your patient in question 780 would include all of the following *except*:

(A) spinal immobilization
(B) decontamination
(C) airway maintenance
(D) oxygenation

782. The patient who has been irradiated by a contamination source is an exposure danger to the first responder.

    (A) true
    (B) false

783. Your patient has been removed from the debris of a large explosion. He has been through a gross decontamination shower and has multiple lacerations and signs of blast injury. HAZMAT responders are reporting high levels of radiation in the blast area. Based on the following, does this patient pose an exposure threat to the Paramedic?

    (A) Yes
    (B) No

784. In responding to incidents which include Radiological materials, responders should use the same rules as HAZMAT events. All of the following are components of this response *except*:

    (A) Isolate the area and restrict traffic.
    (B) Staging is upwind and uphill of the incident.
    (C) Control zones (hot, warm, and cold) are set up.
    (D) Only providers working in the *hot* zone are required to wear personal protective equipment (PPE).

785. The probability that a terrorist organization would use a nuclear device is extremely high in relation to an explosive device or "dirty bomb."

    (A) true
    (B) false

786. Nuclear weapons are impractical because they are too large to be carried by one person.

    (A) true
    (B) false

EXPLOSIVE AND INCENDIARY DEVICES

DIRECTIONS: Each item below contains four suggested responses. Select the one best response to each item.

787. The use of explosive devices accounts for _____% of all terrorist events?

    (A) 70
    (B) 60
    (C) 50
    (D) 40

788. Which of the following does not fall into one of the three explosive categories?

    (A) pyrotechnics
    (B) propellants
    (C) combustible liquids
    (D) dynamite and C4

789. An explosive which goes through almost instantaneous decomposition and produces a shock wave is known as a

    (A) nuclear detonation
    (B) propellant
    (C) high explosive
    (D) low explosive

790. Explosives which go through a slower decomposition rate (less than 3300 fps) are known as

    (A) dirty bombs
    (B) secondary devices
    (C) high explosives
    (D) low explosives

791. You are dispatched to the scene of an explosion at a busy rail depot. On your arrival, police are confirming that there has been an intentional event and that it is suspected that a terrorist or terrorists have exploded one or more bombs in backpacks. Your first concern should be

    (A) setting up a triage area
    (B) directing incoming units to staging areas
    (C) possibility of secondary devices
    (D) broken glass

792. IEDs consist of four components, which of the following is not a component of an IED?

    (A) power source
    (B) switch
    (C) explosive
    (D) clock

793. On close inspection of a scene, the Paramedic can usually identify an IED as they are uniquely shaped.

    (A) true
    (B) false

794. You respond to the scene of an explosion. You are treating a 37-year-old female who was approximately 20 feet from the explosion of a small backpack. Your assessment reveals that she has dozens of small round holes all over her body. You anticipate that this was caused by

    (A) pressure wave
    (B) tattooing from the explosive device
    (C) shrapnel
    (D) flying glass

795. You respond to a large fire in a local drinking establishment, bystanders state that a patron had an argument with the owner and was ejected from the building. About an hour later, he returned and threw a large jar of what appeared to be gasoline with a lighted rag inside the door. This device would be identified as a(n)

    (A) IED
    (B) high explosive
    (C) low explosive
    (D) incendiary device

796. Multiple first responder units are on the scene of a large building fire. While commencing operations, there is a large explosion in a car which is parked across the street from the incident. Several EMS providers in the treatment area are injured and the car is now engulfed in flames, the most appropriate action would be

    (A) Have additional EMS units respond, to assist the injured, and staff the treatment area.
    (B) Have all EMS units retreat from the area and reorganize in a safe area.
    (C) Have the fire department extinguish the fire and continue treatment operations.
    (D) Request police protection in the treatment area, treat the injured providers, and restore the treatment area.

Answers and Explanations

CHEMICAL AGENTS AND DISSEMINATION

755. **The answer is C.** Toxic industrial chemicals are identified as chemicals that are used in everyday industrial settings but have a high potential to be commandeered by terrorists for weaponization. Anhydrous ammonia is used in the farming, as well as other industries. Chlorine is widely available, most commonly as a swimming pool chemical and hydrogen cyanide is used in metallurgy. Sarin agent is not defined as an industrial chemical as it has no useful industrial application.

756. **The answer is B.** Agents which affect the nervous system are classified as chemical nerve agents. Sarin, tabun, soman, and VX are all identified in this category. Nerve agents bind to acetylcholinesterase and prevent the uptake of acetylcholine in the nerve synapses. This results in overstimulation of the parasympathetic nervous system.

757. **The answer is A.** Chemical nerve agents effect on the parasympathetic nervous system result in a syndrome known as "SLUDGEM." The patient will present with the following signs and symptoms:

    S—salivation
    L—lacrimation
    U—urination
    D—defecation
    G—gastrointestinal upset
    E—emesis
    M—miosis

Patients with nerve agent exposure will not present with dry mouth. After treating a patient for nerve agent exposure, the Paramedic should be alert for signs such as dry mouth to confirm that the antidote is beginning to reverse the exposure.

758. **The answer is C.** As soon as the Paramedic, or any emergency responder recognizes the indicators of a hazardous materials exposure, the most appropriate action is to retreat to a safe area and request assistance. The absence of PPE will render the Paramedic crew not only unable to assist, but may endanger them and result in contamination. On arrival, HAZMAT units will set up control zones and begin decontamination. Unless the Paramedic is specially trained and is wearing the proper PPE, he should not attempt to provide care to any patient who is suspected of being contaminated.

759. **The answer is B.** The scenario, history, and patient presentation all indicate that this was an exposure to a riot control agent. Exposure to riot control agents can present with the same forward symptoms as chemical nerve agents; however, they are not nearly as toxic and almost always are self-limiting in their effects. Patients exposed to chemical nerve agents will most likely continue to deteriorate if not appropriately and rapidly treated.

760. **The answer is D.** This patient's presentation is not consistent with a nerve agent exposure. Mark-1 antidote kits are specific to nerve agent, organophosphate, and carbamate poisonings. Riot control agents do not fall in either of those categories and therefore Mark-1 kits are not

indicated. A Mark-1 kit consists of two autoinjectors: one contains 2 mg of atropine and the other 600 mg of pralidoxime.

761. **The answer is A.** Lewisite, a blister agent, creates an immediate effect. Patients who would be exposed, or approach a vapor cloud that consisted of lewisite, would be immediately forced to attempt to retreat from the area. In contrast, Mustard agents tend to have delayed effects which could take from 2 to 24 hours or more to reach effect. Treatment for these exposures is removal from the exposure, decontamination, and supportive care.

762. **The answer is D.** Cyanide, a blood agent, affects the way the body can use oxygen. In enclosed spaces and appropriate concentrations, it can be rapidly deadly. Respiratory arrest can occur in 4 minutes and cardiac arrest within 8 minutes of a toxic inhalation. A telltale sign of cyanide is its bitter almond-like smell. Chlorine, a choking agent can be just as deadly, but chlorine has its own distinct odor like a swimming pool. Carbon monoxide poisoning can also be the case, however, CO is odorless. Illicit drug use is also suspect; however, the history, odor, and scenario lead to a diagnosis of cyanide poisoning.

763. **The answer is B.** The Paramedic can treat the patient who is exposed to cyanide by supporting ventilation and oxygenation. Cyanide antidote kits are rare on ambulances, and would not be plentiful in cases of terrorist dissemination of a cyanide agent. Decontamination is usually not necessary and treatment is aimed at removing the patient from exposure and delivering supportive care.

764. **The answer is B.** IDLH unknown environments identify a situation in which the chemical agent is unknown and its concentration is also not known. Occupational Safety and Health Administration (OSHA) standards for response to IDLH unknown environment calls for level A protective clothing and self-contained breathing apparatus (SCBA) or supplied air respirators (SAR). If a Paramedic is not trained and/or not appropriately attired in the proper level of PPE,

he or she should not operate in an IDLH unknown environment.

BIOLOGICAL AGENTS

765. **The answer is B.** Smallpox, Marburg, and Lassa fever are all caused by viral infection. All three viruses are categorized as class A (high priority) by the Centers for Disease Control. Marburg and Lassa fever, as well as Ebola, are all classified as viral hemorrhagic fevers. There is no cure or established treatment modalities for viral hemorrhagic fevers. There is also no prescribed treatment for smallpox; however, there is a vaccination that is stockpiled in the United States in the case of an outbreak. Historically, smallpox has a 33% mortality rate with its highest effects on the very young, very old, and immunosuppressed.

766. **The answer is A.** Anthrax *(Bacillus anthracis)* is a bacterial agent. Anthrax is caused by a naturally occurring organism that survives for long periods of time in a spore form. Anthrax spores can be inhaled, ingested, or may affect the skin. Cutaneous anthrax is a common disease among animal herds and people who work with the herds have been known to contract it. Terrorists have long attempted to weaponize anthrax into a lethal inhaled form. Inhalational anthrax has a high mortality rate and is difficult to treat once symptoms appear. In the fall of 2001, anthrax-laced letters were sent out through the U.S. Postal Service to news agencies and the state senator of South Dakota. The spores were weaponized to such a fine degree that the entire post office facilities had to be evacuated and decontaminated due to disease transmission.

767. **The answer is C.** This group of people has been infected with chicken pox. Chicken pox is fairly common and highly contagious. Fortunately, chicken pox is rarely fatal and will resolve with just supportive care. The differential diagnosis between chicken pox and smallpox is easy to establish. Chicken pox starts on the chest and moves outward to the rest of the body. Chicken pox also has a series of eruptions, so the patient

will have pox that are fresh and others that are drying and scabbed over. In smallpox, the rash begins on the palms of the hands and soles of the feet and moves to the center of the body. Smallpox will only have one eruption, this means all of the pox will appear in the same stage.

768. The answer is B. This patient has potentially been exposed to anthrax. In most cases, patients who are presenting with symptoms which are consistent with biological agent exposure do not require decontamination. Generally, patients do not develop symptoms for days to weeks after exposure. With this in mind, most patients would have showered and changed clothing many times prior to becoming ill. Proper PPE should always be considered in situations where an infectious disease may be present, but decontamination will not help the patient, or the rescuer.

769. The answer is C. Botulinum toxins are a family of related neurotoxins produced by *Clostridium botulinum*. EMS providers should be alert for the hallmark of this exposure, which is descending flaccid paralysis. Any individual, or cluster of people who are exhibiting afebrile symptoms which include blurred or double vision, dysphagia, dysphonia, and symmetrical descending flaccid paralysis should be suspected of exposure to botulinum toxins.

770. The answer is A. These patients have been exposed to ricin agent. Ricin inhibits protein synthesis at the cellular level and the end result is a rapid onset of symptoms (usually within 4–6 hours) that progress to death in approximately 36 hours generally from pulmonary edema secondary to increased capillary permeability. Rapid onsets (4–12 hours) in large clusters will usually rule out biological agents, which tend to have longer incubation periods. Ricin exposure should be suspected in these circumstances.

771. The answer is A. The only acceptable treatment for exposure to ricin agent is to provide supportive care. Inhaled ricin will cause severe pulmonary edema. This should be treated with high

flow oxygen and medications which you would normally use to treat pulmonary edema (e.g., furosemide and morphine). Ricin can also be ingested and the treatment is gastric decontamination with charcoal and cathartics. Ingestion could also require fluid replacement; however, this case was an inhalational exposure.

772. The answer is D. Smallpox is a highly infectious agent and the Paramedic should take extreme precautions when treating any patient with a suspected case of smallpox. PPE should include barrier protection including gloves and at the least an N-95 respirator mask.

773. The answer is B. Biological events are common as compared to other types of terrorism. In fact, the earliest reported event was in the sixth century B.C. when the Assyrians poised wells with rye ergot. In 1346 in Kaffa, attackers hurled plague-infected corpses over the city walls and forced surrender. It is suspected that refugees fled from Kaffa to Europe and brought with them the disease that was later identified as "black plague." In 1763, smallpox-laden blankets were given to Native Americans at Fort Carillion during the French and Indian war, which resulted in multiple deaths and eventual surrender.

774. The answer is A. One of the late findings in anthrax exposure and subsequent illness is a widened mediastinum on a chest x-ray, which is due to mediastinal inflammation (mediastinitis) and enlarged mediastinal lymph nodes. Early symptoms are flu-like in nature with fever, malaise, respiratory distress, and worsening cyanosis. The disease usually results in death within 36 hours if left untreated. There is pleural effusion in approximately 55% of the cases but it is not a definitive finding. Blood work will indicate an increased white blood cell count in the later stages which will not resolve.

RADIOLOGICAL AND NUCLEAR INCIDENTS

775. The answer is D. There are generally four types of ionizing radiation. They are as follows:

1. *Alpha*: Large heavy particles, which due to size, are heavy and do not travel great distances. Alpha particles are stopped by intact skin—inhalation hazard.

2. *Beta*: Light particles which can penetrate the skin surface, but are generally stopped by clothing—skin and inhalation hazard.

3. *Gamma*: High energy and are not easily blocked, even by leaded shields—absorption and irradiation hazard.

4. *Neutron*: Similar to gamma, they have large mass and can damage atom structure. They can cause up to 20 times more damage than gamma radiation and are only released during a nuclear explosion.

776. **The answer is C.** A "dirty bomb" is an IED that uses conventional explosives to disperse a radioactive material. Generally, terrorist groups will seek out a widely available source of material. This may be medical- or industrial-grade isotopes. Then they will pack it with a regular explosive and detonate. The resulting explosion will spread contamination in two ways: from the pressure wave of the blast and from the environmental wind. The area of contamination is isolated to blast area and wind direction. Buildings, cars, and other obstacles will reduce area of contamination.

777. **The answer is C.** The dirty bomb is constructed from conventional materials and does not involve any type of "reaction" which would create what is defined as a "nuclear explosion." In the absence of a nuclear explosion, there would be no nuclear fallout. Rescuers should be acutely aware of the dangers of responding to an event caused by conventional explosives, such as falling debris. The rescuer should also remain a safe distance away until responders with appropriate PPE survey the area with radiation detection equipment.

778. **The answer is B.** In responding to intentional incidents involving radiation sources, the same rules apply as accidental incidents. Using the time, distance, and shielding formula will prevent large amounts of exposure to radiation. Showering can be used to lessen contamination,

but may have little to no effect on irradiation injuries, since radiation is absorbed through the skin.

779. **The answer is A.** There are typically three types of radiation exposure:

1. *Irradiation*: Exposure to a source which results in a defined absorbed dose. The exposure will cease once the patient is removed from the source. Symptoms and outcome are based on dose.

2. *Internal contamination*: Ingestion or inhalation of a radiation source. A patient either ingests contaminated food or inhales air or dust containing contaminants. The internal exposure continues until all radioactive particles in the body are removed or discharged either by natural means or medical treatment.

3. *External contamination*: External contact with a source from either splash, dust exposure, or embedding of contaminated particles secondary to explosive blasts.

780. **The answer is A.** Based on the time frame alone, this patient is most likely not suffering from acute radiation sickness. Acute radiation sickness usually has an onset of 4–6 hours after exposure and is not an immediate effect. After a blast injury, this patient could surely be nauseous and or vomit from any of the other possibilities listed. The Paramedic should always be alert to treat the causes of traumatic injury before those of radiation sickness.

781. **The answer is B.** Treatment of this patient would include basic airway, breathing, and circulation (ABC) management and spinal immobilization, assessment and treatment for traumatic injuries, and oxygenation. Treatment of traumatic injuries takes precedence over decontamination in the case of radiation exposure. The Paramedic should be careful to avoid personal contamination until the scene is surveyed and cleared of contamination or the patient is subsequently decontaminated. Paramedics should wear appropriate respiratory protective devices and use time, distance,

and shielding measures while attempting to treat patients in this scenario.

782. The answer is B. Patients who have been exposed to a source, and not contaminated by it pose no source threat to the responder. The radiation exposure is absorbed by the patient, but the absorption does not allow the radiation to be emitted from the patient. Noncontaminated patients with irradiation injuries are considered clean.

783. The answer is A. Even after decontamination, the Paramedic should be aware that open injuries can contain remaining particles of contaminant from IEDs. Radioactive agents are mixed with conventional explosives. The resulting conventional pressure wave carries these radioactive particles and they will be embedded in skin as well as inside lacerations and other injuries. These particles are removed by specialized teams during the surgical process. This process would be accomplished at the receiving hospital during treatment and should be done by specially trained personnel. The Paramedic should take great care to avoid contamination and long periods of exposure to these patients.

784. The answer is D. PPE is required in hot and warm zones during any hazardous materials event. This includes events which disseminate radiation. The warm zone is usually the decontamination corridor and anybody working with contaminated patients should be wearing some form of PPE. The determination of PPE level is always dictated by the agent and its concentration. PPE identified for the hot zone may also be different from PPE in the warm zone. In addition, splash protection may be required in the cold zone on the clean side of decon as added protection. Each event will dictate what procedures will be used.

785. The answer is B. It is not probable that a terrorist organization would employ a tactical nuclear device. Weapon-grade nuclear devices are extremely difficult to obtain and even more difficult to construct. While a terrorist organization may attempt to procure one by illegal means, it would be much easier to obtain the

materials to produce a radiological dispersion device (dirty bomb).

786. The answer is B. Due to technologic advances, nuclear devices are now small enough to fit in a briefcase or a backpack. This makes the possibility of a single person being able to detonate a point device extremely feasible, if the terrorist organization could obtain or construct a device. These devices would, however, produce small kiloton output and create as much damage as a conventional truck bomb. Larger devices, which could create mass destruction, would still be difficult to carry.

EXPLOSIVE AND INCENDIARY DEVICES

787. The answer is A. According to FBI statistics, more than 70% of all terrorist events are perpetrated using some form of explosive device.

788. The answer is C. The three categories of explosives are:

1. *Pyrotechnics*: Fireworks, road flares, and smoke-emitting devices (grenades) all fall into this category.
2. *Propellants*: Black powder and rocket fuels.
3. *Explosives*: C4, dynamite, and other forms of "high explosives" fit into this final category.

Although not technically an explosive, combustible liquids are frequently used in the production of incendiary devices.

789. The answer is C. High explosives decompose at an extremely rapid rate (detonate). Explosives which decompose at this rate, produce a pressure (shock) wave of greater than 3300 ft/s and are known as high explosives. High explosives use a shock wave to create their damage path. 2,4,6-Trinitrotoluene (TNT), C4, and dynamite fall into this category.

790. The answer is D. Low explosives tend to decompose at slower rates. This decomposition is known as deflagration. Slower rates result in less of a shock wave and less damage than a high explosive detonation. IEDs using low explosives are generally made from black or smokeless powder, or rocket propellants.

791. **The answer is C.** All first responders need to be aware of the possibility of secondary devices in any terrorist event. There are documented cases of terrorists setting off explosions and then planning secondary explosions, which are specifically aimed at injuring and killing first responders. The Paramedic should be aware of anything that may look out of place at an event and advise the appropriate agency of all suspicious findings.

792. **The answer is D.** Explosive devices consist of four components, they are:

1. *Power sources*: The most popular power source is a battery. The power source provides the initiator with the needed charge to begin the chemical reaction.
2. *Initiators*: These are normally flame-producing devices, which will set off the chemical reaction which can be a blasting cap, fuse, or other improvised device.
3. *Explosive*: The actual medium which decomposes and results in energy release.
4. *Switches*: The actual triggering device. The switch will activate the fuse by allowing the power source to come in contact with it. This creates the necessary reaction to complete the explosive process.

793. **The answer is A.** IEDs can be very difficult to identify. In fact, an IED can be placed in any type of container from a coffee can to a backpack. The Paramedic should exercise extreme caution while operating at the scene of an intentional explosion and avoid any enclosed spaces or areas not secured by law enforcement.

794. **The answer is C.** Terrorists, especially those who use improvised devices, will add projectiles to the devices. In many cases, this could be glass, nails, marbles, or anything which will become airborne after a blast. This will effectively increase the lethality of the device. In this case, it appears that the bomber has added BBs to his device creating the injury pattern described.

795. **The answer is D.** Devices which cause fire, with no blast, deflagration, or detonation are classified as incendiary devices. Incendiary devices are usually made with a combustible liquid and an ignition source. In this case, gasoline and a rag (Molotov cocktail). Incendiary devices are extremely common for terrorist use and are used in small-scale point attacks. Although they lack a pressure or shock wave, they can produce large amounts of damage secondary to the ensuing fire.

796. **The answer is B.** If at any time an EMS provider, or assignment of units is placed in a position of danger, the correct action is to retreat from the scene and restage in a safe area. This incident is clearly a secondary device which was placed to injure or kill emergency responders. Responders, including firefighters, should leave the area until it can be secured by the police department and the HAZMAT/bomb teams.

Bibliography

PARAMEDIC REFERENCES

Bledsoe BE, Porter RS, Shade BR. *Brady's Paramedic Care: Principles and Practice*, 2nd ed. Vol. 1–5. Upper Saddle River, NJ: Prentice-Hall, 2006.

Sanders MJ. *Mosby's Paramedic Textbook*, 3rd ed. St. Louis, MO: Elsevier, 2005.

CBRNE REFERENCES

Note about the Answer References for the CBRNE Section:

Integration of civilian response to CBRNE events began on an extensive scale in the United States around 1996. Since that time, there have been many civilian textbooks developed to assist in the training of first responders. As the quality of these texts has greatly improved, military and Federal government references still provide the greatest amount of technical data regarding the response to CBRNE events.

In an effort to provide the student with the best possible reference information, the rationales for all of the answers in Section VIII come from the military and Federal references listed below.

The CBRNE section in this review book reflects a general awareness level and in no way does it attempt to cover highly technical information that is delivered in advanced coursework. Paramedics, as well as other emergency responders are encouraged to seek out more advanced coursework through their local emergency managers. As the potential for CBRNE events increases, so does the need for trained providers.

You are the first line of defense.

Medical Management of Biological Casualties Handbook, 4th ed. U.S. Army Medical Research Institute of Infectious Diseases.

Medical Management of Chemical Casualties Handbook, 3rd ed. U.S. Army Medical Research Institute of Chemical Defense.

Medical Management of Radiological Casualties Handbook, 2nd ed. Military Medical Operations. Armed Forces Radiobiology Research Institute.

Sidell FR, Takafuji ET, Franz DR. *Textbook of Military Medicine*. Medical Aspects of Chemical and Biological Warfare. Office of the Surgeon General. Department of the Army.

WMD Awareness Level Training Manual (AWR-160). US Department of Homeland Security Office of State and Local Government Coordination and Preparedness. National Domestic Preparedness Consortium.